Introduction to Human Neuroimaging

Developed specifically for students in the behavioral and brain sciences, this is the only textbook that provides an accessible and practical overview of the range of human neuroimaging techniques.

Methods covered include functional and structural magnetic resonance imaging, positron emission tomography, electroencephalography, magnetoencephalography, multimodal imaging, and various brain stimulation methods. Experimental design, image processing, and statistical inference are also addressed, with chapters for both basic and more advanced data analyses.

Key concepts are illustrated through research studies on the relationship between brain and behavior, and practice questions are included throughout to test knowledge and aid self-study.

Offering just the right amount of detail for understanding how major imaging techniques can be applied to answer neuroscientific questions, and the practical skills needed for future research, this is an essential text for advanced undergraduate and graduate students in psychology, neuroscience, and cognitive science programs taking introductory courses on human neuroimaging.

Hans Op de Beeck is a Professor in the Brain and Cognition Research Unit at the University of Leuven (KU Leuven), Belgium. His research in cognitive and systems neuroscience has appeared in top scientific journals (such as *Science, Nature Neuroscience, Journal of Neuroscience,* and *Psychological Science*) and has been awarded and funded by national and international organizations, including the European Research Council and the Human Frontier Science Program. He teaches on topics such as behavioral neuroscience, neuropsychology, and human brain imaging in bachelor's and master's programs of psychology and the biomedical sciences.

Chie Nakatani is a Postdoctoral Fellow in the Brain and Cognition Research Unit at the University of Leuven (KU Leuven), Belgium. She has experience with research and teaching in neuroscience, psychology, ergonomics, and space life sciences at many international institutes, including the University of Massachusetts at Amherst, USA, Leiden University, the Netherlands, and RIKEN Brain Science Institute, Japan. Her specialty is electroencephalography in combination with magnetic resonance imaging, transcranial magnetic stimulation, and eye tracking.

Cambridge Fundamentals of Neuroscience in Psychology

Developed in response to a growing need to make neuroscience accessible to students and other non-specialist readers, the *Cambridge Fundamentals of Neuroscience in Psychology* series provides brief introductions to key areas of neuroscience research across major domains of psychology. Written by experts in cognitive, social, affective, developmental, clinical, and applied neuroscience, these books will serve as ideal primers for students and other readers seeking an entry point to the challenging world of neuroscience.

Books in the Series

Introduction to Human Neuroimaging

Hans Op de Beeck

KU Leuven, Belgium

Chie Nakatani

KU Leuven, Belgium

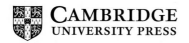

CAMBRIDGE
UNIVERSITY PRESS

CAMBRIDGE
UNIVERSITY PRESS

University Printing House, Cambridge CB2 8BS, United Kingdom

One Liberty Plaza, 20th Floor, New York, NY 10006, USA

477 Williamstown Road, Port Melbourne, VIC 3207, Australia

314–321, 3rd Floor, Plot 3, Splendor Forum, Jasola District Centre, New Delhi – 110025, India

79 Anson Road, #06–04/06, Singapore 079906

Cambridge University Press is part of the University of Cambridge.

It furthers the University's mission by disseminating knowledge in the pursuit
of education, learning, and research at the highest international levels of excellence.

www.cambridge.org
Information on this title: www.cambridge.org/9781107180307
DOI: 10.1017/9781316847916

© Cambridge University Press 2019

First published 2019

Printed and bound in Great Britain by Clays Ltd, Elcograf S.p.A.

A catalogue record for this publication is available from the British Library.

Library of Congress Cataloging-in-Publication Data
Names: Beeck, Hans Op de, 1975- author. | Nakatani, Chie, author.
Title: Introduction to human neuroimaging / Hans Op de Beeck, Chie Nakatani.
Other titles: Cambridge fundamentals of neuroscience in psychology.
Description: Cambridge, United Kingdom ; New York, NY : Cambridge University Press, 2019. |
    Series: Cambridge fundamentals of neuroscience in psychology
Identifiers: LCCN 2018045889| ISBN 9781107180307 (hardback) | ISBN 9781316632185 (pbk.)
Subjects: | MESH: Neuroimaging–methods
Classification: LCC RC349.D52 | NLM WL 141.5.N47 | DDC 616.8/04754–dc23
LC record available at https://lccn.loc.gov/2018045889

ISBN 978-1-107-18030-7 Hardback
ISBN 978-1-316-63218-5 Paperback

Additional resources for this publication at www.cambridge.org/opdebeeck

Contents

List of Figures

Preface

We want to understand the world around us. Society and some of its most brilliant minds invest considerable energy and resources in finding out the laws and the origin of the universe, exposing us to exotic concepts such as big bangs and string theories. For this enterprise, researchers measure all sorts of *signals from outer space* through huge telescopes and satellites. In science fiction movies these devices pick up signals from extraterrestrial beings, but in reality the signals inform us about what physical events happen very far away around other stars and in other galaxies.

Humankind, or at least the physicists among us, is interested not only in the big and the large, such as the borders of the universe, but also in the small and the submicroscopic. We need to know what happens at the smallest as much as at the largest scale before we can truly understand the physical world. For this small scale, scientists make inferences based on *signals from events happening at the subatomic level*. Ironically, the smaller the scale, the larger the apparatus that physicists need to use to detect these events. The current state of the art is the Large Hadron Collider, which detected the signal allowing scientists to infer the existence of the Higgs boson.

This book is about other signals, signals that are perhaps even more interesting. Of course outer space is great, as is picking up signals from an unimaginably small particle using a machine large and complicated enough to make every human nerd drool. However, there is one thing we as humans want to get a grip on even more than our environment, and that is ourselves. We want to understand and control ourselves. For this, we have to look where our "self" is situated, and that is in our head. It turns out that the head, and more specifically the brain, also emits all sorts of signals. This text is about these *signals from our brain* and how to measure them.

We must immediately warn the reader that these brain signals are not simple to understand and not easy to measure. Much must be learned. Measuring signals from outer space is complicated and involves armies of physicists and engineers, but we also need to learn some facts about physics and engineering to understand how we can measure brain signals. We need bits and pieces of knowledge from biology, neurophysiology, electricity, engineering, advanced statistics, radiology, neurology, cognitive science, and even philosophy. Getting the complete picture from brain signals requires you to take a truly interdisciplinary viewpoint. You are, it is hoped, ready for this.

Aims of This Text

The goal of this text is to bring students from a wide background to the point where they can read human neuroscience papers and understand all sections, including methodology – that is, how a technique works and why it was chosen, data analysis, and interpretation of the results. It will take hard work, but it is worth it. We avoid complexity as much as possible, and you should not worry about complicated formulas. For example, you do not need a physics degree to understand the concepts of physics as they are introduced in this book. Rather, our intent is that a motivated student who has successfully obtained an academic bachelor's degree in a scientific discipline should be able to grasp most of this book.

With this knowledge in your backpack, you as a reader will have what it takes to add human brain imaging to your own thinking, in whatever remote subject area you are interested in (e.g., psychology, economics, social sciences, law) and whatever type of neuroscience that might be most relevant to you (e.g., cognitive neuroscience, clinical neuroscience, educational neuroscience, neuroeconomics). And who knows, if you are particularly adventurous, the provision of just enough details about how the techniques are implemented and how the data are analyzed might bring you to the point where you want to do such research yourself. In that case, this book should be a perfect primer.

Key Features

We have included the following features to aid students and instructors in getting the most out of this text:

- **Learning objectives** are listed at the beginning of each chapter.
- **Further reading** suggestions are included, along with explanations of their relevance.
- **Chapter summaries** are provided at the end of each chapter to recap the key points that students should be aware of.
- **Review questions** are included to test knowledge as part of homework or self-study.
- **A detailed glossary** is supplied, with all key words also highlighted in bold throughout the text.
- **Online resources** include lecture slides, answers to the review questions, and links to further tutorials and useful websites.

Choice of Topics

This book covers the most popular neuroimaging techniques at a level of detail that takes into account the following trade-off: On the one hand, we want to avoid unnecessary details to make sure that the book as a whole can be read as part of a normal course or as an introduction to a multi-methods lab environment rather than used as an encyclopedia-style reference. On the other hand, we aim to include sufficient details to provide the student with a relatively in-depth understanding of all the different domains related to human neuroimaging – indeed, also including physics, neuroscience, statistics, and cognition. For example, we do not abstain from a chapter on the physics of MRI, but we focus on the basics needed to understand a typical methods section in a paper and to know the parameters that a *non-physicist* researcher might alter during scanning. As another example, we include many examples of applications of imaging in various research fields in order to illustrate basic concepts, but we do not aim to provide a review of any specific field (no chapter such as "the cognitive neuroscience of attention"). Nevertheless, the knowledge acquired in this book will be tremendously helpful for a better understanding of the many books that focus on specific fields, including many of the contributions in the series to which this book belongs: *Cambridge Fundamentals of Neuroscience in Psychology*.

Our overview of brain imaging does not shy away from criticism. Criticism can be voiced at many levels, from the general level of philosophy of science ("Can brain imaging really help us understand the human mind?") all the way down to very specific criticisms about a particular statistical method. Yet readers will notice that there is no chapter called "Criticisms of Human Brain Imaging." This choice reflects our belief that a thorough, in-depth discussion of the various pros and cons of particular approaches or methods requires sufficient knowledge about conceptual as well as technical issues. Thus, at the appropriate time and place, we present many important discussions, including neuro-hypes, neo-phrenology, brain activity in a dead salmon, reverse inference, open science or lack thereof, the limitations of group studies, the trade-off between spatial and temporal resolution, the relative value of different methods, and why a neuroscientist interested in neurons would measure blood flow, among others. This approach should help the reader not only to become an expert in terms of conceptual and technical knowledge, but also to apply this knowledge to develop a critical mindset when reading about and applying human brain imaging.

Acknowledgments

In the process of writing this book, we received help from numerous people. Naming them puts us at risk of forgetting people, but we will try nevertheless. First, we are indebted to the peers who were involved during the review process organized by Cambridge University Press (CUP), in particular the four peers who read the entire book and provided many helpful comments. Next, several colleagues read almost the whole book (Brendan Ritchie) or important parts of it (Jessica Bulthé, Radha Nila Meghanathan, Lien Peters, Hannah Bernhard, Céline Gillebert, Marcello Giannini, and Kevin Vanbecelaere). We are also grateful to the students who read and commented on precursor texts that we used in our own course on human brain imaging at KU Leuven. Material for figures was provided, in decreasing order of number of figures, by Christine Van Vliet, Céline Gillebert, Nicky Daniels, Jessica Bulthé, Haemy Lee Masson, Ineke Pillet, Brendan Ritchie, Lien Peters, and Michelle Hendriks. Many helpful insights were provided along the full way by Janka Romero and along part of the way by Claire Eudall and Heather Brolly, who all embody the high standards of CUP. Our gratitude to all these special people does not make them responsible for any remaining errors in this book – that curse remains with the authors.

CHAPTER ONE

Introduction and Overview

Learning Objectives

- Understanding why it is important to learn more about brain imaging methods
- Understanding the general basis of the signals emitted by the brain
- Acquiring basic knowledge of how information transfer works in the brain
- Understanding why we can measure brain signals in a noninvasive way
- Acquiring a bird's-eye view of the many different brain imaging methods
- Understanding the basic dimensions on which brain imaging methods differ and the major groups to which they belong

Many paintings depict human figures with an aura of radiation around their head. This tradition dates back to classic Greek and Roman times, continues through early Christian art, and has remained in the art of painters such as Vincent Van Gogh and even pop culture. The depicted aura is typically reserved for figures with a particular status, such as holy saints or, a bit more mundane, the individual painter.

In real life, we cannot see the signals emitted by someone's brain. Nevertheless, the signals are there in every person, saint or not, young or old. Sometimes the underlying physical principles sound very complex, such as "magnetic resonance imaging," but at other times these principles come surprisingly close to an optic signal, as depicted in the painted auras.

In the past few decades, scientists' ability to measure brain signals has improved radically. A first surge came with the advent of electroencephalography (EEG) after 1930. Since about 1970, clinical radiology has been blessed with radiographic methods such as so-called computerized tomography. A third wave occurred in 1980–1990, when brain imaging techniques such as positron emission tomography and functional magnetic resonance imaging were developed, resulting in the Decade of the Brain (1990–2000). The application of these brain imaging methods has only increased in frequency since then, across all scientific disciplines investigating mind, brain, and behavior. This is the case not only in fields such as radiology and neurology, but also psychology, educational science, social science, linguistics, economy, and law have started considering neuroscientific evidence as highly relevant empirical observations. As always, when new methods become popular, this evolution has not been without criticism. Nevertheless, the mere fact that so many disciplines have started to pay attention to brain imaging makes it essential that students in these fields acquire some basic knowledge about the methodology.

In this chapter, we start by explaining why it is important for everyone, including the lay public, to understand a few basic facts about these brain signals, their origin, and how they are measured. We then introduce some important pieces of background knowledge about how the brain works: how neurons communicate, where they find their energy, and how they are organized. We briefly introduce the full spectrum of brain imaging methods discussed in this book and describe the dimensions on which they differ.

1.1 Brain Enthusiasm: The Relevance of Distinguishing Fact from Fiction

Some basic knowledge about brain imaging will allow us to distinguish the actual scientific potential of these methods, which is huge, from science fiction. This is very much needed, not only for students but also for society more generally. Here we give four examples from the popular media in which there is a tendency to get carried away.

In 2009, Willem Verbeke, a professor from the University of Rotterdam, attracted the attention of the mass media by claiming that, in five years, people applying for important jobs would undergo brain scans as an important supplement to traditional job interviews and behavioral testing (Fig. 1.1). According to Verbeke, a brain scan can tell us whether a person is a good fit for a job or whether their behavior might prove detrimental in their potential position. Using brain scans, we could apparently avoid making someone a CEO of a corporation, who through short-sighted behavior might cause a worldwide recession. The statements were backed up by ongoing functional magnetic resonance imaging (fMRI) studies, published in peer-reviewed journals (e.g., Bagozzi et al., 2013). Verbeke claimed his company could help recruiters by providing a brain scan for 5000 euro per person. We are 10 years beyond the point when Verbeke's claims were made. Job interviews and psychometric tests are still standard practice when hiring people; brain scans are not. After reading this book, you should be able to understand why.

As a second example, there has already been an intensive debate about the value of brain scans as evidence in a court of law. A first application is in the context of lie

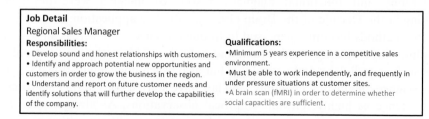

Figure 1.1 Illustration of a job advertisement in the future?

detection, a field in which several private companies are active in the United States (e.g., No Lie MRI). In addition, fMRI has been used to justify claims about the personality of the accused and the degree to which they can be expected to have control over their actions. However, these claims are largely unsubstantiated (Kessler and Muckli, 2011; Parens and Johnston, 2014). As will become obvious upon reading this book, brain scans often lack the validity and reliability to justify strong claims at the level of individual subjects in terms of lie detection as well as personality assessment. Furthermore, the brain scans might be overinterpreted by laypersons (including members of a jury) and as such provide misleading evidence that negatively impacts legal decisions making (see, e.g., Weisberg et al., 2008). For example, a brain scan suggesting a limitation in the degree of free will and self-control does not obviously provide more information than we learn from a psychiatrist who, as an expert witness, comes to the same conclusion based on a battery of standardized behavioral tests. However, will jury members be able to make a rational comparison of such very different types of evidence? We could doubt this, unless all jury members were forced to read a book like this one first!

Third, in the past few years quite a bit of media attention has been paid to research on patients either in a persistent vegetative state or suffering from locked-in syndrome, which suggests that brain imaging can be used to test the state of consciousness of these patients even though they lack the ability to communicate with their environment (e.g., Owen et al., 2006). Indeed, when lack of motor function is complete, brain imaging may be the only way to make such an assessment of conscious awareness. A typical experiment starts by asking the patient to answer yes/no questions by imagining two very different events which are so different that they can easily be distinguished based on elicited brain activity. For example, a patient might answer yes by imagining watching a tennis game and no by thinking of navigating through a house. One surge of media interest in this method arose when it was applied to the late Ariel Sharon, the former prime minister of Israel.[1] Often the results from such scans are not sufficiently conclusive to be the basis for important decisions about life and death, unless they are corroborated by findings from a range of other more standard methods. For the layperson, it is very difficult to judge the potential of this research based on what is written by nonexpert journalists.

Finally, there are high hopes that at some point brain imaging might be an essential and useful tool for the objective diagnosis of a wide spectrum of diseases. This hope fits with reality in the case of many neurological syndromes: the detection and prognosis of tumors, cerebrovascular accidents, presurgical planning for brain surgery. Rapid progress is being made to incorporate brain imaging as part of the diagnostic practice for varieties of dementia (e.g., Alzheimer's disease). Hopefully, this will significantly improve diagnosis and prognosis in the earlier phases of cognitive decline referred to as mild cognitive impairment (see, e.g., Albert et al., 2011). Despite this great progress on neurological diseases, brain imaging has not yet made its way into the everyday diagnosis of psychiatric and mental syndromes such as depression, autism, and schizophrenia. Nevertheless, there is a huge number

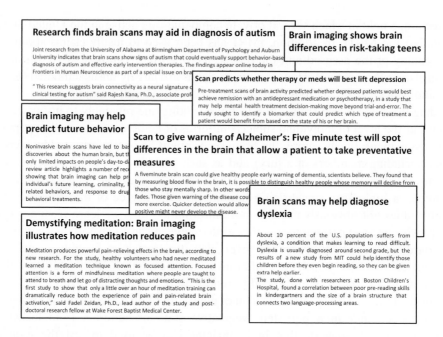

Figure 1.2 A few illustrations of headlines in the popular media about human brain imaging. Examples come from various sources, including the Daily Mail (Fiona Macrae), the MIT News Office (Anne Trafton), and ScienceDaily.com.

of scientific studies showing all sorts of differences between normal and "diseased" brains at the group level! These findings are very exciting and help in understanding the disorders, but the differences have not been large and consistent enough to be useful to help in diagnosis at the individual level. Media reports often do not recognize this nuance when presenting and discussing the results (Fig. 1.2).

These examples have three commonalities. First, the media coverage is based on scientific investigations that appeared in peer-reviewed journals. Second, the science is primarily valid and important in its own right, and the studies advance our knowledge of brain functioning often in a very meaningful way. However, third, the information and claims that make it into the popular media often stretch far beyond the original scope of these reports. Here we recognize an important role of having an in-depth knowledge of the implicated methodology, which is needed to judge the true potential of these techniques. This knowledge is necessary to avoid being a victim of overenthusiasm or, at the other end of the scale, over-skepticism (see Box 1.1).

1.2 The Basis of Neural Signals

The basis of all neural signals can be found in a few fundamental neurophysiological and metabolic phenomena. This section begins with a short primer on neurophysiology in case the reader lacks this background knowledge. Our summary may sound

Box 1.1 Neuroskepticism and Neuroscience

The fact that a lot of science fiction is often portrayed as reality in media reports has created a counter-action from "neurosceptics." The skepticism targets the scientific use of the methods as well as the claims found in the popular press.

In the scientific literature, scholars have attacked the usefulness of brain imaging in the context of many disciplines, including psychology and other social sciences. They argue that brain imaging only informs us about where mental functions are in the brain. The terms "neolocalizationism" and "neophrenology" are often used in this context (e.g., Diener, 2010; Dobbs, 2005; Fotopoulou, 2012; Uttal, 2001), referring to the phrenologists of the nineteenth century who claimed that outer features of the skull were related to mental functions. However, phrenology was a pseudoscience because the claim was never proved empirically, so the comparison is not really fair. Still, it is valid to ask whether knowing where things are is relevant for, e.g., psychology and cognitive science. We would say that it is highly relevant as a first step, because we need to know where a mental function resides in the brain before we can study it further through neuroscientific techniques. However, the next step is to investigate how the mental function is actually implemented through neural networks and circuitry. This next step is very relevant for constraining psychological/cognitive models. Contrary to what is suggested by denoting brain imaging as neo-phrenology, brain scans are not limited to localization in the narrow sense and can also help in this next step, often together with other neuroscientific methods. We hope that the later sections in this book will make this clear.

Currently, another important cause for skepticism arises from claims made in media coverage and public discourse that go further than the actual scientific data allow. Journalists go a long way trying to attract attention by giving a catchy title to an article, but such assertions have attracted a great deal of criticism, and rightfully so. Scientists and universities are also to blame for this situation, because the press releases issued by them already contain simplifications and generalizations (Sumner et al., 2014). This problem is shared by all of science and is not restricted to neuroscience and neuroimaging. Nevertheless, it seems that using the word "brain" or prefix "neuro-" is considered to be a good way to help sell a story or program (e.g., neurolinguistic programming). This "brain" hype might have had its best time, at least according to an analysis of the appearances of the word "brain" in the titles on the *New York Times* Best-Seller list (Box Fig. 1.1A; update of an earlier graph by Daniel Engber at slate.com). In recent years, the number of best sellers on the brain has gone down. This might be a good evolution from the perspective of science. The public trust in what scientists do is not helped by publishing books that tip the balance too much toward fiction and away from fact. Stated otherwise (here we are borrowing some terminology from Brigitte Nerlich's *Making Science Public* blog post, "Making Neuroscience Public"): The neuromania of neurophiles and neurohawks too often leads to neurononsense, neurotrash, and worthless neurobabble. Luckily, the number of scientific papers on the topic "brain" is still steadily increasing year by year, now being close to 60 000 articles

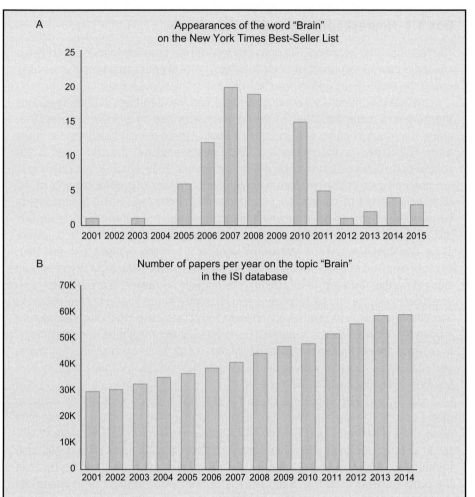

Box Figure 1.1 The use of the word "brain" in best-seller titles (A) and in the specialized academic literature (B).

The idea of counting this word in the best-seller list is credited to Daniel Engber of Slate.com.

per year (see Box Fig. 1.1B; data from the ISI database). Neuroscience in general and human brain imaging in particular are thriving.

This book covers many caveats that have been raised about brain imaging, from very technical and detailed arguments to those that are more conceptual. Nevertheless, a comprehensive overview of the relevance of neuroimaging for behavioral, psychological, and cognitive scientists is beyond the scope of this book. We refer the reader to other sources for the philosophical basis, history, and fundamental assumptions in the study of mind/brain relationships (Cacioppo et al., 2007; Churchland, 2007; Craver, 2007; Shallice, 1988). Here we will suffice by clarifying our position with an analogy. Just like an architect who designs a bridge might not need to know about quantum physics, many domains of psychology and behavioral science might flourish without any reference to brain science. However, the architect will need quantum physics for a full understanding of how gravity works, and psychologists and cognitive scientists will need brain science in order to come to a full understanding of the human mind. In our humble opinion, the aspects of the human mind that we come to understand through neuroscience are also some of the most fascinating.

highly simplistic to students who have had a basic course in neuroscience – and have the luck to remember some of the lessons! However, it is the bare minimum that you should know to understand the basics of human brain imaging that we will be covering.

Next, we provide a short guide on how we can process these neurophysiological signals. We do not aim to turn you into a signal-processing expert, but it is important that you know a few fundamental concepts that are relevant for all brain imaging techniques. Several of these concepts are covered in more detail later in the book. Furthermore, we introduce the presence of additional signals related to the metabolism that correlate with neural processing. Finally, we discuss the features of brain organization that make these signals detectable from outside the skull.

1.2.1 Information Transfer in Neurons

We will limit ourselves to one cell type in the brain, namely, neurons, because neurons have traditionally been seen as the most central cell type for brain function. There are many kinds of neurons that typically have the following parts: a dendritic tree, soma (cell body), and axon (Fig. 1.3). The brain is organized in such a way that the cell bodies of neurons are concentrated in particular structures. Because these structures look grayish in the living brain, this is referred to as **gray matter**. The cerebral cortex is a sheet of gray matter and thus contains cell bodies. Other concentrations of cell bodies beneath the cortex (hence the name "subcortical structures") are often referred to as nuclei. Some neurons have short axons that remain in the gray matter, but many neurons connect to distant neurons through long axons. All these long axons together make up the **white matter**. Underneath the cortex, this white matter takes up a large volume; in the more peripheral nervous system, the axons form nerve bundles and tracts. Here we do not provide a further introduction to neuroanatomy, but it is important to have sufficient knowledge in this domain in order to study human brain imaging. We provide further background literature in the context of Chapter 3.

Figure 1.4 shows at the right a schematic neuron in red with the same major components. This neuron receives input from other neurons, a few of which are shown on the left. The neurons in red are neurons that provide excitatory signals

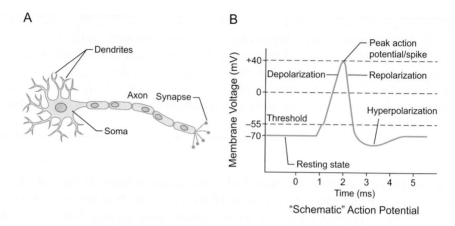

Figure 1.3 Illustration of the main components of a neuron (A) and an action potential (B).

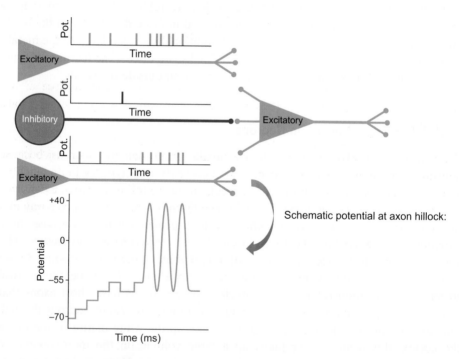

Figure 1.4 Schematic example of communication between neurons through action potentials and changes in the membrane potential. The figure shows three excitatory neurons in red and one inhibitory neuron in blue. The excitatory neuron on the right receives synaptic input (postsynaptic neuron) from the three neurons on the left. For each input neuron, we include a timeline representing the occurrence (time stamps) of action potentials. The plot at the bottom represents the dynamic changes in the membrane potential in the postsynaptic neuron as a consequence of the action potentials in the input neurons.

that make the receiving neuron become more "active." The neuron in blue represents an inhibitory neuron that makes the receiving neuron less active.

Without any input, our neuron is at rest. This resting state is characterized by a resting potential at the cell membrane. This resting potential is an electrical potential difference between the inside and the outside of the neuron. At rest, this potential difference is -70 millivolts (mV). This is the starting point in the schematic potential function shown at the bottom of Figure 1.4.

Our neuron receives input from other neurons by the delivery of a chemical substance referred to as a neurotransmitter at the synapses (contact points between neurons) in the dendritic tree of our neuron. Receptors in the membrane of our neuron react to these neurotransmitters and as such disturb the resting potential. The direction of this effect differs between neurotransmitters and, depending on which neurotransmitter is released, neurons are categorized as excitatory or inhibitory. The neurotransmitter input from an excitatory neuron will make the potential difference less negative (depolarization), so the -70 mV might become -65 mV. The neurotransmitter from an inhibitory neuron will have the opposite effect and make the potential difference more negative (hyperpolarization). In the cerebral cortex, glutamate is an important excitatory neurotransmitter, and a molecule known as GABA is the most prominent inhibitory neurotransmitter.

The changes in the potential difference originate in the dendritic tree of our neuron, but they are transmitted throughout the cell membrane of the soma, toward the point where the axon begins. This point is referred to as the "axon hillock." Something interesting happens when the potential difference reaches a critical level, typically at -55 mV. When the difference between the inside and the outside of the neuron becomes this small, a sequence of events occurs at the cell membrane. This results in a sudden further decrease of the potential difference, an overshoot so that the difference even becomes positive, and then there is a very quick restoration of a negative difference. These rapid changes in the potential take a very characteristic form, which we know as the **action potential**. An action potential is shown in more detail in Figure 1.3B. The schematic potential below Figure 1.4 shows three such action potentials. Given their sharpness, action potentials are sometimes also referred to as "spikes."

The action potentials start at the axon hillock close to the soma, but they are quickly transported through the axon, all the way to the other end where the axon splits into fine branches that end up at synapses. The arrival of an action potential of our neuron triggers the release of neurotransmitters, after which the story repeats itself in the next neuron with changes in its membrane potential.

The postsynaptic neuron will integrate the input that it receives across all the input neurons and across time by the effect that the released neurotransmitters have on the postsynaptic potential. This is also illustrated in Figure 1.4, in which the schematic potential at the bottom shows the effect of each action potential that is "fired" by the input neurons and results in neurotransmitter release.

Each time that there is an action potential in an excitatory neuron (shown in red), the curve of the potential goes up and becomes less negative. If an action potential occurs in an inhibitory neuron (shown in blue), then we see the reverse effect: The curve goes down toward more negative values. Upon receiving excitatory input sufficiently frequently, the membrane potential reaches the critical level, and an action potential is being triggered. Several action potentials follow because more excitatory input is received.

1.2.2 Signal Processing

The changes in the membrane potential across the soma and axon hillock as shown in Figure 1.4 constitute a signal that provides very detailed information of what is happening with our neuron. It summarizes how much input the neuron receives, the relative degree of excitatory and inhibitory input, and when an action potential is triggered. However, it does not provide the complete story. For example, the two red neurons each result in the same effect on the membrane potential and thus cannot be distinguished using this signal. The fact that the postsynaptic neuron fires an action potential does not inform you about which presynaptic neuron caused the depolarization. Nevertheless, as just one signal, the fluctuation in the membrane potential is very helpful to provide a summary of what is happening.

There are methods to directly measure the membrane potential and how it changes over time. One of them is patch clamping, which consists of sucking part of the membrane with the tip of a pipette and then measuring the membrane potential. Obviously, this method is highly invasive. Furthermore, it requires a very stable substrate that is only feasible in a highly controlled animal experiment, and most often even applied to in vitro brain slices rather than living animals. It is not utilized in human research. Nevertheless, patch clamping is the only method by which we can faithfully measure changes in membrane potential. We will use this signal to explain several concepts about signal processing that will be a recurring theme also for signals that we *can* measure in humans.

A first concept is that of **frequency**. Frequency refers to the rate of change in a signal along some dimension, such as time or space. In the time domain, frequency is expressed in hertz (Hz), for which the unit of time is a second. A signal with frequency of 1 Hz is a signal that goes up and down once per second. The full period (going up and going down) takes exactly one second. Biological signals never contain just one frequency. Artificial signals can. For example, a pure tone exists of a sinusoidal sound wave of just one frequency.

Biological signals contain sub-signals or **frequency components**, each having a different frequency, ranging from slow to fast. Each component is determined by three parameters: frequency, amplitude (how much it is going up and down), and phase (when it is going up and down). Apart from the changes that can be induced by altering these parameters, the components are the same. In most methods of signal processing, sinusoidal functions are used, which are indeed characterized by frequency, amplitude, and phase.

The full signal can be seen as an addition of these components. For example, the schematic membrane potential in Figure 1.4 can be approximated by an addition of a slow frequency component and a fast component, which represents the three action potentials. The better we want the approximation to be, the more components we will need. For example, the addition of just these two components will not capture the small indentation caused by the one action potential fired by the (blue) inhibitory neuron.

The range of frequencies in a signal is not infinite. The measured range is referred to as the **frequency spectrum**. The highest frequency that can be measured is ultimately limited by how often the signal is measured, that is, the **sampling frequency**. As an example, suppose that you measure your body weight once per day. With these data, you can capture fluctuations in your weight across days, but not the fluctuations within a day. More generally, we know that with a frequency of once a day you can only faithfully capture fluctuations that are slower than 2 days, or half the sampling frequency. In engineering, this ratio of one half is given by the Nyquist sampling theorem. Here we will not bother you with the mathematics behind it, but it is important that you know about this limit when you work with signals of any kind. To take another example, it is clear that a sampling frequency of 100 Hz, which means that you are getting a sample once every 10 milliseconds (ms), is of not much use for a patch clamp experiment, given that an action potential only takes 1–2 ms to complete.

The lowest frequency that can be detected is limited by how long the signal is measured. If a signal is measured for two seconds at a high sampling frequency, then it is possible to capture frequency components from 0.5 Hz upward, but not frequencies below that. The limit is given by 1 divided by the number of seconds measured.

A final concept to introduce is the notion of **filtering**. In the present context, filtering means that a specific part of the measured frequency spectrum is being attenuated. There are three important types of filtering to know about. First, in low-pass filtering the lower/slower frequencies are not altered, while the higher/faster frequencies are weakened or even completely removed from the signal. This kind of filtering is also referred to as smoothing. Second, in high-pass filtering, the higher frequencies can pass through the filter, and the lower frequencies are attenuated. Finally, band-pass filtering means that only a particular range or "band" of frequencies is allowed to pass through the filter. All frequencies below and above this range are attenuated.

We will proceed with an illustration of signal processing, given in Figure 1.5. The signal on display represents brain activity as measured from outside the skull through a technique known as electroencephalography (EEG). The details of this method are described later. As with the schematic membrane potential, Figure 1.5A shows a signal plotted with time on the X-axis and voltage on the Y-axis. Upon

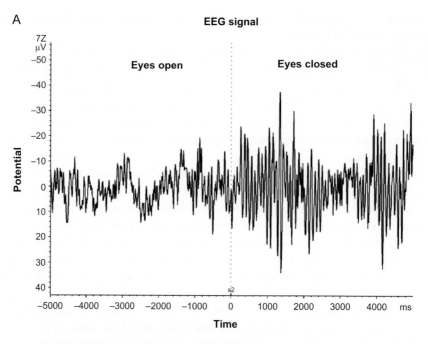

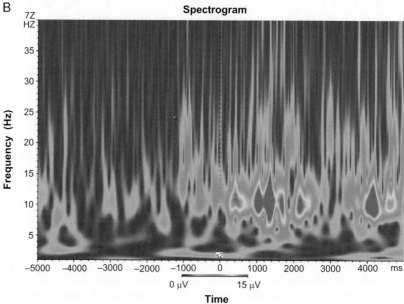

Figure 1.5 Example of signal processing as applied to an EEG measurement. (A) EEG trace (potential as a function of time). Time is counted relative to the point in time (time zero) in which the participant closes the eyes. (B) The decomposition of the signal into frequency components, each with a particular amplitude. Amplitude is represented by the color scale.

inspection of the signal, you might notice that in the first 5 seconds the signal fluctuates relatively slowly, and fast changes are small in magnitude. Using some of the technical terms we just introduced, this is a signal where high-frequency components have a low amplitude and low-frequency components have a higher amplitude. During this time, the person from which this signal was measured had the eyes open. After 5 seconds, the person closes the eyes, and these high-frequency components appear to increase in magnitude.

Thus far, we have referred to these frequency components in a relatively informal and descriptive manner. However, the strength of these components can also be measured in a formal, quantitative way. Frequency-based analyses are widespread in neuroimaging, and we will see many examples and further details in later sections. Here we will limit ourselves to one example that involves analyzing how strong each frequency component is at each moment in time. The result of such a computation is a matrix that contains the strength of each frequency at each moment in time. This matrix is referred to as a **spectrogram**. Spectrograms are often displayed by a colored diagram such as in Figure 1.5B, with time on the X-axis and frequency on the Y-axis. In the color scale, the zero strength/amplitude is shown in blue and the highest amplitude in red. The high-frequency component that we noticed through visual inspection in the EEG signal is visible as a band stretched in time centered on a frequency of 10 Hz. This component increases in magnitude around time zero, when the person closes the eyes.

1.2.3 Other Signals in the Brain: Molecular and Hemodynamic Signals

We have characterized the communication within and between neurons as electrical signals related to changes in the membrane potential. This is an important level of description, and it is the basis of the many techniques that measure the electrical activity in the brain. However, the electrophysiological changes due to neural communication are connected to other kinds of changes that form the basis of yet other methods.

On a smaller scale, the changes in membrane potential only happen because of the movement of chemical substances and molecules in and out of neurons. An action potential is a very elegant and deceptively simple change in the membrane potential, but the underlying fluxes of *molecules* across the membrane are very complex. For example, in the rising, depolarization phase of the action potential there is a strong influx of sodium ions (Na^+), whereas the descending repolarization phase is characterized by an outward current of potassium ions (K^+). At the synapses, there are a lot of molecules involved in many functions, including the release and uptake of the aforementioned neurotransmitters. One particularly relevant molecule is calcium. It is involved in processes such as neurotransmitter release, plasticity, and gene transcription. It moves in and out of neurons through voltage-sensitive channels, and it is an important intracellular messenger.

Interestingly, neurons contain much more calcium when they are electrically active than when they are at rest. For this reason, imaging of the calcium concentration within neurons is a very useful and widespread procedure to measure neuronal activity. This type of imaging is performed with optical devices, such as two-photon calcium imaging. This invasive technique provides single-neuron resolution: The calcium concentration of individual neurons can be determined and differentiated from the concentration in other nearby neurons.

At a larger scale, there are nonelectrical correlates of the electrical activity. Many of them are related to the *energy requirements* of all the processes which are involved in neural activity (for reviews, see Attwell and Iadecola, 2002; Shulman et al., 2004). Cells need energy to stay alive. Neurons need even more energy to perform their function. Up to 20% of our daily energy intake is consumed by the brain. This energy is supplied to the tissue by blood and the glucose in it. The blood supply is adjusted to the current needs and thus changes over time. This is referred to as **hemodynamics**.

The most obvious and highest-amplitude change in the membrane potential is the action potential. However, the amplitude of the potential changes might not be the best predictor of the amount of energy required. In particular, to some extent the action potential itself is a passive chain of events that does not consume much energy. Once the critical threshold is reached at, e.g., the axon hillock, the action potential will proceed even if little energy is present. However, restoring the resting potential after an action potential requires energy (Attwell and Laughlin, 2001). As a consequence, the energy consumption of a neuron can be expected to correlate with the number of action potentials elicited. Several other previously mentioned processes also require energy, including the presynaptic release of neurotransmitters, the functioning of postsynaptic receptors, and the maintenance of a resting potential in the absence of any action potentials or synaptic input. In particular, there has been a lively discussion about the relative importance of presynaptic and postsynaptic factors in the total count of consumed energy (Attwell and Iadecola, 2002).

These issues are not easy to decide. The relative contribution of each of these processes to the total energy consumption by neurons will strongly depend on many factors. As a consequence, it is very difficult to come up with one general scheme. Figure 1.6 shows two results from studies that modeled the anatomical and physiological data (e.g., the consumption of ATP, which is the form energy takes to be used by a cell) in rat (left) gray matter when the mean action potential rate of neurons is 4 Hz (Attwell and Laughlin, 2001). In one case, the change in energy consumption when action potentials occur accounts for 47% of the energy consumption, synaptic transmission for 40%, and the maintenance of a resting potential for 13%. Most of the synaptic energy budget goes to postsynaptic processes, because variations in presynaptic neurotransmitter release (measured through presynaptic Ca^{2+}) account for only 3% of the energy consumption. In the other case, the budget for synaptic transmission takes 64% of the total pie. Note that it is easy to imagine situations in which these percentages might be very different. For

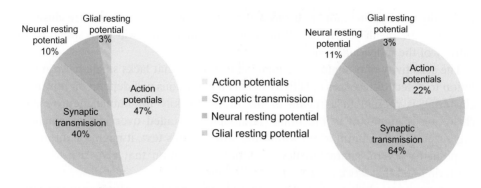

Figure 1.6 The energy consumption by several cellular processes as derived from theoretical modeling and ATP consumption measurements (see, e.g., Attwell and Laughlin, 2001). The two pie charts reflect the outcome of different theoretical models, showing what is common to all models (only part of energy consumption is related to action potentials) and what is not (the exact percentages assigned to different types of processes).
Figures reproduced from Sengupta et al., 2013

example, when a region receives a lot of inhibitory input, then there will be many presynaptic terminals that release a neurotransmitter (e.g., GABA, see Chapter 3) that inhibits the postsynaptic neurons. As a result, there will be very little action potentials fired, and the percentage of the energy consumption related to presynaptic functioning might be much higher overall. In addition, the numbers might depend on species and neuron type.

1.2.4 Maps in the Brain: From the Activity of Single Neurons to Signals without Single-Neuron Resolution

Measuring the electrical activity or metabolism of a single neuron requires direct access to the neural tissue and to be close to the neuron. Techniques can only achieve such resolution when the skull is opened and material is inserted into the brain and thus are highly invasive. Almost all human neuroscience happens with noninvasive techniques that do not have the precision to measure what happens in individual neurons. As a consequence, even the smallest spatial unit of measurement will average the signal from many neurons. For example, even a small cube of 1x1x1 millimeters (mm) centered on gray matter already contains at least 10 000 neurons, of various kinds (excitatory, inhibitory, ...), and in addition to other cell types (e.g., glia cells) and other tissue (e.g., blood vessels).

If the activity of each of these 10 000 neurons were completely uncorrelated with the activity of other neurons in the same cube, then the mean activity of all these neurons would not be very informative about the functional properties of the neurons in the cube. In such a situation, we would say that there is no clustering. **Clustering** refers to the tendency of neurons with similar functional properties to be physically nearby. The more neurons with similar response properties are clustered, the more the mean activity of all neurons in a small cube will correspond to the activity of the individual neurons in the cube.

The sensitivity of a noninvasive imaging technique that lacks single-neuron resolution to detect differences in activity between conditions will depend on how much clustering is present in a region of the brain. Luckily for human neuroscience, clustering is abundant in the brain. Although a detailed overview of functional organization in the brain is not within the scope of this text, it might be interesting to point to several characteristics of brain organization that give rise to strong clustering and that work *at different spatial scales*.

At a small scale below a millimeter, there is evidence for a columnar organization in many brain regions (see, e.g., Mountcastle, 1997; Tanaka, 2003). A column is a cylinder-like volume in the cortex that runs through all cortical layers all the way from the surface of the brain to where gray matter is bordered by white matter. In the human brain, this cortical thickness is 2–4 mm. The radius of the cylinder might be only a few 100 micrometers or less. Within the column, neurons have very similar response properties. Well-known examples of columnar structure are ocular dominance columns and orientation columns in primary visual cortex (which is in the back of your head in the occipital lobe).

At a somewhat larger scale, we find topographic maps that span several millimeters in anatomical space parallel to the cortical surface. Examples of such maps can be found in primary sensory regions: retinotopy (visual), tonotopy (auditory), and somatotopy (somatosensation). In each of these modalities there is a faithful correspondence between the ordering of the receptors and the change in tuning properties of the cortical neurons across the cortical surface. For example, in the case of retinotopy nearby cortical neurons prefer similar and overlapping positions in the visual field, and this preferred position gradually shifts when neurons are further away in the cortex.

At an even larger scale, human neuroanatomy is divided into nuclei (for subcortical structures) and areas (in the cortex). In most standard examples, areas are larger than maps in the sense that areas contain maps. For example, a full map of retinal coordinates is found in several visual areas including and beyond primary visual cortex. In some cases, the neurons in one and the same area tend to have particular functional properties that are different from the properties of neurons in other areas. A textbook example is the middle temporal (MT) area in which neurons show a strong selectivity for the direction of motion of a visual stimulus (Kolster et al., 2010).

Finally, at the largest scale, areas show a preferential connectivity and overlap in functional properties with other areas, usually areas that have a close proximity. As such these areas form cortical systems. Such a system can take up a large part of the cortex. For example, the visual system takes up the whole occipital lobe and extends into the temporal as well as the parietal lobe, occupying close to one third of the human cerebral cortex. Systems can also share areas/regions.

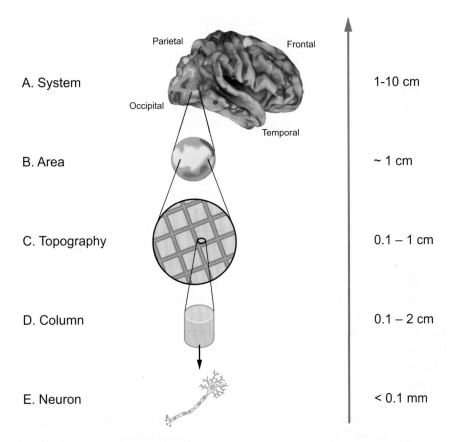

Figure 1.7 Clustering of neurons with similar functional properties at multiple scales. (A) Large-scale activation of cerebral cortex when a participant is navigating through a virtual maze by means of button presses. Prominent clusters of activation are seen in occipital, parietal, and frontal cortex. Red/yellow and blue refer to higher and lower, respectively, activation compared with a rest baseline (data from Op de Beeck et al., 2013). (B) Magnified version of the size of what might be one cortical area in (A). (C) The area might contain a topographic map of visual space, so that a visually presented grid-like pattern might activate the extent of the cortical area in a grid-like manner. (D) At one location in this topographic map, where all neurons have a similar receptive field position, neurons might be further clustered in columns according to their preference for particular visual features. (E) One of the hundreds of neurons in a column.

Figure 1.7 illustrates the different scales of clustering at which we can investigate the neural response during visuospatial navigation. In this condition, strong activity is seen in large regions of occipital, temporal, and parietal cortex. At a finer level, this activity is distributed across multiple visual areas, many of which contain a retinotopic map of visual space. Each location in space is further analyzed in a columnar structure in which single neurons tend to prefer similar visual features.

The smallest spatial unit of measurement of a particular imaging technique will determine which level of clustering can be investigated with this technique.

A technique in which the smallest unit corresponds to a full cortical area will not be able to provide a direct measurement of functional organization at any smaller scale, such as columns and topographic maps. Functional properties that are organized at a smaller scale are missed by such a technique.

To take a specific example, neurons in primary visual cortex are known to be selective for the orientation of small bars that fall in their receptive field. Orientation selectivity is also picked up with invasive optical imaging, which is an invasive technique with a resolution of 20 micrometers (μm). In such an experiment, researchers measure the optical signal when lines are shown with a different orientation. Local clusters of pixels in the resulting image show a clear and consistent orientation selectivity, what we have referred to as a columnar structure. Note that optical imaging would not show any dependency of the signal on the shown stimuli if selectivity for line orientation would not be clustered. This image was obtained in cats, and these animals have orientation columns (as do monkeys). Rodents do not have orientation selectivity: Nearby neurons in the rat or mouse primary visual cortex do not have a similar orientation preference. As a consequence, optical imaging with a resolution of 20 μm would not show much selectivity, because the signal would average across multiple single neurons with a different preference. The nice selectivity at the single-neuron level would be averaged away.

Because of the phenomenon of "averaging away," a technique with a spatial resolution lower than the size of an orientation column would not allow orientation selectivity to be measured easily. A technique with the smallest unit of measurement of 1x1x1 mm would average the signals of multiple orientation columns. The resulting image would be a highly blurred one in which no location would contain the strong selectivity as is actually present at the level of single columns.

1.3 A Short Overview of Methods in Human Neuroscience

The previous paragraph explained that neural activity causes various signals to emerge: local changes in membrane potential, changes in molecular gradients, and hemodynamic changes. Each of these signals has components at multiple spatial and temporal scales. This multitude of signals is measured through a range of methods. Here we will give an overview of these methods. In later chapters we focus on the individual techniques in more detail. The current section will enable you to put each method in the context of many of the main methods used today.

Figure 1.8 provides a graphical summary of neuroscientific techniques in a three-dimensional space formed by the following dimensions: temporal resolution, spatial resolution, and invasiveness. **Temporal resolution** refers to the smallest unit of time that can be differentiated by a method. Millisecond resolution or better is needed to measure individual action potentials, while a resolution of several seconds might be sufficient to measure the aggregated response elicited by a 20-second block of face images. **Spatial resolution** indicates the smallest unit of space that can be resolved. It will determine which scale of organization can be picked up. **Invasiveness** is

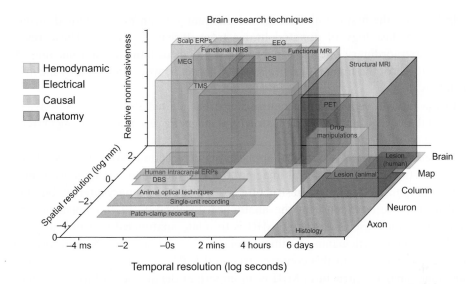

Figure 1.8 Graphical depiction of the spectrum of human brain imaging techniques in three dimensions: temporal resolution, spatial resolution, and invasiveness. The methods are grouped in four classes: hemodynamic methods (pink), electrophysiological methods (light blue), causal methods (orange), and anatomical methods (dark blue). Acronyms for methods are explained in the relevant sections.
The plot is inspired by earlier figures of Churchland and Sejnowski, 1988 and Huettel et al., 2004

primarily a binary factor, because the majority of methods are either fully invasive (skull needs to be penetrated) or not invasive at all.

Each technique is given an approximate location in this space. Similar diagrams can be found in several other sources (Churchland and Sejnowski, 1988; Grinvald and Hildesheim, 2004; Huettel et al., 2004). Later chapters focus on the less invasive techniques because only these techniques can be applied in humans. The diagram in Figure 1.8 includes the full range of techniques because the contrast between invasive and noninvasive techniques forces us to consider what we miss and cannot investigate with noninvasive methods. A visual inspection of the diagram already highlights one big loss by being restricted to the less invasive methods: There are no methods available that have a high (single-neuron) spatial resolution combined with a high (milliseconds) temporal resolution. The lower left quadrant of the space contains only invasive methods.

1.3.1 Techniques to Measure Brain Structure

The traditional method used to investigate brain structure is **histology**. This is an invasive methodology that involves cutting the brain in pieces, such as slices. The slices are further processed chemically in order to visualize the structure of interest. Histology is still a standard method for studying brain anatomy at high spatial resolution in nonhuman animals.

In humans, the first detailed images of the human brain were obtained through postmortem histology of donated brains from deceased persons. These results were of extraordinary interest for the development of human brain imaging. All classic atlases of the human brain (also see Chapter 3) were produced by means of histology.

In the past 30 years, human neuroscience has shifted its focus to noninvasive structural imaging. In these studies, **structural magnetic resonance imaging (MRI)** is the method of choice.

Currently, there are two typical applications of structural MRI. First, studies of brain function include structural imaging to relate the functional findings to brain structure. In these studies, brain structure is often not the primary interest, but it is a tool to increase confidence in the anatomical localization of functional findings. A second typical use of structural MRI is to relate anatomical structure to differences between participants at other levels of description, such as behavior and disease classification. In this context, structural MRI might be performed without functional imaging. Structural MRI is an important diagnostic tool for a variety of conditions, including a cerebrovascular accident (Kidwell et al., 2004) and brain tumors (Weber et al., 2006). For many other clinical conditions, brain anatomy at the group level has been found to differ between patient and control groups. In addition, several aspects of brain anatomy have been related to inter-individual differences in terms of behavior.

Almost any behavior and activity that humans are involved in can be related to brain structure – or at least it sounds reasonable enough to let neuroscientists spend their time searching for such evidence! To highlight one case as an example, Bickart and colleagues (2011) investigated the relationship between neural anatomy and the social network of their participants. For the latter, the authors used a metric known as the social network index, which assesses the size and the complexity (number of subgroups) of the regular contacts with whom a person engages. Neural anatomy was determined using structural MRI. Individuals with a larger amygdala volume had a larger and more complex social network. The same finding extends to online social network size, such as the number of friends on Facebook, which was correlated significantly with gray matter density in several regions including amygdala (Kanai et al., 2012). If even your Facebook usage is related to your brain anatomy, then you might understand the relevance of devoting the first part of this book to structural MRI!

1.3.2 Techniques to Measure Hemodynamic Correlates of Neural Activity

The aforementioned changes in energy consumption by neurons trigger a chain of events. These events can be grouped under the umbrella term "hemodynamic correlates": changes in blood and tissue oxygenation, blood flow, and blood volume. The further down the chain of events, the more distance there is between the location and timing of the neuronal activity and the location and timing of the events caused by this neural activity (see Chapter 4 for more information).

There is a variety of methods to measure one or a combination of these hemodynamic correlates of neural activity. Here we give a brief list. A detailed description of each of the prominent methods in human research is given in Part II of this book, in particular in Chapter 4. A first set of methods uses the effect of tissue oxygenation on the reflection of light that shines on the tissue. In nonhuman animals, this light is directed at the cortical surface to avoid scattering of the light bundle by intermediate tissue. This invasive optical imaging provides a resolution sufficient to measure columnar structure. There is also a noninvasive optical imaging technique used in humans, referred to as **functional near-infrared spectroscopy** (fNIRS). This technique has a very low spatial resolution (centimeters), which is sufficient for studying systems and, in some cases, maps (e.g., a coarse measure of retinotopy, see Chapter 4). Furthermore, the signal is primarily restricted to cortical regions immediately under the skull, and as such cannot be used for the large part of the cortex that is hidden within the sulci (the deeper parts of the folded cortex) or on the medial surface of the hemispheres. Nevertheless, the technique is being used more and more frequently, in particular in infant research, because it is very easy to set up and move.

In the 1980s, there was a surge of studies, some still carried out today, which used radioactive labeling of blood and then measured changes in blood volume through the emitted signal. This technique, referred to as **positron emission tomography** (PET), has a spatial resolution that is often around 1–2 cm and a very poor temporal resolution because the signal is averaged across tens of seconds. Today, PET is primarily used not as a measure of neural activity through blood volume, but as a measure of the distribution of particular molecular markers across the brain. For measuring a hemodynamic correlate for neural activity, PET has for the most part been replaced by **functional magnetic resonance imaging** (fMRI). The fMRI signal reflects multiple hemodynamic correlates of neural activity, as explained subsequently. It is the noninvasive imaging technique with the highest spatial resolution, which explains its popularity as reflected in the high number of published studies in the best scientific journals that use this technique. It is also the brain imaging method that underlies many of the claims that reach the popular press, as illustrated in Figure 1.2.

This short summary highlights that the spatial resolution varies strongly among the different measures of hemodynamic correlates due to the exact correlate being measured (a physiological limit imposed on the resolution) and the physical limits of the measurement device. The range is smaller than for measures of electrical signals: Hemodynamic imaging does not provide the resolution of single-unit recordings, and in most cases it is better than the workhorses of electrical imaging, EEG and scalp event-related potential (ERP). The temporal resolution of hemodynamic imaging is undoubtedly poorer compared with electrical imaging due to the fact that all hemodynamic correlates are temporally smoothed with respect to electrical activity.

1.3.3 Techniques to Measure Electrophysiological Activity

Most of the methods having a good temporal resolution shown in Figure 1.8 measure electrophysiological activity. These methods include patch-clamp recording, single-unit recording, multi-unit recording, local field potentials (LFPs), human intracranial recordings, Electrocorticogram (ECoG) and stereo EEG (sEEG), magnetoencephalography (MEG), and scalp electroencephalography (EEG).

At the same time, techniques to measure electrical activity vary widely in terms of spatial resolution. The spatial resolution of a measurement of electrical activity is related to the distance between the electrode and the source of the signal: the further the distance, the larger the volume that is sampled by the electrode. Another factor is the intermediate tissue, for example, the skull scatters electrical signals and thus is very detrimental for spatial resolution.

The optimal spatial resolution is obtained by **patch-clamp recordings**, the only technique that measures changes in the membrane potential faithfully with only very limited distortions. Alternatively, researchers can insert an electrode into the cortex and bring its tip very close to a single neuron to pick up the action potentials of this neuron. With such an invasive electrode, we might be able to perform **extracellular single-unit recordings**, at least when the electrode has a high impedance so that only signals from very nearby are picked up ("impedance" can be regarded as another word for "resistance"). Alternatively, when a lower-impedance electrode is inserted in the cortex, it can be useful for two types of measurements. First, it could be used for recording the action potentials of many nearby units at once (**multi-unit recording**). Given its very transient nature, an action potential is characterized by fast changes in the membrane potential, and for that reason a researcher would want to filter the incoming signal so that higher frequencies are kept (high-pass filtering). Second, the same signal processed through a low-pass filter would contain information about the slower changes in membrane potential of all nearby neurons, referred to as **local field potentials** or **LFPs**.

All these techniques are very risky in a living organism, because they require opening up the dura that surrounds the cortex and protects it from infections. **Intracranial recordings** still require the opening of the skull (craniotomy) but only to place electrodes on top of the dura which remains intact. The craniotomy allows the researcher to place the electrode much closer to the neural tissue, and it avoids having the skull scatter the signal even further.

All these techniques with a higher spatial resolution are invasive. Without opening up the skull, the distance between electrode and the source of the signal and the further scattering by the skull is so large that the spatial resolution is very poor, more on the order of several or many centimeters. Rephrased in terms of cortical structures and scales of clustering, this means that even brain areas are hard to measure individually and often measurements are related to the activity of multiple brain areas and brain systems. The available methods include **MEG**, which measures electrical activity through the magnetic fields produced by electrical currents, **EEG**, and **scalp ERPs**.

We differentiated between high- and low-frequency signals in the case of electrodes that are inserted in cortex. To some degree, we can extend this distinction to the noninvasive methods. However, the highest frequencies are no longer present in the noninvasive signals. This is another effect of the distance between electrode and signal source. Distance combines with more intermediate mediums (tissue, skull, etc.) through which the signal has to travel, and the scatter occurring because of these mediums is more detrimental for higher temporal frequencies than it is for lower frequencies. For that reason, the long-distance signals with low spatial resolution are also restricted to lower temporal frequencies. This is disappointing, because the different frequency bands contain very different information. For example, the changes in membrane potential that characterize an action potential are very fast – the action potential starts and ends in less than 2 ms – and thus we need to measure frequencies well above 300 Hz to measure an individual action potential. These higher frequencies cannot be recovered through noninvasive methods.

Figures 1.9 and 1.10 represent the full range of electrical techniques that have been used in humans. In very rare cases, primarily in patients with epilepsy, single-unit recordings have been performed intermittently during sessions aimed at determining the site of origin of the epileptic seizures. In an ideal situation with high-quality data, the signal measured by a high-impedance electrode after high-pass filtering looks like what is shown in Figure 1.9B. The continuous signal at the left is composed of a background level (the black band) that represents noise in the signal interspersed with fast transient peaks in the signal that represent the action potentials of a single neuron. All these action potentials are very similar (technically, they have the same waveform), as can be seen when they are plotted on top of each other at the right. Note that this waveform is not the same as the standard temporal profile of the depolarization and repolarization during an action potential, because there are many distorting factors due to the distance between electrode and neuron (only patch-clamp recordings represent the action potential faithfully).

The data in Figure 1.9A come from one of the best-known studies using human single-unit recordings (Quiroga et al., 2005). The authors presented images while recording from single neurons. Each image was presented multiple times. The action potentials recorded from one particular neuron during individual trials are shown below each image as a raster plot (each line is a trial; a blue dot represents the occurrence of an action potential). Below these raster plots are histograms with the summed number of action potentials recorded in each time bin. This neuron is the famous Jennifer Aniston neuron: It fired action potentials each time a picture of the actress Jennifer Aniston was shown. The funny side story is that the neuron did not respond when Jennifer Aniston was pictured together with Brad Pitt (top row on the right), even though at the time of the recordings these two actors were not yet divorced. The serious conclusion of the study was that the human brain contains neurons that are highly selective for particular objects or faces, and often

A.

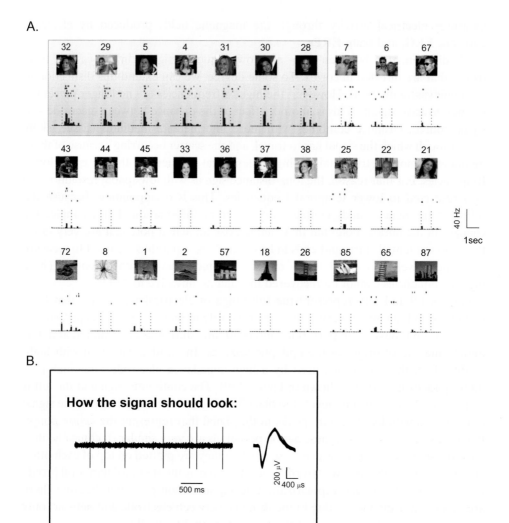

Figure 1.9 Invasive single-neuron recordings in human patients. (A) Action potentials fired by a single neuron when a variety of complex images were presented, including pictures of the actress Jennifer Aniston. Figure reproduced with permission from Quiroga et al., 2005. (B) Visualization of the type of continuous signal (*left*) and template matching (*right*) that underlies the detection of action potentials in (A).

(but not always) retain their selectivity across changes in simple image parameters such as size and viewpoint.

Data like these are impressive, but rare. There are many ethical considerations. The recordings can be done only when the insertion of invasive electrodes is necessary to treat patients who are seriously ill. Invasive recordings cannot be performed in the healthy human brain. Furthermore, even in rare cases in which the recordings are carried out, the quality of the recordings is often much lower than

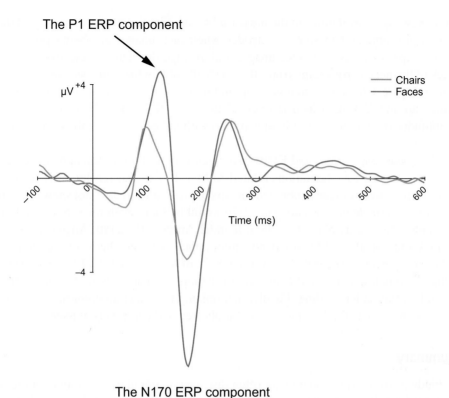

Figure 1.10 reproduced content:

The P1 ERP component

The N170 ERP component

Figure 1.10 Face-selective, event-related potential recorded through EEG. The ERP peaks are larger at two time points, referred to as the P1 and the N170 component, when participants view faces (red) compared with objects (blue).

Figure reproduced with permission from Pitcher et al., 2011

what researchers tend to acquire in animal research with the same methods, as there is less control over where neurons are recorded (often the data contain a mixture of neurons from very different brain areas), and there are fewer neurons recorded, fewer conditions tested, and fewer trials conducted per condition. The ethical and practical complications explain why human single-neuron recordings do not dominate human neuroscience. Still, the data are very thought provoking and influential for formulating hypotheses that can be tested in further experiments using other techniques and other species.

At the other end of the dimension of spatial resolution we have noninvasive methods such as magnetoencephalography (MEG) and electroencephalography (EEG). These techniques are explained in Part III of this book. A method such as EEG involves a number of electrodes (often 32, 64, or 128) placed on top of the scalp. Each electrode measures the accumulated electrical signal from a large volume of the brain. This volume is so large that neighboring electrodes, despite being separated by centimeters, measure an overlapping volume. As a consequence, they show high correlations in the measured signal. Figure 1.10 shows the signal that is typically obtained in some electrodes when face images are being presented. When experimenters show face images and average the signal in electrodes at the back of the head across many trials, they typically obtain the signal shown with a red line in Figure 1.10. This signal goes up and down. A very prominent feature is the valley around 170 ms, which is referred to as the N170. This N170 has a higher amplitude when a face image is shown than with images of other objects (e.g., cars or chairs).

Electroencephalograms and ERPs have been very useful for human neuroscience, but there are obvious limitations related to their low spatial resolution. The signal reflects the activity of many cubic centimeters of the brain and does not show the same selectivity as single neurons do. The N170 would be there, with the same amplitude, no matter the identity of the face: Be it Jennifer Aniston, Brad Pitt, Angelina Jolie, or Barack Obama, the N170 would not differentiate between them. In addition, the relationship between neural activity at the level of neurons and the EEG/ERP signal is highly complex, and even the most complex biophysical models are too simplistic to provide a full understanding. Finally, determining the exact anatomical source of a component such as the N170 is a very complicated and controversial issue.

Summary

- Findings from brain imaging are often discussed in popular media, but a more in-depth knowledge about these methods is needed to differentiate between fact and fiction.
- Information transfer involves slow and fast (action potential) changes in electrical membrane potentials, which in turn change the energy requirements of neurons.
- Even though individual neurons are too small to emit a signal that can be measured noninvasively, they tend to cluster together with other neurons, and as a population they might be large enough to emit a detectable signal.
- Functional brain imaging methods use a variety of physical principles, including electricity, magnetism, optics, nuclear resonance, and radiation, in order to pick up one of two types of signals: electrical and hemodynamic.
- The source of the signals, being either electrical or hemodynamic, has a strong impact on the benefits and drawbacks of the different brain imaging methods.
- Brain imaging methods can be differentiated on three basic dimensions: spatial resolution, temporal resolution, and the distance from the neural tissue that emits the signal to the detector (invasiveness).

Review Questions

1. Describe the extent to which the number of action potentials can be measured through a hemodynamic imaging technique such as positron emission tomography.

2. What is temporal resolution and how is it affected by the source of neural signals (electrical or hemodynamic) and invasiveness?
3. Describe the functional clustering of neurons at multiple spatial scales and how this relates to what can and cannot be measured by a noninvasive brain imaging method.
4. Why do we lose more meaningful signals when we perform low-pass filtering of extracellular single-neuron recordings compared with low-pass filtering (with the same settings) of scalp ERPs?

Further Reading

Cambridge Fundamentals of Neuroscience in Psychology series. (*Introduction to Human Neuroimaging* is a part of this series. We focus on methods more so than on results in a particular domain. The other books in the series contain many applications of these methods in many different domains, illustrating how much these methods have advanced our understanding of how the human brain works.)

Farah, M. J. (2005). Neuroethics: the practical and the philosophical. *Trends in Cognitive Sciences*, **9**(1), 34–40. (The examples of coverage of brain imaging research in the popular media frequently touched on moral and ethical issues, for which this article provides a further introduction.)

Satel, S. & Lilienfeld, S. O. (2013). *Brainwashed: The Seductive Appeal of Mindless Neuroscience*, New York: Basic Books. (An enthusiastic believer in the merits of brain imaging research should not take the universal benefits of this research for granted but be ready to face criticism, which is what this book provides.)

Notes

1 www.telegraph.co.uk/news/worldnews/middleeast/israel/9830203/Comatose-Ariel-Sharon-shows-signs-of-brain-activity.html

PART I
Structural Neuroimaging

Structural neuroimaging investigates the anatomy of the brain. There are good reasons to begin a book on human brain imaging by looking at structural imaging. This might not seem the best place to start to some of the more impatient readers. Unless your ambition is to become a neuroanatomist, odds are high that neuroanatomy is not your favorite domain of study. For example, to a student who wants to understand the determinants of human behavior, techniques that measure brain function might seem far more interesting compared with structural neuroimaging. Why waste time on this and not jump immediately to functional imaging?

We have three major arguments to back up our choice. First, functional imaging data cannot be interpreted properly without knowledge of brain structure. A basis in anatomy is crucial even if the eventual goal is to understand the functioning of the brain. By analogy, when a car is having mechanical or electronic issues, the car mechanic can start fixing the problem only when the piece to repair has been located. It matters whether the engine is in the front or in the back of the car. The same goes for the human brain. Evolution could have come up with a different anatomical structure that would have resulted in more or less the same function – for example, a structure in which visual information would enter the cerebral cortex in the front of the head instead of in the occipital pole. This would even make sense, given that the eyes are also in the front. It is not a coincidence that this is the place given to visual faculties such as form and color by the phrenologists who localized faculties in the head based on intuition rather than science. It could have been true, but it is not. Any neuroscientist who wants to investigate aspects of vision first has to know where visual information is processed in the brain before embarking on further investigations. Correct localization is key before further study of function can commence.

To come to our second argument, given this primordial role of anatomical knowledge, it is not surprising that the majority of functional techniques are implemented in combination with structural imaging. Later on, we will learn about fabulous functional methods such as functional MRI, transcranial magnetic stimulation, and magnetoencephalography, all of which are by default combined with structural imaging.

As a third and final argument, neuroanatomy by itself, without functional data, can be surprisingly relevant for understanding behavior. Marked behavioral differences between people can sometimes be traced to relatively subtle differences in neuroanatomy. Such findings should be incorporated into theories of human behavior.

Given that the most relevant data for these three arguments chiefly come from the method of magnetic resonance imaging, this technique will be the focus of interest. In Chapter 2, we first explain the physics behind MRI. In Chapter 3, we introduce specific methods, in particular T1-weighted imaging and analyses, diffusion tensor imaging, and magnetic resonance spectroscopy. In each case, we provide illustrations of correlations between such structural data and human behavior.

CHAPTER TWO

The Physics behind Magnetic Resonance Imaging (MRI)

Learning Objectives

- Understanding the principles of nuclear magnetic resonance
- Understanding how these principles can be used to obtain images of the brain
- Acquiring basic knowledge of the hardware and parameters available to researchers
- Understanding the factors that determine contrast in MRI images

In this chapter, we aim to provide a basic understanding of what happens at the physical and biological levels when someone is placed into a nuclear magnetic resonance (NMR) scanner. This aim fits with the overall goal of this book: understanding typical research papers in the literature. We do not refer to highly technical papers in dedicated NMR journals; to understand those papers, an entire text on NMR physics would be a more appropriate background. Still, even the simplest papers that include magnetic resonance imaging contain a technical section that is as unintelligible to the naïve reader as Shakespeare's *Hamlet* in sixteenth-century English would be to a ten-year-old present-day French native.

As a very representative example, we here provide the technical section from an MRI experiment published in the respected journal *Psychological Science* (Kubilius et al., 2011):

Functional MRI (fMRI) data were obtained using a 3-T Philips Intera scanner with an eight-channel SENSE head coil using an echo-planar imaging sequence. We recorded 38 slices from the first 2 participants and 37 slices from the remaining 6 participants. Slices were oriented downward for full inferotemporal cortex coverage and covered almost the entire brain (voxel size = 2.75 × 2.75 × 2.75 mm, interslice distance = 0.2 mm, acquisition matrix = 80 × 80). Each run consisted of 168 measurements; the interval between measurements (repetition time) was set to 2,000 ms with an echo time of 30 ms. The T1-weighted anatomical scan had 0.85- × 0.98-mm in-plane resolution, 1.37 mm between the slices (acquisition matrix = 256 × 256), a 9.6-ms repetition time, a 4.6-ms echo time, 182 coronal slices, and a duration of 383 s.

This journal is targeted at an audience of behavioral scientists; nevertheless, having a basic understanding of this technical section would help them enormously to understand the ins and outs of what happened in this research and to infer what can be concluded from it. After studying this chapter, the technical section reproduced here will be understandable. The reader will have some understanding of the meaning of the parameters, why certain parameters were chosen, and how these parameters might influence the results of the imaging experiment. Given that the physical background of MRI is shared between structural and functional MRI imaging, most knowledge conveyed in this chapter will also be relevant when functional MRI is introduced in Chapter 4.

2.1 The Effect of Magnetic Fields on the Human Body

Magnets and the magnetic field they generate have obvious and visible repulsion and attraction effects on a range of materials. For a brain imager, these effects can be a matter of life or death. It cannot be stressed enough how important it is to consider these phenomena (Kanal et al., 2007), even though they are not relevant for the images that are obtained. Many other facts that you will learn in this and the following chapters are highly relevant for determining whether experiments will succeed or fail, but a failed experiment is typically not deadly. In contrast, a fire extinguisher or a screwdriver that contains ferromagnetic metal and that is brought into a scanner room could very well do serious harm to a person in the scanner. Similarly, the magnetic field would interfere with the functioning of a pacemaker in the body of a participant, with dramatic consequences. Instead of spending a thousand words on this point, we suggest conducting an Internet search for the term "MRI safety," and the importance will soon be obvious.

In contrast to magnets' strong effect on particular materials, it is not immediately clear that they have any effect on biological tissue. For example, we can stand next to an MRI scanner or slowly slide into it and feel nothing. Nevertheless, there is an influence on the nuclei in the body. These are not the types of effects to cause alarm, you will not become ill in the short term, and there is no evidence for effects at the long term. Anecdotally, a scientist had himself scanned during 84 sessions for just one experiment (Shine et al., 2016), and he remains healthy. This technique is sometimes referred to as *nuclear* magnetic resonance (explained subsequently), but in this case the term "nuclear" does not imply radioactivity or any increase of cancer risks (in contrast to other imaging techniques such as X-rays).

The most pronounced effects of a magnetic field on biological tissue have to do with changes in the magnetic field over time. At higher magnetic field strengths such as those generated by many MRI scanners, for example, 3 tesla (T) or preferably even higher, it does not take much effort for a person to feel at least some effects. Making a series of fast movements with your head might be enough to start feeling nauseous. This effect is due to the fact that these magnetic fields are not perfectly homogeneous and differ depending on where you are in the field. When you move your head, it will experience a magnetic field that changes over time, and this is what causes nausea. You will typically not experience this as a participant in an experiment with scanners of 1.5T or 3T, because this effect is small at those field strengths and because you do not make fast and abrupt head movements.

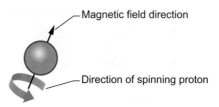

Figure 2.1 A schematic drawing of a proton, the magnetic momentum of which is aligned with a magnetic field and which spins at a particular frequency.

It all starts with a property of atomic nuclei, hence the term *nuclear*. The protons and neutrons in these nuclei spin among other protons/neutrons. In nuclei with an odd number of protons/neutrons, these spins do not cancel out, and as a consequence the nucleus has a nonzero magnetic momentum. When placed in a magnetic field, this magnetic momentum will align with the direction of this field, hence the term *magnetic* (Fig. 2.1). In addition, the nuclei with an odd number of protons/ neutrons spin around at a particular frequency. This frequency is referred to as the Larmor frequency. When the magnetic field is changing periodically, thus oscillating, it will make the nuclei absorb energy from the field if the oscillation frequency matches the Larmor frequency of the nuclei. This is also referred to as the *resonance* frequency. This explains why this phenomenon is known as nuclear magnetic resonance (Bloch et al., 1946, Purcell et al., 1946).

The most relevant element for brain imaging is hydrogen (^{1}H), which is the most abundant atom in biological tissue and as such also provides the strongest signal. In an NMR scanner, the oscillating magnetic field is applied, while a static magnetic field is present all the time. The Larmor frequency depends linearly on the strength of this static field (Schick, 2005). For hydrogen, it is 63.76 MHz at 1.5T, 127.7 MHz at 3.0T, and 298.0 MHz at 7.0T. These frequencies are in the range of radio waves. If the other magnetic field oscillates at that frequency, then it will have most effect on the energy state of the ^{1}H atoms. Hence, the oscillating magnetic field is often referred to as an RF pulse (RF stands for "radio frequency").

The oscillating magnetic field has two effects on the spin of the affected atoms (Fig. 2.2). First, the spins get in phase, meaning that they are in the same position on the cycle when they spin around. Second, the spin changes direction and will be flipped in the direction of the oscillating field. This flip goes together with an increase in energy state (the nucleus absorbs energy). The angle of this flip depends on the difference in angle between the static magnetic field and the oscillating field. In Figure 2.2 the angle is 90 degrees. When the oscillating radio frequency field is no longer applied, then these two effects gradually disappear. Each of these effects has a certain time constant, which determines the time it takes before the effect is diminished by a certain amount. The smaller the time constant, the faster the effect changes over time. First, the nuclei get out of phase again: dephasing. Second, the nuclei **realign** with the static magnetic field by flipping back in the direction of this

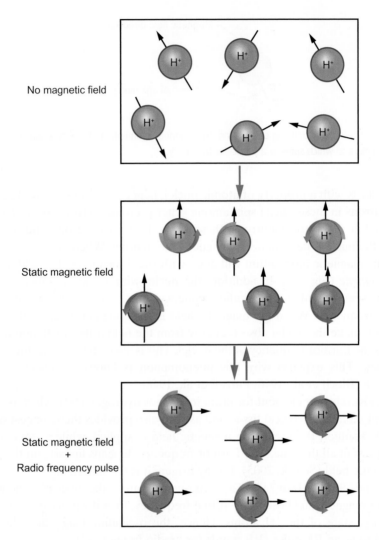

Figure 2.2 The effect of a static and an oscillating magnetic field on the phase and spin direction of protons. The direction of the magnetic momentum and of the spin is indicated by the black arrows, and the phase in which a proton is spinning by the position of the red arrow.

static field. Each time a nucleus realigns, it emits energy that by itself is a very small signal in the radio frequency range. These small signals integrate over all the nuclei that realign, and the resulting signal is stronger the less dephasing has happened. If too much dephasing has happened, then the signals of different nuclei will largely cancel out and no net signal will remain.

Note that the absorption of energy by biological tissue is coupled with a slight increase in temperature. The larger the tissue, the more energy it can absorb without a significant increase in temperature. This is taken into account in a safety index known as the specific absorption rate (SAR). The parameters and safety settings used with scanners for human imaging take this index into account (ICNIRP, 2004). To calculate these safety margins, we need to include the weight of a participant, the reason the weight of a participant is always requested by experimenters prior to scanning.

2.2 From Resonance to Imaging

Over the years, physicists have come up with highly ingenious methods to use nuclear magnetic resonance to obtain two-dimensional and three-dimensional images of the brain. Here they use the fact that the Larmor frequency depends on field strength. If field strength differs across space according to a particular gradient, then nuclei will have a Larmor frequency that depends on their position in this static field gradient. For example, if the gradient increases from left to right, then nuclei on the left will have a slower Larmor frequency compared with nuclei on the right. The application of a radio frequency (RF) wave will then only affect those nuclei that are in a spatial position where the static field gradient gives them a Larmor frequency that matches the frequency of the RF wave.

To use this phenomenon to obtain two-dimensional (2D) and even three-dimensional (3D) images, scientists apply gradients of field strength on top of the overall stationary field. For the most part, these gradients are linear (more accurately: one tries to make them as linear as possible). The gradients are often applied for only short periods of time, but when applied they are stationary (they do not oscillate).

A first gradient is referred to as a slice-selection gradient. It is applied during the RF pulse, as illustrated in Figure 2.3A. The total field strength B_{net} experienced by a nucleus corresponds to the static and, hopefully, homogeneous magnetic field (often referred to as B_0) plus the magnetic field G, which is characterized by the linear gradient. The RF pulse will primarily affect those nuclei of which the Larmor frequency matches the frequency of the pulse, and as such influence those nuclei that experience a B_{net} within a small range. This volume of excited nuclei is referred to as a "slice." For example, at 3T with an RF pulse of 127.7 MHz and a slice-selection gradient going from superior (top) to inferior (bottom) in the brain, the RF pulse will only affect the nuclei in a horizontal slice where the summed field strength is 3T. In two-dimensional imaging, one slice is typically recorded per RF pulse. In that case, scanning a full 3D volume will require as many RF pulses as the number of slices needed. Often slices are excited in an interleaved manner (interleaved slice acquisition) to minimize cumulative effects due to cross-slice excitation (an RF pulse will partially excite neighboring slices as well). Now that these nuclei are excited, the signal they emit will be affected by the two other gradients.

A second gradient is the phase-encoding (PE) gradient. This gradient is applied after the RF pulse. The PE gradient will change the spin resonance frequencies of the excited nuclei, causing differences in phase depending on where nuclei are along the PE gradient. When the PE gradient is removed, the resonance frequencies will

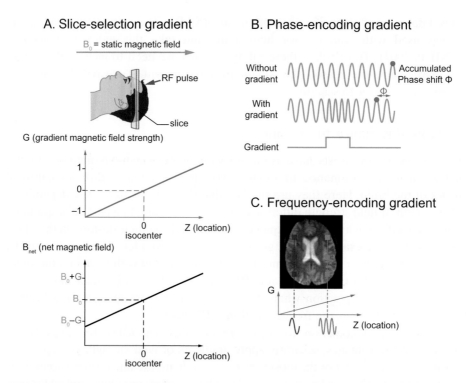

Figure 2.3 The use of magnetic gradients to determine the spatial origin of signals in three-dimensional space. (A) A slice-selection gradient allows the selection of one slice by matching its net magnetic field strength to the strength needed to be excited by the radio frequency (RF) pulse. (B) The phase-encoding gradient affects the resonance frequency, resulting in a phase shift that is different for nuclei at different positions along the gradient. (C) The frequency-encoding gradient affects the resonance frequency during readout, resulting in a resonance frequency that depends on the position of nuclei along the gradient.

be the same again but the differences in phase will persist. This series of events is illustrated in Figure 2.3B. All nuclei at a certain position in the PE gradient (a row perpendicular to the gradient) will have the same phase, thus the phase is informative about where the nuclei are.

A third gradient is the frequency-encoding (FE) gradient. This gradient is turned on during data acquisition and is for that reason also referred to as the "readout gradient." As illustrated in Figure 2.3C, all nuclei at a certain position in this gradient will have a particular resonance frequency that deviates from nuclei at other positions. For this reason, the resonance frequency at the time of acquisition is informative about where these nuclei are.

The timing and duration of the gradients, together with the RF pulse, form a pulse sequence (Bernstein et al., 2004). A schematic example is given in Figure 2.4. This sequence is known as a gradient-echo echo-planar imaging (GE-EPI) sequence. As part of this sequence, we see the basic sequence of events that is shared by many pulse sequences: an RF pulse (first line) applied together with a slice-selection

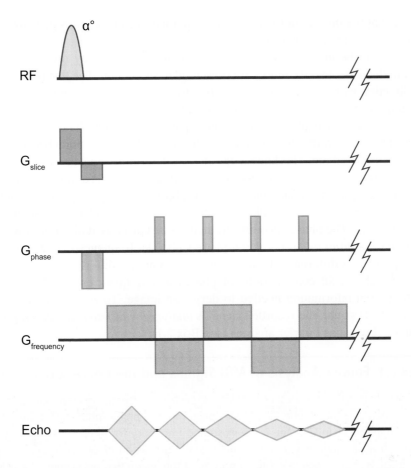

Figure 2.4 A schematic example of the pulse sequence related to gradient-echo echo-planar imaging. From top to bottom: the RF pulse, the slice-selection gradient, the phase-encoding gradient, the frequency-encoding gradient, and the signal that is acquired. This signal consists of a series of echoes elicited by the gradient reversals. A gradient reversal is depicted by a sign reversal of the rectangles that define the timing of the gradients. The duration of the gradient is reflected by the length of these rectangles.

gradient (G_{slice}, second line), followed by a phase-encoding gradient (G_{phase}, third line), and ending with a frequency-encoding gradient at the time of readout ($G_{frequency}$, fourth line). This is a simplified diagram of an actual pulse sequence. Pulse sequences can differ in a number of ways, such as what happens prior to the RF pulse, the form and amplitude of the RF pulse, the direction and the amplitude of the gradients, and the occurrence of one or multiple so-called **gradient reversals**.

A gradient reversal is a change in the direction of the gradients, which is illustrated in Figure 2.4 by a flip of the sign of a gradient. The gradient reversal will undo the effect of the initial gradient. For example, the dephasing caused by a gradient is corrected by applying the reverse of that gradient. The acquired signal is illustrated at the bottom of Figure 2.4. It is characterized by a series of echoes, each of them caused by a gradient reversal.

Echoes can be induced by reversing gradients, as well as by reversing the RF pulse. In that case, two RF pulses are presented in succession. The first pulse tilts the spin direction with a particular angle, while the second pulse tilts it in the opposite direction. Such a sequence is known as a spin-echo sequence.

The pulse sequence allows us to obtain a spatial image from the characteristics of this signal. We know that the signal comes from one slice in the brain because of the slice-selection gradient. This knowledge already determines one dimension of space. The two other dimensions, horizontal and vertical in the slice, are related to the frequency components in the signal and their phase. The pulse sequence as shown in Figure 2.4 runs through multiple durations and directions of the phase-encoding gradient G_{phase}. The phase-encoding gradient causes protons at different rows in the slice to have a different accumulated phase shift. The frequency-encoding gradient causes protons at different columns in the slice to have a different frequency. With sufficient echoes, all combinations of phases and frequencies are characterized, resulting in all information needed to derive an image. To reconstruct this image from the MRI signal, the recorded signal is *analyzed with frequency-decomposition techniques* known as Fourier analysis (see Box 2.1).

Box 2.1 Fourier Analysis of MRI Signals and the Concept of *k*-Space

Fourier analysis decomposes a signal into a spectrum of frequency components, each with a particular amplitude (amplitude spectrum) and phase (phase spectrum). (See also Chapter 11.) In Chapter 1, we illustrated frequency for temporal signals, but it works in an analogous way for spatial signals such as an image. A low-frequency modulation in an image refers to a property of the image that only changes slowly if you move across the image. An example is the brightness of the sky half an hour after sunset: brighter in the west and then gradually darker and darker when moving toward the east. A high-frequency modulation would be characterized by large differences between nearby regions in the image, such as would be seen in a photograph of a zebra.

Each image, be it a scan of the brain or a selfie on a cell phone, can be decomposed in that way. The process can also be applied in the other direction (inverse Fourier transform): Given an amplitude and a phase spectrum, one can construct an image. In MRI, Fourier analysis is first done on the acquired temporal MRI signal in order to construct an amplitude and phase spectrum. Next, inverse Fourier analysis is performed to create the actual spatial image from this amplitude spectrum and phase spectrum.

The amplitude spectrum is expressed in polar coordinates as shown in Box Figure 2.1 (images to the left). In this space, each point represents the amplitude of a particular frequency component running in a particular direction/orientation in the image. The midpoint in this spectrum refers to frequency zero, and its brightness represents the overall luminance (brightness) of the image.

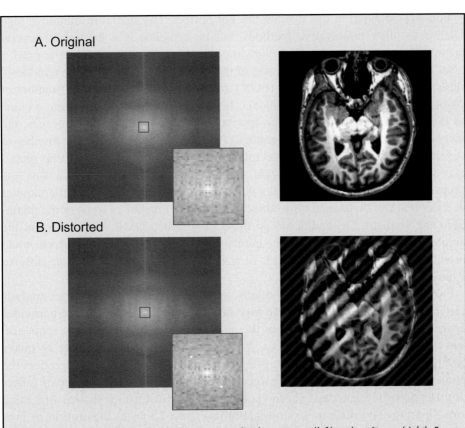

A. Original

B. Distorted

Box Figure 2.1 The relationship between an amplitude spectrum (*left*) and an image (*right*). See text for more explanation.

The distance from this midpoint determines the frequency of the component, with higher frequencies represented more distant from this midpoint. Finally, the orientation of a point from this midpoint determines the direction in which the spatial frequency modulation goes (the orientation of the sinusoidal modulation in the image/slice). Magnetic resonance physicists refer to this spectrum as k-space.

Box Figure 2.1 contains a few examples to help in reading such a spectrum and its relationship to an image. Box Figure 2.1A shows on the right the brain slice that corresponds to the amplitude spectrum on the left. The amplitude spectrum has a characteristic hill-shape form with highest amplitudes in the middle. This reflects the general property of most images in which lower spatial frequencies, which are represented near the middle, have a higher amplitude. In Box Figure 2.1B, we see what happens if one particular point in the amplitude spectrum is distorted with an unusually high amplitude (look for the white dot in the inset). The consequence is the appearance of a sinusoidal modulation in the anatomical images. The frequency and the orientation of this modulation depend on, respectively, the distance and orientation of the affected point compared with the midpoint of the frequency spectrum.

Volumes obtained in this manner are not perfect. The spatial resolution is high relative to other noninvasive methods, but nevertheless it is limited by several factors. The unit of space in the volumetric image is a voxel (A volumetric pixel: a pixel with a third dimension). The size of this voxel is determined by the number of slices, the maximum field of view (FOV), and the matrix size per slice (number of voxels per row and column in the slice). The in-plane (or in-slice) voxel size is equal to the field of view divided by the matrix size. In classical pulse sequences, the number of slices depends on the number of (sequential) RF pulses. The number of voxels per row/column in the slice relates to the number of steps of the phase-encoding gradient, which are again implemented sequentially. Obviously, the shorter the time is in which a total volume has to be taken, the lower the number of slices that can be imaged, as well as the lower the number of steps of the phase-encoding gradient. Depending on all these parameters, NMR images vary in the number of steps per dimension. The number 256 is already a high one, which would provide a three-dimensional matrix of size 256x256x256 and resolution close to 1 mm in each direction.

Furthermore, several steps in the pulse sequence, readout, and Fourier analysis can introduce noise to the data. To give just a few examples, there are particular artifacts related to imperfections in the magnetic fields, the used pulse sequence, and the Fourier spectrum analyses. MR users refer to these artifacts as spikes (white points in the image that are often repetitive in space and as such reflect the point in k-space where something went wrong), ghosting (the presence of reflections/shadows of the actual anatomy), and geometric distortions such as stretching and shearing. The didactic example in Box Figure 2.1 is an illustration of how specific events that affect the obtained frequency spectrum can alter the reconstructed anatomical image. Box Figure 6.1 in Chapter 6 provides a few further examples of possible artifacts.

2.3 How Do These Physical Principles Give Rise to an Image with Anatomical Structure?

After the RF pulse (or later at the time of an echo), a signal is measured that decays over time. The strength of this signal depends not only on several parameters, for example, the flip angle and the echo time, but also on the properties of the biological signal. This is why we see interesting structure in the resulting images.

A first important characteristic of biological tissue is the density of ^{1}H protons at each position in its volume. Given that we use an RF frequency that matches the Larmor frequency of ^{1}H protons, the signal in each voxel is proportional to the density of these protons.

Next, the decay of the signal over time follows an exponential curve that depends on two time constants. First, there is the speed at which the spins realign with the direction of the static magnetic field, also referred to as the recovery of the longitudinal orientation or T1 recovery. Second, there is the loss of transverse magnetization as a result of the loss in phase coherence. This is also known as T2 decay. "T1" and "T2" are terms that refer to the time constant of the function determining the recovery and decay as a function of the time: the lower the number, the faster it goes.

Proton density, T1 recovery, and T2 decay differ between tissue types. These differences give rise to signal contrast: the difference in signal between different tissue types. The pulse sequence and the choice of its parameters can determine which factor will have the most weight. A careful choice of parameters can result in images in which the contrast is almost exclusively determined by one of the afore-mentioned factors, giving rise to proton density imaging, T1-weighted imaging, and T2-weighted imaging.

T1 recovery is related to how easily individual spins give off their energy to the surrounding environment ("spin-lattice relaxation"), which depends on how the atoms are embedded in the tissue. Figure 2.5A shows the recovery of longitudinal magnetization in cerebrospinal fluid (CSF) and fat as a function of the time since excitation. The plot illustrates that this recovery spans a relatively long time, going up to several seconds in the case of CSF. Cerebrospinal fluid has a long T1 and a long T2, while fat has a markedly shorter T1. The T1 contrast will be heavily

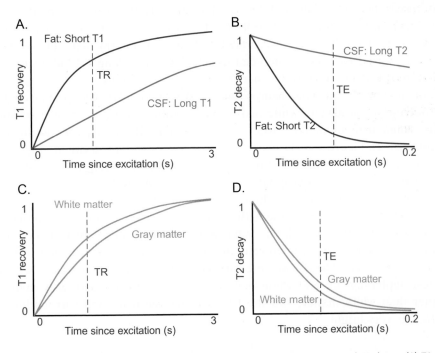

Figure 2.5 Schematic illustration of differences between tissues in T1 recovery and T2 decay. (A) T1 recovery of fat and cerebrospinal fluid (CSF); (B) T2 decay of fat and CSF; (C) T1 recovery of gray and white matter; (D) T2 decay of gray and white matter. The dotted lines give an indication of the repetition time (A and C) and echo time (B and D) that maximizes tissue contrast (see text for further information).

influenced by the time between successive excitations, the repetition time (TR). For example, if a second pulse follows a previous pulse after only 1 second, then most tissues except fat will not yet have recovered longitudinal magnetization at the time of the second pulse.

T2 decay depends on spin-spin interactions between the spins of neighboring atoms, which differ between tissues. For example, CSF has a longer T2 compared with that of fat. Nevertheless, overall, T2 decay occurs much faster than does T1 recovery. Figure 2.5B shows the signal (= transverse magnetization) in fat and CSF, again as a function of the time since excitation. Given the speed of T2 decay, it depends markedly on the time interval between excitation (or refocusing by a gradient switch) and data acquisition, the echo time (TE).

By the composition of the pulse sequence and adjusting parameters such as repetition time and echo time, we can determine to what extent we pick up proton density, T1-weighted contrast, or T2-weighted contrast. To have the optimal measure of one of these three factors, we aim to find a regime in which one factor gives the strongest difference in magnetization between different tissues and in which the effect of the other factors is minimized. If (for simplicity) we ignore the additional complexity of the exact pulse sequence used, we can derive from the plots which combination of parameters will in general provide maximal T1 and minimal T2 differences between CSF and fat: an intermediate TR (big difference in T1 recovery) and a very small TE (hardly any T2 decay). T2-weighted imaging typically uses a long TR (all tissues have recovered) and an intermediate TE (maximal contrast in T2 decay). For proton density imaging, a very long TR (all tissues have recovered) and a very short TE (hardly any T2 decay) are used.

For anatomical imaging, neuroscientists are often interested in the contrast between gray matter and white matter. Gray matter and white matter are much more similar in tissue characteristics than are fat and CSF (see, e.g., Narasimhan and Jacobs, 2002). Figure 2.5C,D illustrates T1 recovery and T2 decay in gray matter and white matter as a function of time since excitation. The differences are sufficient to obtain contrast with appropriately chosen values of TR/TE.

As an illustration, Figure 2.6 shows a T1-weighted and a T2-weighted image. On the T1-weighted scan, the tissue with the fastest recovery of longitudinal magnetization has the highest signal. This is fat. White matter is relatively white because it contains fat in the form of the myelin that surrounds axons. Gray matter is darker and CSF is black. The T2-weighted image is the reverse: The tissues with the fastest dephasing, fat and white matter, have the lowest signal, gray matter is whiter than white matter, and the CSF (in the ventricles and surrounding the cortex) is very bright.

2.4 The Hardware of a Scanner

A diagram of an NMR scanner is shown in Figure 2.7. The static magnetic field is generated by a large superconducting electromagnet of which the wires are cooled

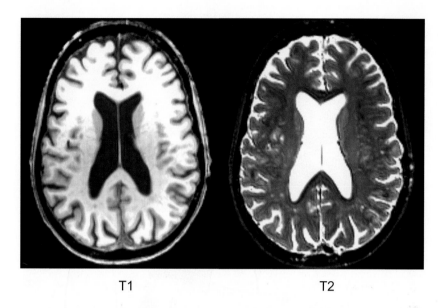

T1   T2

Figure 2.6 Comparison of T1-weighted and T2-weighted images.

by liquid helium in order to obtain superconductance. Inside this magnet there are gradient coils. A coil is a loop of wire. The gradients are generated by electrical currents running through the coil. Finally, there is a radio frequency (RF) coil around the head of the participant. Often one and the same coil is used for emitting (transmitting) the excitation pulse and for recording (receiving) the resulting signal. In the previous sections, we did not mention how the MRI signal is measured. Importantly, what we refer to as the recorded MRI signal (e.g., the bottom line in Figure 2.4), are the electrical currents that are induced in the receiver coil because of magnetic field changes related to the realignment of nuclei after an RF pulse. Dedicated hardware outside the magnet is responsible for the programming of the RF pulse and gradients and for detecting and processing the signal.

The hardware of the scanner has a significant impact on what can be done and the signal that is measured. Here we will restrict the overview to three important factors: the static field strength, the gradient coils, and the RF coil. First, scanners vary widely in terms of the strength of the static magnetic field. For research purposes, 3T (tesla) scanners are the current workhorse. In clinical settings, there are still many 1.5T scanners. Higher fields such as 7T are used less frequently for human imaging, because they are far more expensive to buy and to construct, they require a lot of expertise, often have more downtime for repairs and technical service, and have an occurrence of stronger image artifacts. Nevertheless, higher fields can have marked benefits, such as a higher signal, more contrast (differences in signal), higher spatial resolution (if the signal is higher per unit of space, the units of space can be made smaller while retaining signal per unit of space), and often a more specific localized signal (see Chapter 4 on hemodynamic imaging).

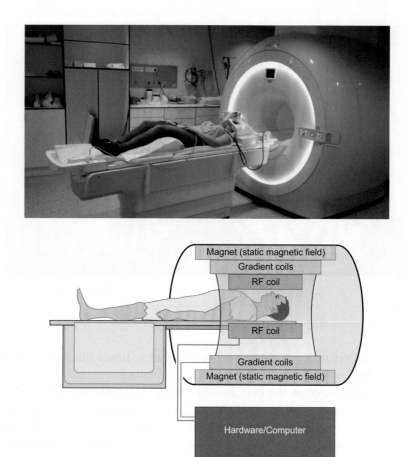

Figure 2.7 A photograph and a schematic illustration of the hardware of an NMR scanner.

Second, many pulse sequences require gradient coils, which can generate strong gradients that can ramp up and shut down in very little time. The steeper the gradients are, the higher the spatial resolution which can be achieved.

Third, there is a large variety of RF coils. Traditional coil designs include volumetric head coils wherein one coil surrounds the head and surface coils. A volume coil gives a homogeneous sensitivity in the whole volume. In the case of a surface coil, there is much higher signal near the coil but a strong drop as the distance to the coil increases. Surface coils are commonly used for receiving the signal (the transmission of the RF pulse happens through another coil) in experiments in which researchers are interested in a particular region of the brain. Currently, many scanners include multi-channel phased-array coils, which combine the benefit of a volumetric coil (more homogeneous signal) with the benefit of the surface coil (high sensitivity near the coil). In a phased-array coil, multiple surface coils are placed around the head. Each of them provides a very good signal near its center, and the drop-off at a larger distance is compensated for by combining the signal across multiple coils. The overall signal quality increases with the number of channels, but in a sublinear manner (twice as many coils provide an improvement by less than a factor of 2). Coils with 16 or 32 channels are very common. The presence of multiple coils is also used by manufacturers to speed up image acquisition time. Knowledge about how coils differ in where they are most sensitive can compensate for a less dense sampling of k-space. Of the main manufacturers of MR scanners, Philips refers to this approach as sensitivity encoding (SENSE); Siemens uses acronyms such as GRAPPA, mSENSE, and iPAT (integrated parallel acquisition technique); and GE refers to ARC.

2.5 Parameters That Are Chosen by the User

When a new fMRI study is begun, the researchers have to make several choices. In an experienced facility/lab, pulse sequences might already exist, and one might employ most of the same parameters used in previous experiments. Even then, it is useful to consider why one might select different options.

First, researchers have to select which volume they want to cover: Do they want full brain coverage, or do they want to zoom in to specific regions? There is often a trade-off between coverage and spatial resolution because of the maximum matrix size and number of slices.

Second, the orientation of slices has to be chosen: coronal, horizontal, oblique (in between horizontal and coronal). The required coverage might determine the optimal orientation so that all the regions of interest are included in the volume. In addition, there can be artifacts in the images that are more problematic in some orientations. The exact positioning of the slices is often done manually at the start of each individual scan session. In contrast, most of the choices in the following paragraphs are made once for a whole study and then applied for all scan sessions.

Third, the number of slices has to be determined. In many sequences, the number of slices is equal to the number of required RF pulses, thus the amount of time needed to acquire a volume increases linearly with the number of slices. In structural imaging, it is standard to image the complete head. In functional imaging it used to be the case that time constraints forced researchers to restrict the number of slices, resulting in the imaging of much smaller sections. However, in recent years, methods have become available that allow the imaging of multiple slices after one RF pulse. These methods are referred to as multiband or multi-echo imaging, because multiple echoes are elicited (e.g., by repeating gradient reversals). With such sequences, there is an extra acceleration parameter that determines how many slices are obtained per RF pulse. Often there is little or no loss of signal to noise as long as the acceleration factor is relatively small (e.g., 2 or 4).

Fourth, **slice thickness** and **inter-slice gap** are chosen, often together with the in-plane resolution to get voxels of which the different dimensions are not too different in size (isotropic voxels). The inter-slice gap helps to get more coverage with the same number of slices and to avoid interference between adjacent slices (cross-slice excitation).

Fifth, the field of view (FOV) is the spatial extent of each dimension in a slice. The larger the field of view is, the more voxels are needed to obtain the same voxel size. Typically, researchers try to have the slices extend outside the brain at all sides to avoid warping effects where the regions outside the slice field of view intrude/warp into the imaged volume (e.g., the tip of the nose touching the back of the head).

Sixth, the matrix size is the number of voxels in each dimension of a slice. Again, there is an upper limit imposed by the pulse sequence and time constraints. Furthermore, for computational reasons related to the Fourier analyses, the possible matrix sizes are limited to certain numbers (such as 64, 96, and 128) and combinations (most often square matrices, such as 96x96). The in-plane voxel size will be the field of view divided by the matrix size. Note that a smaller voxel size is not always better. The smaller the voxel size is, the better the spatial resolution appears to be. However, the volume in space across which the signal is sampled is smaller, which will be detrimental to the signal-to-noise ratio in individual voxels.

Seventh, the repetition time (TR) is the time between RF pulses which excite the same slice.

Eighth, there is the echo time (TE), which is the time interval between excitation (or refocusing by a gradient switch) and data acquisition. As we discussed in Section 2.3, TR and TE are very important parameters that determine contrast between different tissue types.

Finally, the flip angle is the degree to which the spin direction is flipped by the RF pulse. A flip angle below 90 will reduce the signal strength compared to 90 (less energy absorbed by the flipped atoms), but it will also reduce the time needed before the tissue returns back to equilibrium after the flip. As such there is often a trade-off with TR, as a larger flip angle can be used when the TR is longer.

After reading this chapter, the reader should be ready to return to the technical description taken from Kubilius and colleagues (2011), now with a better understanding of their methods section.

Summary

- Nuclei and in particular protons behave in a very predictable manner in the presence of stationary and oscillating magnetic fields.
- A proper combination of a uniform stationary magnetic field, magnetic field gradients, and an oscillating radio frequency magnetic field allows for the acquisition of images.
- This pulse sequence determines the extent to which the contrast in these images is determined by spatial differences in proton density, speed of recovery of longitudinal magnetization (T1-weighted imaging), and/or decay of transverse magnetization (T2-weighted imaging).

• Many hardware considerations and parameter settings influence the properties of the obtained images.

Review Questions

1. Explain which physical phenomenon is described by "nuclear magnetic resonance."
2. Describe the three gradients that are used in magnetic resonance imaging and how they help in obtaining images.
3. What is the difference between T1- and T2-weighted imaging in terms of the underlying contrast mechanisms and in terms of how the resulting images look?
4. A researcher aims to obtain T1-weighted images of a small brain structure with an anatomical resolution as high as possible. Which choices are relevant in terms of hardware and parameter settings of the pulse sequence?

Further Reading

Huettel, S. A., Song, A. W. & McCarthy, G. (2004). *Functional Magnetic Resonance Imaging*. Sunderland, MA: Sinauer Associates. (The book includes 100 pages on MRI physics.)

Narasimhan, P. T. & Jacobs, R. E. (2002). Neuroanatomical micromagnetic resonance imaging. In A. W. Toga & J. C. Mazziotta (Eds.), *Brain Mapping: The Methods*. New York: Elsevier. (This chapter contains a more quantitative description of the underlying physics.)

www.imaios.com/en/e-Courses/e-MRI (This online resource provides interesting and partially interactive tutorials of key concepts of MRI.)

www.cis.rit.edu/htbooks/mri/inside.htm (This is a link to a very in-depth online tutorial of the physics of MRI.)

CHAPTER THREE

Structural Imaging Methods

Learning Objectives

- Understanding structural T1-weighted imaging and the main analysis approaches
- Acquiring knowledge about diffusion tensor imaging and how structural connectivity is related to behavior
- Understanding the basics and the relevance of magnetic resonance spectroscopy

Noninvasive imaging of the detailed structure of the living human brain can be extremely challenging. It is a very different perspective compared with the histological approaches available for the fine examination of tissue postmortem.

Historically, structural neuroimaging in its modern form started with X-ray imaging. A derivative of X-ray imaging is still widely used in a clinical context, often referred to as CT (computerized tomography) scans. A CT scan involves a multitude of X-ray images that, as a whole, provide a three-dimensional structural image of a body part, such as the head, and can easily differentiate hard tissue, in particular bone, from soft tissue. In addition, by targeting specific contrast ranges typically covered by soft tissue, it also provides some contrast between the different kinds of soft tissue in the head, such as gray matter, white matter, and cerebrospinal fluid. Nevertheless, this contrast is much less clear compared to the contrast which is typically obtained in MRI, as illustrated in Figure 3.1. For this reason, CT is rarely used in the cognitive and behavioral neuroscience literature. It is useful, however, to aid in the diagnosis of a wide range of diseases (see, e.g., Lebby, 2013), such as inflammation, demyelination, infection, and vascular conditions (as revealed by contrast-enhanced [CE] CT) as well as traumatic head injuries, strokes, and various tumors (often involving non-enhanced [NE] CT). Many examples of the combination of CT and MRI in the context of such diseases can be found in Osborn and colleagues (2016).

Most cognitive neuroscience studies do not include CT scans but perform structural imaging based on the principles of magnetic resonance imaging. In this chapter, we introduce the three main methods: structural T1-weighted MRI, diffusion tensor imaging, and magnetic resonance spectroscopy.

| CT scan | T1-weighted | T2 (FLAIR) |

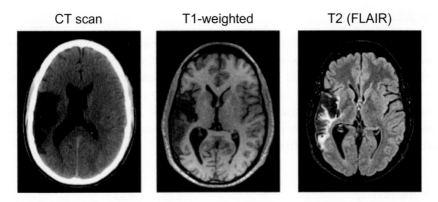

Figure 3.1 A comparison of three imaging modalities that are frequently used for clinical diagnosis: CT, T1-weighted MRI, and T2-weighted fluid-attenuated inversion recovery (FLAIR) imaging.

3.1 Structural T1-Weighted MRI

Structural T1-weighted MRI is a component of the vast majority of human brain imaging studies. Almost all hemodynamic imaging studies (see Part II) include a T1-weighted anatomical scan in order to pinpoint the anatomical location of functional activations within an individual and/or group of individuals. The same goes for electrophysiological imaging studies when researchers aim to localize the source of signals (see Part III), and for the more sophisticated causal methods mentioned in Part IV. In these studies, the structural T1-weighted MRI is often referred to as "anatomical imaging," which is how we will refer to this image modality in the remainder of this chapter.

The physical principles behind anatomical imaging and the concept of T1 contrast were introduced in Chapter 2. The most important concepts needed to understand the acquisition of T1-weighted MRI have been covered already. In the current section, we focus on the further image processing steps, give a short overview of the most important statistical analyses, and end with some illustrations of reported relationships between anatomy and behavior.

3.1.1 Quality Check

Before embarking on a complicated and quantitative analysis of the anatomical volume, a researcher should first engage in a quality check of the image as it was obtained. Often this step has already been completed during the scan session when the image was reconstructed and put up for display immediately after acquisition. A few examples of possible problems that might warrant follow-up are discussed in the following sections.

Image Artifacts

The most common artifacts have to do with the presence of objects that distort the magnetic field. Some objects, such as a hairpin, can be removed, readily solving the problem. Other objects might be fixed in place – for example, orthodontic devices. (See Chapter 6, Fig. 6.2, for an example image.) Most of the bolts, wires, and other dental machinery that a participant might carry in the mouth are not a contraindication for scanning, but they do affect the resulting image, in particular in nearby regions such as the ventral frontal cortex.

Incidental Findings

Even though study participants who are selected have no prior neurological history, and the scans for a research study are not conducted for diagnostic purposes, the resulting images still might reveal an unexpected abnormality. The problems can range from tissue that should be there but is absent (lesions, gross asymmetries in anatomy) to tissue that should not be there (e.g., tumors). The follow-up procedure for the participant will depend on the local institutional guidelines. For the researcher, the incidental finding will often result in the need to remove the participant from the experimental sample.

Image Acquisition Problems and Constraints

Anatomical scanning is based on routine pulse sequences and is relatively robust for acquisition problems as long as no unwanted objects are present and the head does not move. However, in particular studies there might be circumstances that would diminish data quality. A first example is the use of a high-field scanner such as a 7T. High-field scanning can be beneficial for anatomical imaging in order to visualize particular brain structures in fine detail. However, the image will typically be optimized at a very local level, with very inferior images of other parts of the brain. A second example is the use of surface coils, again to optimize image quality in a particular region of interest close to the coil, but with the side effect of inferior data quality further away from the coil. In such circumstances, the anatomical images might not be appropriate for some, or even most, of the following analyses steps.

3.1.2 Finding Structure in Anatomical Images and Normalization

Volume-Based Normalization

Normalization refers to the procedure used to bring the data of an individual participant into a common spatial reference space. In volume-based normalization, this alignment is done in a way that preserves the basic three-dimensional volumetric structure of the neural anatomy.

As is true for all of the following, whether or not a researcher performs this analysis step depends on the research questions. Normalization is needed when a researcher wants to compare or pool the brains of different individuals in ways that assume that a particular point in the volume of participant X corresponds to a point in the volume of participant Y.

Suppose that we have an anatomical volume of two individuals and we want to match the two as thoroughly as possible. First, we would restrict the matching to the organ of interest by performing **brain extraction**, during which the brain tissue is delineated in the images. Other tissue such as the dura (a thick membrane around the brain visible in brain scans) is stripped away (virtually) from the images. Then one of the volumes is taken as reference and the second volume undergoes a transformation to optimize the correspondence with the first. The simplest approach is a **rigid transformation** in which the second volume can be translated (shifted in position) and rotated (turned around). To account for differences in size, we can also add scaling (made smaller/larger). The full transformation can be summarized by nine numbers: three scale factors (one in each direction), three translation parameters (one in each direction), and three rotation parameters.

This simple rigid transformation can be expanded to improve the match. A rigid transformation will never bring the two anatomical volumes in perfect alignment because individual brains differ in local characteristics, such as the exact form for cortical sulci, the size of gyri, and the exact shape of brain structures. To accommodate all these differences, we would need to give the normalization procedure more degrees of freedom to transform the anatomy, not only with more global parameters (e.g., with affine transformations), but even by allowing local deformations with a multitude of parameters at a local level (optimized by a local fitting procedure such as nonlinear regression or spline fitting).

Most studies transform the individual anatomies into a standard template space, which is shared between studies. As explained further in Box 3.1, several coordinate spaces or "templates" have been used over the course of time.

Segmentation and Segmentation-Based Normalization

A lot of information is not used when the anatomical volume is considered as a volume without any further structure. The steps described in this section are used to reveal an increasing degree of structure in acquired images, with the aim to improve normalization and the amount of information that can be obtained from a structural scan.

An important step is **tissue segmentation**. The brain is separated into white matter, gray matter, and cerebrospinal fluid (CSF). This separation can be made partially based on the T1-weighted MRI signal value of voxels, with larger values for white than for gray matter, and very low values for cerebrospinal fluid. However, by itself this would not work very well. Several problems have to be solved. First, not all voxels of a particular tissue have exactly the same value. Second, low values

Box 3.1 Template Reference Spaces for Normalization

Historically, the most famous template is the Talairach atlas, which is based on the histology of one elderly woman (Talairach and Tournoux, 1988). The atlas provides a series of coronal, horizontal, and sagittal slices together with a procedure to normalize other brains to the atlas. This procedure uses several landmarks: the anterior commissure (AC), the posterior commissure (PC), the orientation of the midline, and the superior and inferior (temporal lobes) boundaries. The resulting X (left-right), Y (anterior-posterior), and Z (ventral-dorsal) coordinates are all zero at the AC.

More recently, the Talairach atlas has been replaced by templates that are based on anatomical MRI scans of large representative samples of participants, such as the MNI templates developed by the Montreal Neurological Institute. The new templates use the same coordinate frame as the old Talairach brain, although at a detailed level the coordinates do not exactly match. Figure 3.2A shows the ICBM152 template (based on 152 individuals) as it is used by several software packages, and which is constructed by normalizing and averaging the images of all 152 individuals. Because of the large intersubject variability in anatomy, this template is blurry.

Not all studies use this MNI-152 template. First, it is not representative of the general human population. For example, it does not include a good racial mix. For that reason, most studies performed in Asia use a different template based on Asian participants. Even more specific, many studies on particular sub-populations have investigated the use of population-specific templates for children or the elderly or even worked with study-specific templates. Such templates can improve the results for the sub-population of interest, but might compromise direct comparisons between different populations or at least require an additional step to normalize the study-specific template with a more generally used template.

would also be abundant at the outer edge of the cortex, where no CSF is present. To solve such problems, segmentation routines are a bit more complicated than just taking three tissue values, and several additional steps are incorporated in the analysis pipeline. The exact ranges of tissue values can be optimized, possibly including manual adjustment. Furthermore, prior knowledge is used concerning where a particular tissue is typically located. As a final solution, manual corrections of remaining segmentation errors are often needed, although over the years software packages have improved considerably in terms of fully automatic segmentation.

The segmentation results in a volume of each tissue type. In order to proceed with segmentation-based normalization, we can construct tissue-specific anatomical volumes and register each of them with tissue-specific template images, so-called tissue probability maps. Figure 3.2B shows the tissue probability maps associated with the ICBM152 dataset. Clearly, these maps contain much more detail than the blurry template in Figure 3.2A. As such, it is not surprising that segmentation-based

A. T1-weighted template

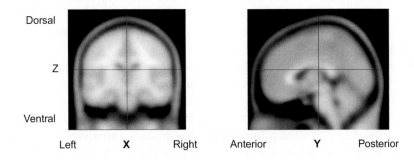

B. Tissue probability maps

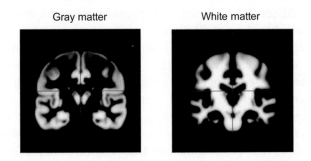

Figure 3.2 Templates used for volume-based (A) and segmentation-based (B) normalization.

normalization overall gives better results compared with volume-based normalization without segmentation.

Surface Extraction and Surface-Based Normalization

Segmentation can also be used to extract and render the cortical surface. Once we do this, we move away from volume-based procedures toward surface-based analyses. Some software packages, such as FreeSurfer, are very much tailored to surface-based analyses.

The exact definition of the cortical surface varies. It would make sense to define it as the outer edge of the cortex, where layer 1 of the cortical gray matter ends. Often it is alternatively defined as the edge between white matter and gray matter. When the analyses include a "cortical thickness" parameter, the dichotomy between these two alternatives disappears, and the surface might in fact be an average of all values between the outer and the inner edge of the cortical sheet. What all these definitions have in common is that the original three-dimensional position of each point on this surface is transformed into a two-dimensional position in this sheet. We have one sheet per hemisphere, and the sheet itself is composed of vertices, not voxels. Note that the value of a vertex is a weighted combination of the signal value of neighboring voxels; thus, it is possible to switch back and forth between a voxel and a vertex/surface space.

This cortical sheet can be visualized in several ways, as illustrated in Figure 3.3. Surface-based representations thus take many forms: inflated brains, brain spheres, and flattened brains. A common variant is to **inflate** the cortical surface, by which the massive indentation of the surface is neutralized by bringing all the sulci to the surface (Fig. 3.3A). You can understand this process intuitively by seeing what happens when you flatten a wrinkled piece of paper. In this variant, the two-dimensional surface is still represented in a three-dimensional format (e.g., there still is a medial-lateral direction in the view). Some software packages go somewhat overboard with the inflation and create a balloon-like representation of the surface, referred to as spheres. This step is typically only taken as a means to put together the surfaces of different individuals in a common reference frame, which is an example of **surface-based normalization**.

A further step is to obtain a two-dimensional view by **flattening the surface** (Fig. 3.3B). To obtain a flattened surface, a few cuts need to be defined. To return to the paper metaphor, you can create a flat piece of paper from a wrinkled paper because the original paper was flat. But imagine that your paper was brought into a hat-like formation by using a few staples, and then you had it wrinkled. With inflation, you remove the wrinkles. To proceed with flattening, you also have to remove the staples. After defining the cuts (the position of the imaginary staples in the brain), we obtain a flat surface.

The best format for visualization depends on the purpose. When the anatomical images are used to visualize data from functional imaging, often inflated brains are used. Inflated brains show all activity, including activity within sulci, in a manner that is faithful to the topology of the cortical surface and that at the same time retains a straightforward relationship to the original three-dimensional layout. Flattened brains, or so-called flatmaps, are more difficult to read for the less-experienced researcher because the original three-dimensional layout is no longer available to help orienting in the image. It feels a bit like looking at a map of the Earth if the cuts on the globe were made at random positions, rather than at the poles, and if East were "up" rather than North. For this reason, the use of flattened brains is restricted to specific domains that use very particular landmarks. For example, in studies of visual perception, the calcarine sulcus is a useful landmark because it is a standard cut to generate the flattened surface and it predicts the layout of the retinotopic organization in the visual cortex (Fig. 3.3C,D).

There are some problems associated with surface renderings. The most general caveat should be obvious once we take a few seconds to consider what we have learned. Surface-based analyses pick up only cortical activity. Subcortical activity disappears from the data when results are looked at on the surface. There is no use

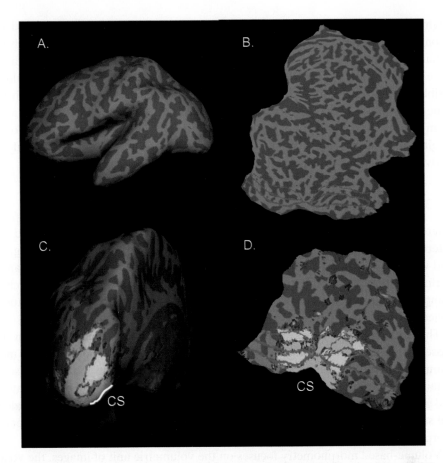

Figure 3.3 Inflated and flattened visualizations of the cortical surface. (A) Inflated surface. (B) Flattened surface. (C) Inflated surface with visual activity from a contrast of vertical-horizontal, with vertical representing stimulation of the visual field above and below the point of fixation (the so-called vertical meridian) and horizontal stimulation of the visual field left and right (the horizontal meridian). (D) Part of the flattened surface with visual activity in the contrast vertical-horizontal. Purple lines indicate the approximate delineation of visual areas V1–V3 based on anatomical normalization. The color map for functional activity ranges from blue for negative values (more activity for the horizontal meridian) to red and yellow (more activity for the vertical meridian). CS, calcarine sulcus.
Visualizations were generated with FreeSurfer

for surface-based cortical analyses if you would happen to be interested in hippocampus, amygdala, thalamus, or basal ganglia, to just name a few subcortical regions.

As a more subtle variant of the above, surface-based analyses are also subject to the need for a good correspondence between the definition of the surface (e.g., edge of white and gray matter) and the variable of interest. Take the example of functional activity that would be displaced a bit, because it is primarily measured in a vein that runs next to the surface and not in gray matter. A first consequence might be that it does not intersect well with the surface edge. If it is a relatively strong and spatially extended activation, it could also intersect too much with the surface: It could intersect twice, once with the closest surface edge, and with the edge of the surface at the other side of the sulcus. Two clusters of activity would be visible on the surface representation. We can summarize these caveats with the general observation that surface-based analyses bring the researcher further away from the original data format. Whenever this is done, it is worth returning to the original data format to check whether final conclusions are backed up not only by derivative analyses but also in the original data.

3.1.3 Approaches to Investigate Brain Morphometry

There are two general purposes for anatomical images. First, they are acquired as a reference for the application and analysis of other methods, such as to coregister and visualize functional data or to guide brain stimulation. Second, analyses can be performed directly on the anatomical images. For this second goal, researchers compute indices that are meant to quantify specific properties of the anatomy, collectively known as brain morphometry.

The analysis of brain morphometry includes many steps, which have been discussed in previous sections, such as various forms of normalization. Because morphometry typically requires an extra level of accuracy for some of the steps, some details of the procedures differ systematically depending on the goal of the anatomical processing. In general, the methods for brain morphometry can be divided along the same lines as for normalization: volume-based morphometry and surface-based morphometry (Greve, 2011).

Volume-based morphometry focuses on the volumetric unit of images, the voxel, which is why this method is typically known as **voxel-based morphometry** (VBM). Analysis steps for VBM include normalization and segmentation. Extra care is taken with the normalization, which involves nonlinear registration to a group template separately from normalization of the group to a standard template (e.g., MNI). The registration to the group template also provides information about which deformations (compression, stretching) happened to each voxel to bring it in alignment with the group, also known as the "jacobian map." The segmentation specifies for each voxel in the normalized image the probability that it belongs to a particular tissue. Such a probability map is obtained for individual subjects for each tissue of interest. To allow a comparison across subjects, it is necessary to first smooth the data of individual subjects in order to compensate for remaining differences in the location of anatomical landmarks. The better the normalization is, the less smoothing is needed.

In **surface-based morphometry**, the cortical surface is reconstructed first for each participant and aligned across participants. Afterward, analyses are performed on surface properties. For gray matter in particular, the surface-based analyses allow the calculation of very specific indices, such as the thickness of the surface, the curvature (amount of folding), and the volume. These indices can be computed for each individual, but further normalization (e.g., by creating a surface sphere reference frame) is necessary before data can be compared between individuals and groups of individuals.

3.1.4 Statistical Analysis and Interpretation

Statistics are applied to whatever property has been computed (e.g., a gray-matter probability map) on whatever units have been used (voxels or vertices). The statistical approach to determine whether any significant differences in morphometry are observed between two groups of participants (e.g., participants with and without depression) is very similar for the two methods and similar to the statistical approach used in other imaging modalities. The statistical details are described more fully in Chapter 7 in the context of functional imaging. In short, many studies apply a **voxel-wise (VBM) or vertex-wise (surface-based) random-effects analysis**. In its simplest form, this analysis comes down to the calculation of a simple statistical test such as the student's t-test for each voxel or vertex. The value of this test statistic would simply be the difference between means of the two subject groups divided by a measure of the error variance in the data. In a further step, the probability of observing this value is typically corrected for multiple comparisons, taking into account that many tests are run in parallel (many voxels/vertices).

There are a few general concerns when performing morphometric analyses, which are relevant to pay attention to during the analyses and when interpreting the results. First, the outcome is very sensitive to problems with normalization. For example, a lower gray matter value in a particular voxel or region in a first group of subjects compared with a second group could be interpreted as a difference in gray matter density between the two groups, but it could also be caused by a less accurate normalization in the first group. One possible solution would be to obtain a measure of the quality of normalization in each participant and use this variable as a covariate in the statistical analyses. Quality of normalization is just one example of a range of confounds that might affect the values calculated locally for voxels/vertices. A second important factor is the total brain volume. Different approaches are followed to take into account this total brain volume, such as including it as a covariate in the aforementioned second-level analyses or, alternatively, by adjusting the calculated indices on which statistics are done. If an effect is robust, then it should not matter which method is followed to consider such confounds. It is good practice to check this, because the interpretation of findings is complicated when effects depend on the analysis method. To give an illustration, several brain regions have been shown to be larger in men than women when total brain volume is not considered, including the hippocampus. This effect goes away when total brain volume is controlled for by using it as a covariate, and it even reverses, with larger relative hippocampal volumes in women, when the indices are adjusted (Perlaki et al., 2014). Clearly, when considering the relationship between hippocampal volume and sex, the outcome of the analysis is not robust to the way in which analyses are performed.

3.1.5 Voxel-Based Lesion-Symptom Mapping

The aforementioned methods for brain morphometry are appropriate when the inter-individual differences in brain anatomy are small. In neuropsychological patients, there might be clear lesions at the individual level. In such cases, we might wonder how the characteristics of a voxel, in this case whether it is within or outside the lesion zone, correlate with behavioral symptoms. This question is addressed through voxel-based lesion-symptom mapping (VLSM) (Bates et al., 2003). First, the lesion zone is delineated, which can be performed manually "by hand" or automatically (the latter possibly with further manual correction), using images as shown in Figure 3.1. Next, the anatomical images with the lesion delineation are normalized. In this step, special attention is given to the possibility that large lesions will complicate the normalization. Finally, statistical analyses are performed to determine for each voxel whether the lesion status of voxels is related to differences in symptom severity – that is, whether patients with a lesion in a voxel show more deficit compared with patients without a lesion in that voxel.

A specific example of this method is shown in Figure 3.4. Lesions were delineated in aphasic stroke patients. For each voxel, patients with lesions in that voxel were compared with those without lesions in that voxel using a two-sample t-test on several behavioral symptoms.

3.1.6 The Relevance of Brain Structure for Behavior and Mind

Structural MRI can reveal neuroanatomical abnormalities with devastating effects on behavior. Famous examples are the medial temporal lobe damage underlying anterograde amnesia in patient HM (Corkin, 2002) and the lateral occipital lesion related to agnosia in patient DF (Steeves et al., 2006). These neurological cases, with very specific behavioral fallout, are rare. However, many people are confronted at some point in life with various debilitating neurodegenerative and neurovascular diseases. Major cerebrovascular accidents can affect large parts of the brain and the consequences will be visible on a structural MRI (see Fig. 3.1). The same goes for later stages of dementia. Methods such as voxel-based morphometry can quantify the structural changes caused by these diseases.

Apart from structural changes resulting from such major events, there are numerous studies that investigate the "normal" brain that is not affected by disease, or diseases that are not typically viewed as being associated with major structural abnormalities. In these studies, quantitative aspects of brain structure are related to various behavioral variables to find out how inter-individual or inter-group differences in anatomy relate to inter-individual or inter-group differences in

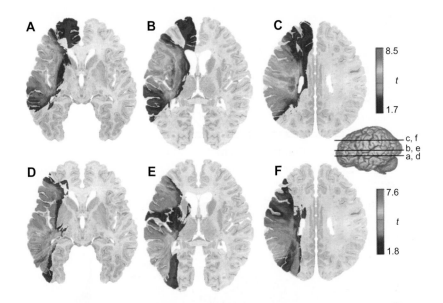

Figure 3.4 Voxel-based lesion-symptom mapping in aphasic stroke patients for two behavioral measures: fluency (A–C) and auditory comprehension (D–F). High *t*-scores indicate that a lesion to a voxel is associated with a large effect in behavior. Deficits in fluency are associated with lesions in the insula (B) and parietal white matter (C), whereas problems with comprehension were related to more posterior lesions in the middle temporal gyrus (D).
Figure reproduced with permission from Bates et al., 2003

behavior. Many relationships have been found (Kanai and Rees, 2011). Psychologists have ranked their fellow human beings on various dimensions, including general intelligence (the intelligence quotient or IQ), more specific forms of intelligence (e.g., performant IQ and verbal IQ), and dimensions that characterize personality such as the "big five" personality traits (extraversion, neuroticism, openness, conscientiousness, agreeableness). Neuroanatomical studies have attempted to relate each of these dimensions to measures of neural anatomy, most often with success. Indeed, higher gray-matter density in various cortical regions (including frontal areas) is related to IQ (Frangou et al., 2004), and extraversion, conscientiousness, and neuroticism (DeYoung et al., 2010). The same goes for other prominent distinctions such as sex (Joel et al., 2015).

It should be noted, however, that the effect size of these relationships is often not very large, and it is nowhere near the effect size observed in well-characterized neurological case studies. With a large effect size, the intelligence or personality of an individual could have been predicted fairly well by measuring anatomy. To give a benchmark, the relationship between sex and height is relatively strong. Knowing about someone's height will allow you to guess his or her sex reasonably well. To put it in numbers, suppose we have a few hundred men with a mean height of 174 cm and a standard deviation of 7 cm, and we want to distinguish them from a

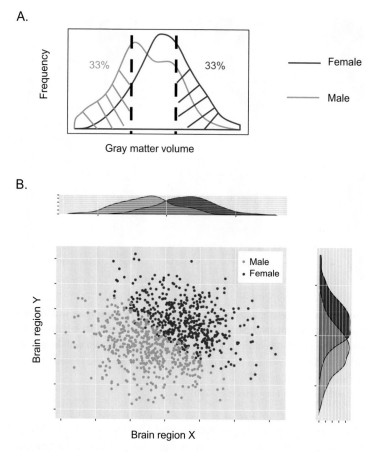

Figure 3.5 The relationship between gray-matter volume and sex. (A) Typical distribution of gray matter volume in males and females in the left hippocampus. According to the data of Joel et al. (2015), the difference in gray matter volume in this region is associated with a Cohen's *d* of 0.7 at best. Figure adapted from Joel et al. (2015). (B) Schematic (not actual data) to illustrate why the combination of information from more than one brain region can improve the ability to discriminate between males and females based on gray matter volume data. Orange and purple dots refer to hypothetical individuals, male or female, respectively. The marginal distributions of values show high amounts of overlap in each single brain region, but the distinction is clear in the bivariate distribution.
Figure adapted from Rosenblatt, 2016

few hundred women with mean height 164 cm and standard deviation 7 cm.[1] Cohen's *d*, a typical measure of effect size that normalizes the difference between the means by dividing this difference with the standard deviation, equals 1.4 for these data. We can convert this number to a more intuitive measure: What is the maximum performance that we could get when we would try to categorize individuals as man or woman when we just have their height? With a *d* of 1.4, guessing accuracy would be 75% correct.

The effect size of the relationship between anatomical measures and behavior is often much smaller. It is always possible to find individual research studies that report large effect sizes, but most often the average effect size across multiple replications and in meta-analyses is relatively small. For example, Cohen's d for the relationship between gray matter density values and sex is 0.7 or lower (Joel et al., 2015)(see also Fig. 3.5). With a d of 0.7, you would perform at 64% correct when trying to predict sex from gray matter density. Note that most replicated effect sizes are notably smaller than this example. This is the situation for simple correlations between individual brain structures and sex. However, the two sexes differ in anatomical characteristics in more than one region of the brain. Depending on the region, sometimes the male brain shows a larger gray matter density, and sometimes the female brain does. As a consequence, better discrimination, up to 80%, is possible in the same dataset with more complex multivariate methods that take into account the relatively small differences not just of one brain structure but of many brain regions (Rosenblatt, 2016). We further discuss the potential of such multivariate methods in the context of functional imaging in Chapter 8. We can conclude that macroscopic anatomy, such as that revealed through structural imaging, is to some degree related to behavior and various diseases, but it is a complex relationship and also not the whole story.

3.2 Diffusion Tensor Imaging (DTI)

All neurons communicate through action potentials. However, an action potential by itself is a meaningless entity. An action potential (or in the real brain, a particular pattern of action potentials fired by many neurons) could signal danger, safety, feeling worried, seeing your dog, the memory of your grandmother, and so on. The action potentials have meaning because of where they come from (the input of a neuron) and where they go to (the output). As mentioned in Chapter 1, the roads taken by action potentials on their path are referred to as axons. A complete wiring diagram of a brain would require tracing the path of each individual axon.

Such an enterprise is not entirely unheard of. In small animals with a low number of neurons (such as *Caenorhabditis elegans* with approximately 300), all the neurons and connections have been traced and labeled. In the mouse, invasive methods are allowing researchers to fully reconstruct the so-called connectome of small volumes of tissue. However, in humans, the grand-scale application of the implicated invasive methodology is out of the question. As such, we are limited to noninvasive brain imaging techniques. This is where diffusion tensor imaging (DTI) comes into the picture.

As mentioned, the restriction to noninvasive methods has grave consequences for the level of the spatial detail that can be obtained. With noninvasive methods such as DTI, we cannot image individual axons. At best, we get an idea of the properties of large bundles containing many thousands of axons. Luckily, we are again helped by the tendency of the brain to put or keep together things that somehow belong together. We already know that this is true for neurons with a similar function (see Chapter 1), and with neuronal connectivity the same tendency pops up. Axons that start in each other's vicinity, e.g., coming from neurons of one and the same brain region, and that end nearby, tend to stay together and form larger white matter pathways or tracts. As it turns out, DTI is able to provide us with estimates of the properties of such larger tracts.

3.2.1 Data Acquisition

Diffusion tensor imaging is based on the previously explained nuclear magnetic resonance principles. It also involves an NMR scanner, and the application of pulse sequences that are characterized by a succession of radio frequency (RF) pulses and multiple magnetic gradients. In DTI, the pulse sequence is adapted so that it becomes particularly sensitive to a biological process referred to as diffusion and is called **diffusion-weighted imaging (DWI)**. What is diffusion and how does it teach us something about brain structure?

Diffusion refers to the phenomenon in which molecules tend to move around in a medium. The molecules spread out as evenly as possible in the medium, moving from parts with a higher concentration to parts with a lower concentration. From the information in Chapter 2, the reader can infer that such movement would typically decrease the magnetic resonance imaging (MRI) signal. Indeed, the movement would cause dephasing because it would change the magnetic field experienced by a molecule and make it different for each molecule. We learned about methods to refocus dephasing, which was induced on purpose, but the dephasing caused by diffusion is chiefly random – at least in a simple medium.

The brain, however, is not a simple medium. It is a complex environment, with many barriers for molecules. In the current context, the most relevant barrier is the cell membrane around axons and how it constrains the mobility of protons. For a proton, it is easier to move back and forth within an axon than it is to move from inside to outside the axon. In more technical terms, we obtain an anisotropy in the diffusion. When many axons are aligned with one another, we get relatively large volumes of tissue, one or even multiple cubic millimeters, in which proton mobility is constrained primarily to the direction parallel to the axons. Such volumes fall in the order of magnitude that we can resolve with noninvasive imaging.

Diffusion tension imaging is typically based on a spin-echo echo-planar imaging (EPI) sequence. In such a sequence, a 90° RF pulse is followed by a 180° refocusing pulse, resulting in a spin echo. In addition, the echo-planar imaging involves multiple phase- and frequency-encoding gradients. With a regular spin-echo sequence, the MRI signal would be degraded by the total amount of diffusion, independently of the direction of diffusion or the anisotropy.

With DTI, we augment the spin-echo EPI with an additional pair of gradients (see, e.g., Alexander et al., 2007). These gradients have a particular direction in 3D space, which is a linear combination of the X, Y, and Z directions. The first gradient in the pair occurs before the 180° RF pulse, the second after this RF pulse. The first gradient dephases the protons, while the second rephases the protons, at least if protons have not moved since the first gradient.

With this "pulsed gradient" spin-echo (PGSE) sequence, it suddenly matters in which direction protons move. If they have moved in the direction of the gradient, the so-called encoding direction, the magnetic field experienced by the proton is not the same during the first and the second gradient, and rephasing will not be successful. Returning to the anisotropy of diffusion with an axon bundle, the greater diffusion along the axons in a white matter tract will result in MRI signal loss as a result of incomplete rephasing when the pulsed gradients align with the axons. A larger MRI signal will be preserved in encoding directions orthogonal to the axons, because little diffusion happens in these directions. The anisotropic diffusion results in a dependence of the obtained signal on the gradient direction in the PGSE sequence.

To quantify the amount of diffusion in each possible direction in 3D space, the diffusion is typically viewed as a three-dimensional ellipsoid (more or less the shape of a rugby ball) of which the shape is described by a symmetric 3x3 matrix in which the diagonal elements describe the variance (length) in the X, Y, and Z directions. The three off-diagonal elements describe the covariance between these three directions. This matrix is referred to as the **tensor**. With a mathematical trick called matrix diagonalization, this matrix and its six values are converted into a matrix of which the columns describe the three axis directions of the ellipsoid and a diagonal matrix with diagonal elements that describe the length of these three axes, from the longest ($\lambda 1$) to the shortest ($\lambda 3$) (Alexander et al., 2007). In more intuitive terms, these numbers describe in which direction the ellipsoid points and how thick it is (Fig. 3.6).

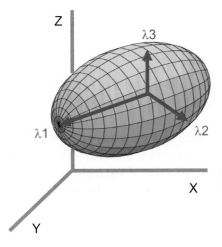

Figure 3.6 The diffusion in three dimensions is characterized as an ellipsoid. The orientation and axis lengths $\lambda 1$ to $\lambda 3$ of this ellipsoid are determined in each voxel.

All these numbers have to be determined in each voxel. Given that we have six numbers to estimate, we need to include at least six encoding directions during image acquisition covering the full space of directions as equally as possible. In practice, DTI sequences often include tens of encoding directions. In addition, a reference image is obtained without diffusion weighting.

Diffusion tensor imaging is sensitive to several types of artifacts, in particular because of field inhomogeneities, so-called eddy currents related to the relatively long duration of the gradients, and subject motion. Intuitively it makes sense that DTI would be highly sensitive to motion. The contrast of interest is related to the mobility of molecules; thus, we have designed a sequence that is particularly sensitive to how much stuff has moved. The use of EPI helps to restrict this sensitivity because it allows imaging of complete slices in a short amount of time. Various strategies exist to already minimize artifacts during acquisition and image reconstruction.

3.2.2 Data Analysis

The data analysis of DTI data is often performed with dedicated software packages. A (long) list can be found in (Soares et al., 2013).

Preprocessing

As with all imaging modalities, data analysis starts with a control of the quality of images. By scrolling over the full set of images, large artifacts and other major problems can be detected. In extreme cases, this might result in the removal of the full dataset or of particular encoding directions. Smaller problems can be taken care of with further preprocessing. Eddy current artifacts as well as small degrees of subject motion can be corrected with registration to the obtained reference image without diffusion weighting (Rohde et al., 2004).

Tensor Estimation

The diffusion-related changes in the MRI signal have been characterized per encoding direction. A model with six parameters is fitted to these empirical data. After this model fitting, we know the three vectors describing the direction of the three axes of the 3D ellipse, as well as the length of these vectors/axes. Images can be created with the values of each of these six parameters (Fig. 3.7). A more comprehensive picture is obtained by plotting the direction of the main axis of diffusion with a color scale. This picture already involves a comparison between parameters.

Tractography

The map with the direction of the main axis of diffusion for all voxels is a possible basis for delineating white matter tracts in individual brains. The simplest, and most manual, approach is to define a particular seed region as the starting point of the tract and follow the tract by a path of voxels with smooth changes in the main diffusion direction. This is a time-consuming enterprise even for just one tract. Automatic algorithms exist to delineate tracts, and for multiple tracts at a whole-brain level. After applying such an algorithm, a color map can be created in which the color of voxels represents the tract to which they belong

Tract delineation requires several parameters to be set, such as the size of the seed region, the minimal anisotropy threshold, and the maximal difference in diffusion direction between neighboring voxels on the tract. It is underdetermined where fiber tracts cross. A voxel in which a $0°$ oriented tract crosses with a $90°$ oriented tract will not show a high anisotropy, because the two diffusion anisotropies at the microscopic level cancel each other out at the macroscopic voxel level. Automatic algorithms for tractography try to bring in extra knowledge to solve such problems (e.g., identify crossings from the local environment of voxels and predict how anisotropies would be mixed at the crossing).

Useful Indices

The six numbers obtained through tensor estimation provide a multivariate dataset that together fully describes the 3D diffusion profile. In most DTI studies, these numbers are converted to a few indices which are more directly related to what this diffusion profile might tell us about the underlying neuroanatomy. All indices are computed based on the lengths of the three vectors, starting with the length along the direction of maximal diffusion $\lambda1$, followed by $\lambda2$ and $\lambda3$. Example coronal images of these lengths and derived indices are shown in Figure 3.7. A first index characterizes the overall amount of diffusion, independent of direction, and is computed as the mean of the lengths of the three vectors, known as **mean diffusion (MD)**. The second index refers to the anisotropy of the diffusion and is computed by taking the difference between the length of each diffusion axis and the mean diffusion, followed by a further normalization for the total diffusion. The resulting scalar, referred to as **fractional anisotropy (FA)**, is 0 when the diffusion is isotropic and 1 when there is only diffusion along the main axis. Finally, there are two further indices that capture the amount of diffusion along the direction of maximal diffusion, **axial diffusivity (AD)**, or along the other two directions, **radial diffusivity (RD)**. In Figure 3.7, AD is equal to $\lambda1$ and RD to the average of $\lambda2$ and $\lambda3$.

Statistics

Typically, DTI is performed to search for differences in white matter properties between sets of scans, such as two groups of subjects (e.g., a clinical group versus controls). Several statistical approaches to analyze DTI data are inherited from other imaging modalities and are described in more detail elsewhere. One approach is to take whole-brain maps of a particular index, such as FA, and perform a

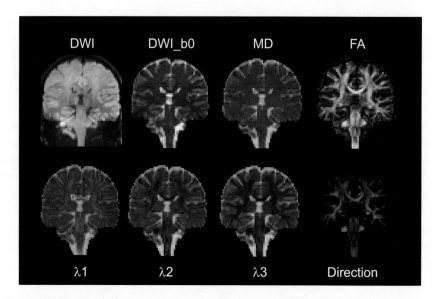

Figure 3.7 Illustration of various images and indices that can be computed from DTI: a diffusion-weighted image DWI with nonzero pulsed gradients (which is consequently weighted for T2 as well as diffusion), a T2-weighted reference image when the pulsed gradients have zero strength (DWI_b0) mean diffusivity (MD), fractional anisotropy (FA), the amount of diffusion along the three axes ($\lambda1$–$\lambda3$), and the direction of maximal diffusion in a color scale (red: left/right; green: anterior/posterior; blue: superior/inferior). Images were created with TrackVis software

random-effects analysis followed by correction for multiple comparisons to assess the significance of differences in this index between the two groups (for more details, see Section 3.1.4 and in particular Chapter 7).

A second approach is to average the values of such an index across a region of interest (ROI; for other examples of ROI analyses, see Chapter 7). This average provides one value per subject per ROI. A between-group comparison could be as simple as an unpaired t-test on these values, possibly combined with correction for multiple comparisons if many ROIs are involved. The ROIs could be defined based on various criteria. One common variant is first to identify particular white matter tracts of interest and then average indices such as FA across all voxels belonging to such a tract.

Interpretation

In optimal circumstances, changes in DTI measurements reflect changes in diffusion, without being compromised by artifacts such as subject motion. Changes in diffusion can be the result of different phenomena, and the different indices described above can show a differential sensitivity to some of these phenomena. As such, the indices can show partial dissociations. The overall diffusion can go up while the

FA goes down, such as when we compare white matter (low MD, high FA) with cerebrospinal fluid (high MD, low FA). When white matter tracts are compromised, FA could go down by a decreased AD, an increased RD, or a combination of both. In some neuropathological conditions, the exact changes are well known, such as diseases that affect myelination or neurodegeneration, and specific predictions can be made about which indices should be affected and how. For example, with decreased myelination, and otherwise intact axons, it makes sense to find that fractional anisotropy goes down because radial diffusivity goes up (less of a barrier for molecules) while axial diffusivity is less affected (Song et al., 2002).

3.2.3 The Relevance of Anatomical Connectivity for Behavior and Mind

Sometimes a distinction is made between two major types of hypotheses: hypotheses that refer to the decreased functioning of particular mental processes and the brain regions relevant for these functions on the one hand, and so-called disconnection hypotheses that refer to changes in the connectivity or access between mental processes and the underlying brain regions on the other hand (Boets et al., 2013). Diffusion tension imaging is particularly relevant in testing disconnection hypotheses. However, when articulated these hypotheses seldom specify the nature of the underlying biological mechanism. Connectivity could be decreased by many mechanisms, some of a structural nature such as smaller or less numerous axons, lower myelination, and problems with the integrity of axons, and the other of a more functional nature such as synaptic deficiencies. As far as structural changes are involved, the most common operationalization of hypothesized decreased/increased connectivity is to look at an expected decrease and, respectively, increase in fractional anisotropy, without much further expectations for the other indices.

Diffusion tensor imaging measures of connectivity have been found to be related to numerous aspects of behavior and mental functioning. Before discussing them, we will mention one an important caveat. Small differences in DTI values do not have much meaning at the level of individual subjects. In clinical cases, very strong abnormalities can be visualized with DTI, e.g., during presurgical mapping, but such massive effects are not present in studies of the normal brain or even in most psychiatric disorders. Research studies typically do not speak about significant connectivity for an individual subject, but rather about differences in connectivity between groups of subjects. Given this reliance on between-group comparisons, the confidence in the conclusions is strongly related to group sample size.

Given the importance of group sample size, we will give examples of relationships between DTI measures and behavior from meta-analyses that have combined findings from multiple studies and thus are based on relatively large sets of participants.

Meta-analyses have primarily been applied in the context of prominent mental disorders, for which many studies have already been performed, and for the most frequently studied index, fractional anisotropy. For example, schizophrenia has been linked to lower FA values in deep white matter in the left frontal and left temporal lobes (Ellison-Wright and Bullmore, 2009). To interpret these findings, one has to consider the white matter tracts that cross these locations. This implicates lower connectivity in many candidate tracts that connect frontal regions with other cortical and subcortical regions. In the case of major depression, a comparison of patients with controls revealed only regions with decreased fractional anisotropy, again implicating a variety of white matter tracts (Liao et al., 2013).

Note that it is not very obvious how to relate the reduced fractional anisotropy in the diverse set of possibly affected tracts to the diverse set of symptoms in the studied syndromes and the diverse parameters on which the patients and controls differ as a group (diagnosis, anamnesis, long-term use of medication, etc.).

Diffusion tensor imaging has also been performed in the context of rarer or more specific syndromes or to study specific behavioral functions or tracts. In such cases, we are confronted with a huge number of possibly interesting relationships to study, and thus there is typically only a small number of studies that have investigated a particular relationship between a behavioral function/deficit and brain regions/tracts. Many individual studies exist, but often it is too early to tell which findings are replicated consistently and which are not, and they tend to show some differences between individual studies, suggesting a complex pattern of deviant connectivity. For example, if we compare the findings from the most cited studies on differences in anatomical connectivity between patients with autism spectrum disorder and controls (Barnea-Goraly et al., 2004; Lee et al., 2007; Thomas et al., 2011; Weinstein et al., 2011), then the convergence between the actual findings is not high. Therefore, we have to conclude that the pattern of findings is far more complex than can be predicted in a straightforward way from the dominant theories of autism spectrum disorders (Vissers et al., 2012).

3.3 Magnetic Resonance Spectroscopy (MRS)

Thus far, we have defined brain structure as the spatial distribution of different tissue classes: which voxels contain which tissue classes and to what extent. However, there are also other biological components that have a distinctive spatial distribution, and that together are implicated in the processes that make the brain a living organ. These processes are known as our metabolism, and the biological components as metabolites, and include all the molecules involved in neural functioning.

Any basic course in neuroscience introduces students to a range of metabolites. Particular attention is given to neurotransmitters because they are essential for the chemical information transmission from one neuron to the next. In addition, there is also a high number of other molecules keeping neurons and other cells alive and kicking. For a small minority of these molecules, it is possible to quantify their concentration and spatial distribution in the brain in a noninvasive manner through a method referred to as **magnetic resonance spectroscopy (MRS)**.

A large proportion of behavioral scientists moving into neuroscience might not immediately be confronted with MRS and are more likely to have been exposed to the other methods introduced in this book. Nevertheless, it is appropriate to cover MRS for several reasons. First, in some fields of behavioral neuroscience, such as animal work, it is very common to perform molecular analyses. A combination of methods such as immunohistochemistry and in situ hybridization allows researchers to characterize the presence of a wide range of specific molecules in neural tissue. Magnetic resonance spectroscopy comes nowhere near the potential of such invasive methods, but it is useful to know what is and is not possible in humans for a scientist trying to relate animal and human work. Second, MRS is an interesting variant of the principles behind magnetic resonance imaging, making it relatively straightforward to explain the method given what the student knows already from previous sections and to use MRS as a test of the depth of understanding of these principles.

3.3.1 Data Acquisition

From Biological Structure to a Frequency Spectrum

Spectroscopy refers to a wide range of methods in which a signal is decomposed into its frequency components. As such, a **spectrum** is formed where the strength or amplitude of each frequency component is determined. All of us have literally seen spectroscopy at work in nature each time we spotted a rainbow. A rainbow comes about when sunlight is reflected by raindrops. Light of different frequencies, which we refer to as wavelengths, is separated because different frequencies are reflected at a different angle. Thus, through a rainbow we see the frequency/wavelength spectrum of sunlight.

We have seen before that magnetic resonance is also characterized by variations in frequency. Here we will focus only on MRS of protons (also indicated as H-MRS) because it is probably the only type of MRS that the reader might be confronted with, but as with other domains of MRI the same principles can also be applied to image other nuclei. In structural MRI, there are variations in signal frequency that are intended by the researcher as well as unintended frequency variations. The intended variations are induced by the frequency gradient that is applied during the readout of the signal. Thanks to the frequency gradient, protons in different positions on the gradient experience a different magnetic field strength and give rise to a signal with a different frequency. As a consequence, the frequency of a signal becomes informative about the spatial location of the protons that elicit the signal.

In addition, there are several natural sources of variation in frequency that are not introduced by the experimenter. One of them is the **local chemical environment of protons**. Many protons are embedded in a complex molecular structure (Govindaraju et al., 2000). In Figure 3.8, we illustrate this complexity by showing the chemical structure of two well-known brain metabolites, the excitatory

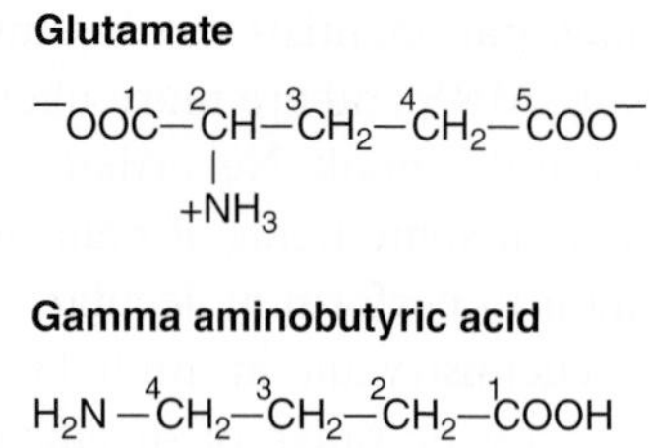

Glutamate

$$^-OOC-\overset{2}{C}H-\overset{3}{C}H_2-\overset{4}{C}H_2-\overset{5}{C}OO^-$$
$$|$$
$$^+NH_3$$

Gamma aminobutyric acid

$$H_2N-\overset{4}{C}H_2-\overset{3}{C}H_2-\overset{2}{C}H_2-\overset{1}{C}OOH$$

Figure 3.8 Chemical structure of glutamate and GABA.

neurotransmitter glutamate and the inhibitory neurotransmitter GABA. This local chemical environment influences the spin frequency of the protons. In structural MRI, this unintended variation in frequency can induce systematic artifacts. In MRS, we use this variation in frequency to our advantage to measure the chemical composition of brain tissue. Note that it is absolutely critical to minimize other unintended sources of variation in frequency, such as problems with the homogeneity of the magnetic field. For that reason, the preparation for MRS includes extra procedures to improve this homogeneity specifically in the volume of interest. This process is typically referred to as **shimming**, which is also done for other NMR imaging modalities but is particularly important for MRS.

Single-Voxel MRS and MRS Imaging

There are several approaches to MRS (for a longer introduction, see Bertholdo et al., 2013). The simplest form of MRS, **single-voxel MRS** or **single-voxel spectroscopy (SVS)**, images one volume of interest or voxel. The position of the volume/voxel is typically determined by first performing a structural T1-weighted scan. To determine the three-dimensional position of the volume of interest, three RF pulses are applied, each simultaneously with a magnetic gradient in one of three orthogonal directions. Each pulse-plus-gradient determines the position in one direction. We have seen this principle before, when a pulse applied simultaneously with a slice-selection gradient determines the slice that is imaged.

No gradient is applied when the signal is measured. In other types of MRI, this is the time at which the frequency-encoding gradient is applied so that spin frequency becomes informative about spatial position. Magnetic resonance spectroscopy also uses the frequency spectrum during readout, but in MRS the frequency variations reflect the chemical composition of the imaged brain tissue. Thus, no frequency-encoding gradient is needed. There are several types of single-voxel MRS that are all based on this simple scheme. They are known by acronyms such as PRESS and STEAM. A simple introduction to these methods can be found elsewhere (Bertholdo et al., 2013).

In addition to single-voxel MRS, there are also methods used to obtain three-dimensional images with MRS. This approach is known as **magnetic resonance**

spectroscopy imaging (MRSI). In MRSI, phase-encoding gradients are applied in up to three dimensions to obtain information about spatial location.

Nevertheless, many studies still resort to single-voxel MRS instead of MRSI. As one might expect, single-voxel MRS takes less time, typically a few minutes per voxel. Many single-voxel MRS studies also include at least one control volume, and the total scan time goes up linearly with the number of independent volumes. Magnetic resonance spectroscopy imaging scan time can be shortened by using various fast imaging techniques, such as echo-planar imaging, but often only by compromising the accuracy of the quantification of the obtained frequency spectrum. This brings us to the main benefit of single-voxel MRS: It provides a frequency spectrum that is less deteriorated by various artifacts. You measure only one or a few voxels, but you measure them well. In particular, for the investigation of metabolites with low signal-to-noise ratio, such as GABA, most experiments use single-voxel MRS.

Water Suppression and Editing

In both single-voxel MRS and MRSI, we are confronted with the problem that, by far, protons are most abundantly found in water. However, water is typically not the chemical compound of interest in H-MRS. Without suppression of the signal from water, the frequency spectrum as obtained from MRS would be dominated by water, and the signals from other protons would be washed away. For this reason, MRS applications include techniques for **water suppression**. The most frequent method is known as CHESS and includes a 90° pulse prior to the actual pulse sequence. The frequency of this additional pulse is adjusted to match with the resonance frequency of protons in water. As such, water protons are saturated, and their effect on the obtained frequency spectrum is greatly diminished.

Figure 3.9 shows a typical frequency spectrum for one voxel as obtained by MRS before and after suppression of the signal from water. The shifts in frequency are typically expressed in units of parts per million (ppm). This is a unit that normalizes for the change in frequency as a consequence of magnetic field strength. As a result, the scale is the same no matter the field strength of the scanner. Several peaks are seen, each at a different chemical shift. Most of them are related to metabolites that do not sound familiar after a basic course in neuroscience. Nevertheless, the peaks of several of these metabolites show an altered amplitude in several neurological diseases and thus are potentially useful for differential diagnosis.

A prominent application of MRS focuses on the neurotransmitter **GABA** (Puts and Edden, 2012). GABA is related to multiple peaks, because the GABA molecule contains multiple protons that differ in their local chemical environment (see Fig. 3.8). Each of these individual peaks overlaps in frequency with the peaks of other prominent metabolites, including glutamate/glutamine and N-acetylaspartate (NAA). These other metabolites are more abundant and thus largely obscure any effects due to GABA at the individual peaks. There are several ways to overcome

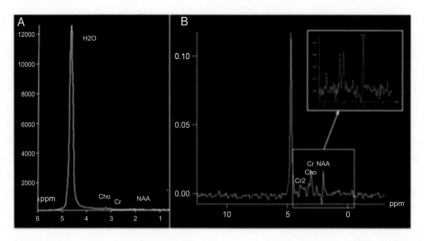

Figure 3.9 MRS frequency spectrum (A) before and (B) after suppressing the signal from water.
Cho: choline, Cr: creatine, NAA: N-acetylaspartate.
Adapted (with permission) from Bertholdo et al., 2013

this problem. The most popular solution involves the addition of a second sequence that includes a frequency-specific RF pulse to suppress one of the peaks. For most metabolites, this will not affect the signal and thus not their peaks. However, for GABA the different peaks are coupled, and thus the suppression of one peak will also affect the peak at other frequencies. By comparing the results from sequences with and without the suppression of one GABA peak, we can estimate the contribution of GABA at other peaks. This method is referred to as the edited detection of GABA through an **edited spectrum**.

3.3.2 Data Analysis

The processing of MRS data involves specific software packages. The software tools that are useful in general for a broad spectrum of imaging methods, such as SPM and Brainvoyager, do not contain any functionality for MRS. This is related to the fact that MRS data require a very specific processing stream that is different from other imaging methods.

The data analysis starts with the MRI signal treated as a one-dimensional frequency spectrum on which a Fourier analysis is performed to capture the amplitude of different frequencies in this signal. Several artifacts can compromise the signal (Bertholdo et al., 2013). Some of them, such as eddy-current artifacts due to gradient switches and remaining signals from water protons, are typically removed prior to applying the Fourier transform. After the Fourier transform, there might be a further need to adjust the obtained baseline and to put the peak amplitudes on an interpretable scale. Most often, the peak amplitudes are arbitrary values in an absolute sense, and only obtain meaning when they are compared with other values that are used as a normalization factor. For example, the peak amplitude values of a diseased volume of interest could be normalized by the values of a control region. Another common solution is to normalize by the peak amplitude of metabolites that are known to be particularly stable, such as creatine.

Magnetic resonance spectroscopy is also sensitive to subject motion, which should be avoided as much as possible during acquisition. In MRSI, there is some possibility for realigning the data during processing. In single-voxel MRS, this is not possible, and we do not have a measure of the degree of motion that can be used as a control variable in later analyses. Magnetic resonance spectroscopy applications that rely on edited spectra, such as GABA MRS, are particularly sensitive to motion because at least two scan sequences have to be compared, each of which is obtained at a different point in time. Interleaved data acquisition can help, but, needless to say, the best approach is prevention.

3.3.3 The Relevance of Molecular Indices for Behavior and Mind

Magnetic resonance spectroscopy offers the exciting opportunity to relate the concentration of particular molecules to diseases and to behavioral variability in the healthy population.

When used as a clinical tool, what matters most is the specificity and sensitivity of the amplitude of a particular frequency peak in the MRS spectrum for a particular type of disease. Stagg and Rothman (2014) illustrate the wide variety of diseases in which some of the most prominent peaks in the MRS spectrum are affected, such as the differentiation between classes of brain tumors, stroke, and inflammation.

However, a downside of this approach is that these peaks are related to metabolites or, in most cases, several metabolites together, that have a rather general function for cellular biology. It is not uncommon to find a complex combination of peaks, each deviating slightly between patients and controls. As an example, mild cognitive impairment has been related to reductions and increases of several peaks in a number of brain regions (Tumati et al., 2013). The peaks might reflect the integrity and general "healthiness" of the tissue, secondary consequences of diseases such as inflammation and neuroenergetics, and compensatory mechanisms, rather than capturing specific aspects of neural processing.

This is the reason why neuroscience researchers often opt for more difficult approaches and decide to measure less prominent and more noisy peaks, such as for GABA, with MRS. The prospect of measuring GABA, a neurotransmitter with a specific function in the central nervous system, sounds much more exciting to a neuroscientist compared with the prospect of measuring creatine, to name one example.

We will illustrate this potential of GABA MRS with a study by Yoon and colleagues (2010). In a first section of their study, Yoon et al. investigated orientation-specific surround suppression. In this paradigm, participants have to indicate the contrast of a local pattern of lines that is surrounded by another larger

A.   B.

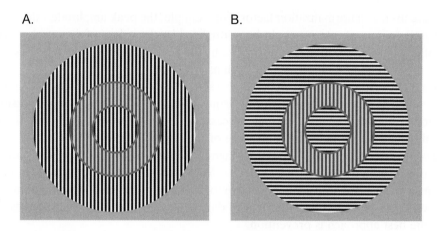

Figure 3.10 Orientation-specific surround suppression. In reality, the contrast of the black and white lines is the same in panels A and B, but the contrast is perceived to be stronger in panel B. The strength of this perceptual effect varies between observers. Yoon et al. (2010) showed that this inter-individual variability in perceptual surround suppression is correlated with the GABA signal as measured through MRS.

pattern of lines that are either oriented in the same direction (Fig. 3.10A) or in a different direction compared with the local pattern of interest (Fig 3.10B). The surround modulates the perceived contrast of the local pattern of interest, with a reduction in the perceived contrast when the lines of both patterns are in the same direction. Years of human psychophysical and animal research have already suggested that this surround modulation is related to intracortical inhibition through GABA. This literature was nicely corroborated by Yoon and colleagues, who found that the strength of this orientation-specific surround suppression at the behavioral level was related to the strength of the GABA signal as measured through single-voxel GABA MRS focused on the primary visual cortex in the calcarine sulcus.

Half of the participants in this experiment were schizophrenic patients. It has been hypothesized that reduced GABA-related functioning would be responsible for cognitive deficits in schizophrenia, and this hypothesis was confirmed by the findings: lower GABA levels in MRS in the schizophrenic patients compared with healthy controls.

No matter how interesting such findings may sound, it is important to emphasize an important caveat when interpreting the outcome of GABA MRS. A scientist with a basic education in neuroscience will immediately think about the function of GABA as explained in textbooks. GABA is an inhibitory neurotransmitter that is present around synapses and of which the concentration is modulated by its release in presynaptic terminals. When we read and interpret findings such as those of Yoon and colleagues, it is this function of GABA that we have in mind. However, the biology of the real brain is far more complex than we learn in textbooks. Stagg and colleagues (2011) identify at least two other functions of GABA apart from its inhibitory and relatively phasic (short-term) role at the synaptic level. GABA is also present extracellularly outside synapses, where it might have a more tonic inhibitory effect through extrasynaptic receptors. Even more remote from the first function, GABA is also present in the cytoplasm throughout a neuron, which is probably related to a general role in metabolism. While the correlation with specific behaviors, as in the results of Yoon et al., suggests that at least part of the measured signal is related to the first function of GABA as an inhibitory modulator of neural activity, it is possible that the findings also reflect other pools of GABA.

Summary

- Nuclear magnetic resonance–based methods can be used to measure a variety of structural brain properties.
- Structural T1-weighted MRI obtains images that are useful for coregistration of other imaging modalities, for normalization between subjects, for segmentation of different tissue classes, and for various forms of brain morphometry.
- Diffusion tensor imaging measures structural brain connectivity through the local anisotropy in proton diffusion, which is related to various properties of white matter tracts.
- Magnetic resonance spectroscopy provides unique opportunities to determine the concentration of several metabolites important to brain function.

Review Questions

1. Describe the differences in the pulse sequences used for T1-weighted MRI, for DTI, and for magnetic resonance spectroscopy.
2. Explain how fractional anisotropy (FA) might be related to changes in axons, such as myelination, and to what extent other confounds might complicate measures of FA.
3. To what extent can we state that brain anatomy as measured with T1-weighted MRI can be a reliable source of information to infer differences between people in terms of intelligence and personality?

Further Reading

Mai, J. K., Majtanik, M. & Paxinos, G. (2015). *Atlas of the Human Brain*. London: Academic Press. (Access to a good atlas is necessary for structural neuroimaging. This book also has very useful online resources that are even accessible if you do not buy the book, see www.thehumanbrain.info/brain/sections.php.)

Soares, J., Marques, P., Alves, V. & Sousa, N. (2013). A hitchhiker's guide to diffusion tensor imaging. *Frontiers in Neuroscience*, **7**, 31. (This article is a practical guide to DTI with a lot of useful references.)

Stagg, C. & Rothman, D. L. (Eds.). (2013). *Magnetic Resonance Spectroscopy: Tools for Neuroscience Research and Emerging Clinical Applications*. London: Academic Press. (Chapters 1, 2, and 5 of this book contain more than 100 pages with detailed technical information about the three methods that we summarized here.)

Notes

1 Such a sample would be the height reported by 1259 Italian individuals in 1966; see www.econ.upf .edu/docs/papers/downloads/1002.pdf.

PART II
Hemodynamic Neuroimaging

In Part II, we describe the human brain imaging techniques that measure hemodynamic signals. These methods are responsible for a large part of the hype around neuroscience since the 1990s. The unprecedented spatial resolution offered by these methods allowed a detailed picture of the functional organization of the human brain. In order to grasp the enormous impact of these methods, and of methods in neuroscience in general, it is useful to go to a university library and check the section on human neuroscience. Try to find a textbook from around 1980, and a recent one. One good example is the book *Principles of Neural Science* by Eric Kandel and colleagues, which has had five editions spanning the interval between 1981 and 2012. The difference in the amount of knowledge is amazing!

This part is structured as follows. First, in Chapter 4, we provide a general overview about the hemodynamic events that are triggered by neural activity, and we introduce the three imaging methods that measure these hemodynamic events: functional MRI, positron emission tomography (PET), and functional near-infrared spectroscopy (fNIRS). Chapter 5 contains an introduction to a range of considerations that are relevant when designing experiments for hemodynamic imaging. Chapter 6 introduces the steps of image processing that are necessary before any statistical analyses can be performed. Chapter 7 then explains the most basic statistical analyses and caveats for the interpretation of the findings, followed by an introduction of more advanced statistical approaches in Chapter 8.

CHAPTER FOUR

Hemodynamic Imaging Methods

Learning Objectives

- Understanding the relevance of hemodynamics as a signal for human brain imaging
- Acquiring knowledge about the components of the hemodynamic response function
- Understanding the principles behind each of the three main hemodynamic imaging methods: functional magnetic resonance imaging (fMRI), positron emission tomography (PET), and functional near-infrared spectroscopy (fNIRS)

Using hemodynamics to learn something about neural processing is not an obvious thing to do. As described by Raichle (2000), the general relationship between neural activity and blood supply was first observed by Roy and Sherrington (1890), but dismissed later before becoming more universally accepted. This history contains several odd approaches to studying this relationship, including observations that the temperature of the brain rises during mental exercise, and even a case study where the auditory noise made by blood flow in an arteriovenous malformation was correlated with effortful visual processing! Many experiments have been performed in order to reach the current state of affairs in which hemodynamic imaging of neural activity is virtually ubiquitous in cognitive neuroscience. Nevertheless, this approach is still not without its critics (see Box 4.1).

In this chapter, we first describe the characteristics of the hemodynamic signal that underlies all hemodynamic imaging methods. We discuss how these hemodynamic events are correlated with neural activity. Next, we provide further details on the principles behind the three hemodynamic imaging techniques that are commonly used in human neuroscience: functional magnetic resonance imaging (fMRI), positron emission tomography (PET), and functional near-infrared spectroscopy (fNIRS). We present the three techniques at the same hierarchical level. Nevertheless, the section on fMRI is longer despite the fact that much of its physics has already been covered in Chapter 2. Furthermore, most of the discussion and examples in later chapters refer to fMRI. This bias is warranted given the massive difference in the frequency with which most readers will likely encounter these three methods.

Box 4.1 Why Neuroscientists and Behavioral Scientists Measure Blood

Hemodynamic imaging methods are not only popular but also highly criticized. High trees take more wind.

Two important criticisms are of a methodological nature (Farah, 2014). First, the strength of these methods is related to the measurement of hemodynamics, and this is also their Achilles' heel. Sometimes it seems that almost every time that a brain imaging study makes it into the media, there must be someone cited saying, "Remember, these researchers are not measuring neural activity, no, they just measure blood supply. Imagine!"

Indeed, why would a neuroscientist care about blood supply? Most neuroscientists do not. Nevertheless, hemodynamic imaging is widely accepted in the scientific community as providing insights into brain function. The reason is explained in this chapter: Overall, there is a good correlation between various aspects of neural activity and hemodynamics. The relationship is complex, further work is needed, and caveats do exist, but when properly interpreted, it is possible to make reasonable inferences about neural activity based on hemodynamics.

In addition to pointing to the reliance on hemodynamics, a second frequent point of criticism refers to the complexity of the methods and the analyses. The reasoning seems to be that whatever is complex cannot be trusted. However, that is not how scientists think. A better argument is this: If something is complex, then scientists should understand it at a deep enough level so that they can reliably discriminate between valid and invalid ways of using the complex methods. Chapters 5 through 8 are intended to provide the knowledge and understanding that are needed to promote a valid use and interpretation of hemodynamic imaging methods.

To put the two main criticisms into perspective, let us consider the analogy with empirical physics. No matter whether a physics lab is interested in the infinitely small or the infinitely large, it will often rely on indirect measurements and on complex procedures. To find the Higgs boson, researchers did not measure the boson itself but rather the radiation resulting from it. Furthermore, to do so they used the Large Hadron Collider (LHC), which is substantially more complicated and expensive than any scanner used for human brain imaging. Likewise, to explore the farthest parts of our universe, again scientists rely on relatively indirect signals picked up with very powerful and complex telescopes and antennas. A new Earth-like planet is typically inferred from slight and periodic dimming of the light measured from the star around which it circles, which relies on very heavy image processing and data analysis. No one has ever directly seen a Higgs boson, nor has anyone ever seen an Earth-like planet; nevertheless, we trust that the inferences of physicists about their existence based on complex analyses of indirect correlates are correct.

We do not dare to imply that the inferences made from a typical human brain imaging experiment are as solid as the work coming out of worldwide empirical physics experiments. However, the analogy is useful to make the point that the use of indirect measurements and complex procedures does not necessarily invalidate an approach. What is critical, though, is the understanding of the measurements made and procedures conducted by the scientists who use these methods and by everyone else interested in the implications of human neuroscience. We need to know to what extent, how, and under which conditions hemodynamic changes are correlated with neural activity. Biology is messy, at least from the point of view of physicists and mathematicians, so it is not a surprise that our understanding of these matters is still far from complete. It will depend on our experimental question whether this partial understanding is sufficient to be able to achieve interpretable results for a hemodynamic brain imaging experiment.

4.1 Hemodynamics and Its Relationship to Neural Activity

4.1.1 The Hemodynamic Response Function

With hemodynamic imaging we measure a hemodynamic signal that changes in response to neuronal activity, which is a hemodynamic response. After a short pulse of neuronal activity, this hemodynamic response unfolds over time and is known as the **hemodynamic response function (HRF)**. The HRF is an example of what is more generally known as an impulse response function: a response over time occurring after an input pulse.

We explained in Chapter 1 that the link between hemodynamics and electrical brain activity is present because blood circulation is responsible for providing the neuronal tissue with the energy needed to sustain and modulate the membrane potential of neurons. The energy supply depends on a series of biological processes. Energy takes the form of adenosine triphosphate (ATP), which can be produced from glucose. To function, neurons require a continuous supply of glucose and oxygen, which is the function of blood circulation. Blood enters the brain through the arteries and arterioles (small arteries). The exchange of glucose and oxygen with other cells happens in capillaries where oxygen molecules are removed from hemoglobin, turning it into deoxyhemoglobin. The deoxygenated hemoglobin moves to venules and from there to larger veins.

When energy consumption increases locally because of neural activity, several parameters change in this scheme, as summarized in Figure 4.1. We provide only a brief sketch, as more details about these processes can be found elsewhere (Huettel et al., 2004). The major parameters are blood volume and blood oxygenation. The local increase in energy consumption causes a slightly delayed local increase in oxygen consumption. As a consequence, the ratio of oxygenated to deoxygenated hemoglobin (**blood oxygenation**) will decrease. This will generate a signal through a **neurovascular coupling** mechanism that triggers an increase in the supply of blood. This increase in blood volume and blood flow is accompanied by a marked increase

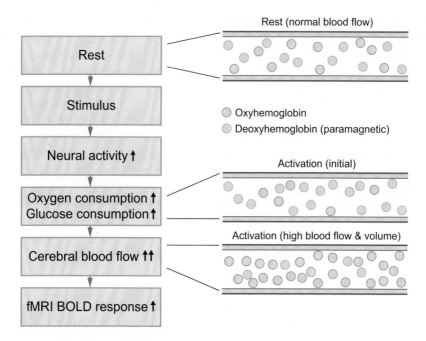

Figure 4.1 Hemodynamic events during and following neural activity (*left*) and a graphical illustration of their effect on oxy- and deoxyhemoglobin (*right*).
Figure inspired by Miyapuram, 2008

in blood oxygenation and is much larger than in the initial decrease because much more blood flows in than is needed. The peak in the increase in blood supply and blood oxygenation occurs up to 6 seconds after the oxygen consumption that triggered the increase. Furthermore, these later events expand across a larger territory than the region in which oxygen was consumed (even including blood vessels, which are relatively remote). After the peak, the blood volume and oxygenation decay again, with the latter even showing a negative overshoot to below-baseline levels (Zhao et al., 2007).

This short summary makes it clear that there are several processes that characterize the hemodynamic changes related to neuronal activity. It is important to know about these processes and their characteristics because they will influence the signal that is measured by a hemodynamic imaging technique. We differentiate two factors that will influence this hemodynamic signal. First, the signal will be different depending on which process and parameter dominates the measurement, such as blood volume, blood flow, blood oxygenation, or a combination of these. Second, the signal will depend on whether we only measure the hemodynamic changes very near to the site of neuronal activity or, alternatively, average across a larger area.

As a first example, we consider how the hemodynamic signal evolves over time when a measurement is proportional to blood oxygenation very near to the site of

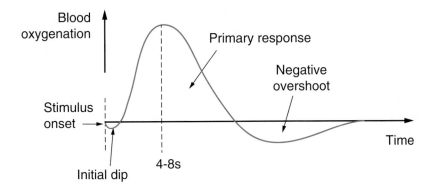

Figure 4.2 The hemodynamic response at the site of neural activity.

neuronal activity. The expected signal is shown in Figure 4.2. Immediately after neuronal activity, there is the local oxygen consumption, which results in decrease of blood oxygenation and thus a decrease in the measured signal. This decrease is also referred to as the "initial dip" (Thompson et al., 2003). Next, there is an influx of oxygenated blood, resulting in a strong increase in the measured signal. Afterward the blood oxygenation decreases again, resulting in a decrease of the signal, even to below-baseline levels.

After this first example, we can consider how this signal would be different if we vary one of the two factors mentioned above. First, suppose that we would not measure blood oxygenation but instead blood volume. In that case, the resulting signal would be simplified, primarily showing the positive peak but no initial dip and less negative overshoot. Second, suppose that we would average the signal across a larger region by using a technique with less spatial resolution. In this case, the initial dip would most likely be missed, while the positive peak and negative overshoot would remain. The next sections provide more information about the hemodynamic parameters picked up by the different hemodynamic neuroimaging methods, which will thus determine the signal.

Thus far, we have dealt with the HRF related to a single burst of neuronal activity. This is, of course, an artificial situation. In reality, our brain is constantly bombarded with sensory stimulation. Even though lab researchers tend to simplify reality a great deal and go for a reductionist approach, most experiments are also more complicated than a single and very short stimulus presented just one time. What happens when multiple stimuli are presented, or one stimulus is presented for a longer time interval? This will complicate the neuronal activity, with multiple bursts of activity that might continue for a while. The typical default assumption in neuroscience is that the brain behaves like a so-called linear system. In a linear system, the response to a complex stimulus can be estimated from the responses to the simple stimuli that make up the complex stimulus. Schematically, if a complex stimulus AB is composed of two simple stimuli A and B, then the response to AB would be the sum of the response to A and the response to B. This property is referred to as **additivity**. This assumption of additivity is not taken for granted, and many studies have already investigated to what extent it holds and in which conditions it does not. Overall, the evidence in favor of additivity is relatively clear (Boynton et al., 1996), and some of the conditions under which it breaks are also known. As an example, we expect from the principle of additivity that increasing the number of presented stimuli increases the total hemodynamic response. If the amount of stimuli per unit of time goes up by a particular factor, then the measured response will be increased by the same factor (e.g., a two times stronger response when there are twice as many stimuli). However, if the stimuli are presented very frequently, faster than one stimulus per second, then the total hemodynamic response becomes less than the sum of the responses to individual stimuli (Mukamel et al., 2004). Note that in this case the cause of the nonlinearity might not be a nonlinearity in how hemodynamic changes are related to neural activity, but instead a nonlinearity in the neural activity itself.

4.1.2 The Relationship between the HRF and Different Aspects of Neural Activity

In the previous paragraphs, we suggested that the hemodynamic response (HR) is related to "neural activity," up to some deformations (e.g., some hemodynamic effects extend to a larger volume than the neural activity). However, we have not specified what this "neural activity" would be. In the present context, it would be all processes that happen in a neuron and that influence how much energy is consumed by neurons. We have seen in Chapter 1 that many processes influence energy consumption: maintaining the (negative) resting potential, restoring this negative potential after an action potential, processes at the level of the synapse such as neurotransmitter release, and so on.

When we record the action potentials of a single neuron, we know exactly what we are measuring: the output of a neuron. When we record the HR in a region, we are not sure whether and to what extent the signal represents the overall action potential output in the region. Theoretically, it is easy to think of situations in which the overall energy consumption of a region could increase, while the action potential output might not change. For example, a region could receive inhibitory input. In such cases, the inhibitory activity might cause increased energy consumption and an increased HR, while the action potential output across the region might not change or even decrease. This thought exercise suggests that the HR might, in some cases, be related to other aspects of neural processing than to action potential output. It is unclear how often it happens that clear dissociations would exist, but it is more than just a theoretical possibility and it can happen in practice.

Whether this is a problem for the interpretation of findings obtained with hemodynamic imaging depends on the conclusions that researchers want to draw from them. When two conditions are compared and found to be associated with a different HR, then it remains appropriate to conclude that something about the neural processing is different between the two conditions. However, it might not be warranted to conclude that the action potential output is different between the two conditions.

Attempts have been made to measure the relationship between the HR and different components of the electrical potential changes as they are picked by an electrode (see Chapter 1): single-unit action potential activity (SUA), multi-unit action potential activity (MUA), and local field potentials (LFPs). Given the fast transients in membrane potential related to action potentials, SUA and MUA are measured by filtering the incoming signal to retain the higher temporal frequencies (high-pass filtering), and then counting the number of action potentials. Local field potentials include the slower changes at frequencies below 200 Hz. Little is known about what exactly is measured through LFPs, although it is a widely distributed belief that LFP amplitude is very much related to the relatively slow changes in postsynaptic membrane potential summed across all neurons in the neighborhood of the electrode (Kajikawa and Schroeder, 2011). As such, LFP is believed to be a measure of the synaptic input of neurons, while SUA and MUA can be considered a measure of the action potential ("spiking") output of neurons.

The most important experiments in this context were performed in animals –in rodents and cats, more often in monkeys. Without such experiments, the HR as it is used in so many human imaging experiments would not have sufficient empirical support. In this respect, animal experimentation is crucial even for noninvasive human brain imaging. Given these dependencies, it is not correct to regard human brain imaging as an alternative for animal experimentation. Without animal experiments, the development, validation, and further progress of human imaging would be slower, more difficult, and for some aspects even impossible.

The first and most famous experiment to relate the HR to specific neural correlates was performed in monkeys and published by Logothetis and colleagues (2001). These authors simultaneously measured electrical activity from neurons and the HR through fMRI (more specifically, BOLD fMRI, as is further explained in Section 4.2.1). Figure 4.3A shows part of their results. In Figure 4.3A, one can see a brain slice with an electrode inserted into area V1. Voxels with an increased fMRI signal after visual stimulation are shown in color. In Figure 4.3B, the raw unfiltered signal from the electrode is shown in black, and the variance or amplitude of changes in this signal (root mean square [RMS]) are shown in orange. It is clear that this unfiltered electrical signal increases as soon as and as long as a stimulus is shown (the blue line represents the stimulus timing; in this case, the stimulus is shown for 12 s). The temporal profile of the fMRI signal change is different – it starts later, reaches a peak after 12 seconds, and then slowly decreases again. This temporal profile is expected given the HRF and its additivity.

To find out to what extent the HR is related to different components of the electrical signal, the latter signal was further processed to obtain MUA and LFP.

A

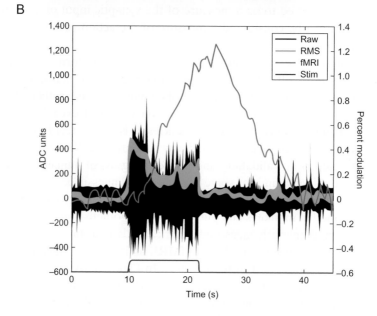

B

Figure 4.3 Simultaneous fMRI and invasive extracellular recordings in monkey primary visual cortex to investigate the neuronal basis of fMRI. (A) Visualization of the location of the electrode together with the fMRI activation elicited by visual stimuli (color map with red-yellow-white = moderate to high activity). The green dotted line indicates the area across which the fMRI signal was averaged for further analyses. (B) Percent signal change (compared with prestimulus baseline) elicited by a 12-second visual stimulus (Stim), as a function of time. Three signals are shown: the raw electrophysiological signal measured by the electrode (black), the root-mean-square (RMS) variance of this signal (orange), and the fMRI signal (pink). (C) The fMRI signal change, local field potentials (LFPs), multi-unit activity (MUA), and single-unit spike-density function (SDF) for three stimulus durations: 24, 12, and 4 s.
Adapted with permission from Logothetis et al., 2001

C

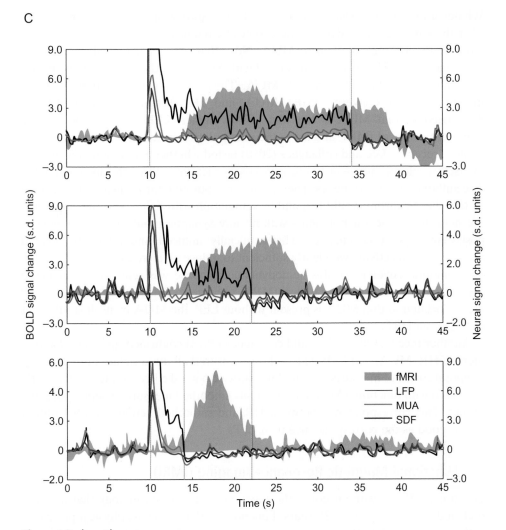

Figure 4.3. (*cont.*)

This is shown in Figure 4.3C. In most circumstances, MUA and LFP would be correlated almost perfectly; then the fMRI signal would be correlated highly with each of them. Thus, the authors needed to create a special circumstance. This was done by including very long periods of visual stimulation. The top panel represents the findings for a stimulation of 24 s. In such a situation, MUA and LFP diverge. After a while, MUA (pink line) falls back to the baseline spontaneous activity when there is no stimulation at all. In contrast, LFP (black line) remains higher than the baseline. If the HR is related to MUA, then it would be expected to also fall back to baseline before the end of visual stimulation. The findings are very different.

Whatever the length of visual stimulation, the HR stays well above the baseline until after the stimulus has ended. In these special circumstances, the HR corresponds more to the LFP signal than to MUA. Note that overall, across all data in the experiments, the HR was also correlated with MUA, and the correlation with LFP was only slightly higher than with MUA. Thus, in a typical situation, all three measures tend to converge: fMRI, MUA, and LFP. When MUA and LFP are dissociated so that MUA is low and LFP is higher, LFP seems to be a more important driver of fMRI, at least in the manipulation tested in this experiment.

More recently, Lee and colleagues (2010) tested whether action potential activity by itself would be sufficient to elicit an HR as measured through functional MRI. The authors used optogenetics: They engineered output neurons in a cortical region so that these neurons would respond to stimulation with light. With this approach, the neurons fire action potentials without any synaptic input processing or slow postsynaptic potential changes. This artificially induced and relatively isolated action potential activity was clearly sufficient to induce an increase in the HR signal. The temporal envelope of this hemodynamic response was remarkably similar to the HRF as it is observed in a typical fMRI experiment. Thus, when MUA and LFP are dissociated so that MUA is present without LFP, the MUA by itself is sufficient to trigger an HRF.

Another recent study by Issa and colleagues (2013) confirmed the general agreement of HR, MUA, and LFP. The authors measured all three signals in the inferior temporal cortex of monkeys. The findings showed a good correspondence of the HR measured with functional MRI and a spatially smoothed measure of action potential output. This correspondence between HR and smoothed action potential output was as good as the correspondence with LFPs.

4.2 Functional Magnetic Resonance Imaging (fMRI)

Functional MRI is without doubt the functional imaging technology that has sky-rocketed in use in the past 25 years. Functional MRI shares its physical principles with structural MRI, already introduced in Chapter 2. The following question is addressed in the current chapter: How can we use the physics of magnetic resonance to measure hemodynamics?

We said in Section 4.1 that several hemodynamic parameters are changed in relation to neural activity, including blood volume, blood flow, and oxygenation. Each of these changes can have an influence on the MRI signal. The relative weight of the different parameters on the fMRI signal changes depends on the pulse sequence (e.g., spin-echo versus gradient-echo) as well as hardware considerations (e.g., field strength).

Here we first focus on the approach that is most prevalent in behavioral and cognitive neuroscience, namely, the measurement known as the blood-oxygenation-level dependent **(BOLD)** fMRI signal. Then, we introduce arterial spin labeling (ASL).

4.2.1 Blood-Oxygenation-Level Dependent fMRI

Blood Oxygenation and the Physics of fMRI

The oxygenation of blood has an impact on MRI signals because deoxygenated hemoglobin is paramagnetic (the molecule has a magnetic moment), while oxygenated hemoglobin is not. The paramagnetic nature of deoxyhemoglobin will alter spin-spin interactions and result in a faster T2 decay (see Chapter 2). As a result, an increase in oxygenation will cause an increased fMRI signal picked up after a radio frequency (RF) pulse in a sequence that is sensitive to T2 decay. One such sequence is spin-echo echo-planar imaging (EPI), which was introduced in the context of structural imaging. This is one way to obtain BOLD fMRI signals.

However, one can use other sequences that, on top of T2 decay, are also sensitive to all the other side effects of paramagnetic particles and thus generate even larger signal changes depending on blood oxygenation. Together, these effects speed up the transverse magnetization decay compared with T2 decay. A spin-echo sequence compensates for these effects by controlling the dephasing related to them by its use of a 180° pulse signal. This spin echo is needed to get proper T2 weighting. However, in addition to the spin-spin interactions underlying T2, there is dephasing due to more macroscopic differences in the local magnetic field experienced by the nuclei. There are several factors that contribute. A first factor is local **field inhomogeneity**. Even if the scanner hardware establishes a perfectly uniform magnetic field, the placement of biological tissue in this magnetic field will cause small spatial variations in this field. As a consequence, different nuclei will experience a different field strength, spin at a slightly different frequency, and as such get a difference in phase and thus dephasing. A second factor is **tissue susceptibility**. The Larmor frequency of the same nucleus, such as protons, depends slightly on the type of tissue it belongs to (water, fat, etc.). Again, these differences in frequency will result in dephasing. The total dephasing as a consequence of all these factors (spin-spin interactions, field inhomogeneity, tissue susceptibility, etc.) is known as **T2* decay**. T2* decay is always faster (more dephasing) than T2 decay.

Measuring the BOLD Contrast

Pulse sequences that are T2* weighted give more signal when blood is more oxygenated. This was first verified in rodents by Seiji Ogawa and his colleagues (Ogawa et al., 1990). Most BOLD fMRI studies are based on **T2*-weighted functional imaging**. The most popular sequence to obtain T2* weighting is **gradient-echo echo-planar imaging (GE-EPI)** (see Fig. 2.4). The word "echo" again refers to the fact that multiple echoes of the signal are elicited, in this case by reversing the direction of the frequency-encoding gradient. This reversal realigns the dephased protons, which gives rise to a strong signal at the moment of realignment.

Most BOLD fMRI studies in the literature perform GE-EPI imaging with a 3T field strength, an echo time (TE) close to 30 ms, a repetition time (TR) between

1 and 4 seconds, and a more or less isotropic voxel size between 1.5 and 3.3 mm³. Each of these parameters has particular effects on the properties of the obtained signal and might be relevant to reconsider for projects with particular goals. A first important property of interest is the spatial resolution. Spatial resolution is often derived from the so-called **point-spread function (PSF)**, a function that characterizes the broader spread of signal when a very small point in the brain is activated. The PSF of GE-EPI at 3T is about 2–3 mm. A second property of interest is the size of the BOLD signal changes.

These two properties, spatial resolution and BOLD signal change, are affected by the aforementioned parameters. As a first example, GE-EPI at 3T measures a spatially less specific signal (13% broader PSF) than spin-echo EPI, but provides a larger and less noisy signal (Parkes et al., 2005). As a second example, scanning at higher field strengths (e.g., 7T) increases the BOLD signal considerably, and in addition increases the weight of small local changes in smaller capillaries compared with the weight of more global changes in larger blood vessels (Shmuel et al., 2007). Combining the information from these two examples, suppose that a researcher would want to measure the initial dip in the HRF, then spin-echo fMRI at high field strength would be much better compared with gradient-echo EPI at lower field strength.

With the more default parameters mentioned above, the HRF is expected to look very much as illustrated in Figure 4.4. This HRF does not include a clear initial dip, because the BOLD signal changes with gradient-echo EPI at 3T are spatially not specific enough. In addition, for each individual trial or even in the experiment as a whole, this HRF will only be sampled sparsely. In Figure 4.4, this sparse

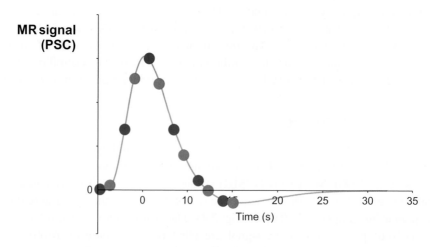

Figure 4.4 A typical hemodynamic response function in a BOLD fMRI experiment. In each trial, this function is sampled with a sampling rate that depends on the TR. Two sample schemes are shown with a TR around 2.75 s – one in which the first sample occurs exactly at stimulus onset time zero (blue circles), and one in which it occurs later (pink circles).

measurement is illustrated for a TR around 2.75 seconds for two trials (blue and pink circles) with two different offsets between start of the trial and the first sample. The samples of each trial allow the capture of part of the continuous function, but not fully. For example, the offset in the pink circles causes us to miss the peak of the function.

The echo time is another important parameter. Its value is important to consider when researchers are interested in brain structures that are located in or near regions with known signal dropout due to massive dephasing (e.g., related to field inhomogeneity or tissue susceptibility). This is the case in regions of the medial temporal lobe and ventral frontal cortex. More dephasing means that the transverse magnetization is decaying much faster, which we can compensate for by taking a shorter TE. In this example, it also helps to increase spatial resolution in order to avoid having too many tissue types be covered by single voxels.

4.2.2 Arterial Spin Labeling fMRI

Arterial spin labeling (ASL) (perfusion) fMRI measures blood flow by indexing the displacement of water molecules. This displacement is referred to as **perfusion**. Perfusion should not be confused with diffusion. Diffusion is a passive movement of molecules, while perfusion is an actively triggered fluid displacement, in this case of blood induced by the function of the heart.

To make the MRI signal in an imaged volume sensitive to perfusion-related displacement, the spins of protons in a nearby location, such as an adjacent slice of the brain, are magnetized or "labeled" by an RF pulse prior to signal acquisition. Depending on the characteristics of this RF pulse, the labeling leads to either saturation (no more magnetization possible of the magnetized spins) or inversion (magnetization in the opposite direction). Molecules that have moved from the nearby location targeted by the labeling pulse will contribute less to the obtained MRI signal than they would have done without the labeling. The more blood has flowed from the labeling time point at the labeled site to the site imaged at the current time, the lower the MRI signal will be. To quantify these effects, the signal with ASL is compared with a stationary image that did not involve ASL.

Arterial spin labeling has existed for some time and has many clinical applications. However, in cognitive neuroscience it has been used much less than BOLD fMRI, which is easier to implement. Nevertheless, ASL also has advantages, and its popularity is increasing as a result of recent improvements in ASL imaging sequences (Borogovac and Asllani, 2012). Compared with BOLD, the physiology behind ASL is simpler, because ASL depends (at least theoretically) on blood flow only, while BOLD depends on additional processes. Furthermore, owing to this simplicity and the availability of a stationary reference image, ASL can be used for quantitative imaging. Statements such as "blood flow was twice as large" can be meaningful.

4.2.3 The Relevance of fMRI for Behavior

Functional MRI was one of the major methods responsible for the large increase in neuroscience studies in the 1990s, the years known as the Decade of the Brain. Functional MRI provided an unprecedented spatial resolution for noninvasive imaging, and as such allowed the investigation of the functional organization of the human brain with unprecedented detail. The current end point of this enterprise has been the recent publication of an atlas of the cerebral cortex with 180 parcels (Glasser et al., 2016).

In parallel, fMRI has helped to differentiate the neural processing related to a wide range of mental processes. We will give further insight into the incremental progress over the past 25 years for some of these domains through some selected examples in the next chapters. For full overviews, we refer the reader to other books in the *Cambridge Fundamentals of Neuroscience in Psychology* series, many of which illustrate the impressive contribution of fMRI to deepening our understanding of the biology of mental functioning.

In the ensuing chapters, we show how the progress in knowledge has been facilitated by an ever-increasing sophistication in experimental design and statistical analysis. One consequence has been the transition of the field beyond mere localization of function into a more computational approach that addresses not only where but also how mental functions are implemented in the human brain. This is an important evolution, as fMRI has in the past often been criticized for giving undue attention to localization, localization-focused hypotheses, and oversimplistic views of how the brain works (Farah, 2014).

These innovations, many of which are discussed in the following chapters, have boosted the role of fMRI in furthering our understanding of the neural basis of human behavior. However, many behavioral scientists want to move a step further, not only to understand but also to predict human behavior. Functional MRI studies have identified many correlations between brain activity and behavior. Nevertheless, the size of these effects has sometimes been overestimated (Vul et al., 2009). In this respect, the situation for fMRI is not very different from that of structural imaging (Chapter 3), with large effects being restricted to particular neurological applications. Functional MRI has been shown to have a good sensitivity for investigating characteristics of information processing that are shared between individuals and also for picking up differences between groups of individuals. However, these group differences are often not consistent enough between subjects to allow near-perfect prediction at the individual subject level.

In the next chapters, we will see many examples of the application of fMRI and discuss further which inferences can be made from the findings.

4.3 Positron Emission Tomography (PET)

At the end of the 1980s, we were still in the early days of functional brain imaging. At that time, positron emission tomography (PET) was the dominant hemodynamic imaging method. Convincing results had been obtained with PET, but the first landmark papers introducing functional MRI were yet to come. The findings resulting from PET triggered the imagination of many. In 1994, two of the pioneers of that period, Michael Posner and Marcus Raichle, published the book *Images of Mind*, which disseminated the early results to a large audience of scientists and laypeople (Posner and Raichle, 1994). The content of their book highlights how much the evidence in those days was dominated by the technique of PET rather than fMRI. Since then, the situation has changed radically, at least for studies that aim to obtain an index for local neural activity. However, there are other goals for which PET has made a much more unique contribution, such as for measuring metabolism and for the detection of biomarkers and neurotransmitter concentrations.

Here we introduce the physics of PET, we describe how PET can be used to measure correlates of neural activity, with attention to the benefits and drawbacks in comparison with fMRI, and, finally, we describe the use of PET for other kinds of measurement.

4.3.1 The Physics of PET

A schematic illustration of the PET measurement is shown in Figure 4.5. Positron emission happens in the presence of radioactive tracers. Given that such tracers are not naturally present in the human body, they have to be injected into the body. The tracer is not injected as an isolated isotope, but in a form in which it is attached

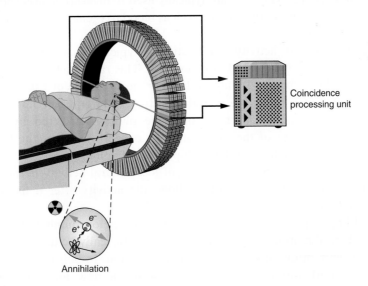

Figure 4.5 Illustration of the setup and measurement of positron emission tomography. The top left photograph shows a PET machine. The schematic in the middle illustrates the principle of positron emission and coincidence detection.

Based on an image created by Jens Maus.

to a molecule with a specific biological action. After injection, the tracer spreads to a broader area through mechanisms that partially depend on the site of injection and the molecule to which the tracer is attached.

For PET, the radionuclides are those having a relatively short **half-life**, which is the time it takes before half of the radionuclide transforms into the more common nonradioactive form. This transformation is referred to as "positron emission decay" because it involves the emission of a positron. The positively charged positron is an antiparticle of the negatively charged electron. The positron will interact with an electron, at which point the electron and positron annihilate. This **annihilation** produces a pair of photons that travel in opposite directions. These photons are detected by the scanner by means of photosensitive tubes or diodes. Two such photons have to be detected at the same time (**coincidence detection**), as single photons are ignored. Given the opposite direction of the two photons, the original position of the annihilation event can be localized along a straight line between the two detected photons. Tens of thousands of such coincidences are detected and localized, and together they allow for the reconstruction of an image.

The application of PET with radionuclides with a short half-life requires the ability to create the radionuclides near the PET machine. This production implicates a cyclotron.

4.3.2 Using PET for Measuring Neural Activity

Human brain imaging techniques are typically used to measure neural activity or a correlate as a proxy for neural activity, such as blood oxygenation. PET can also be used for this purpose.

To measure neural activity, PET studies typically use the radionuclide **oxygen-15,** which is administered intravenously. This radionuclide has two useful characteristics. First, oxygen-15 has a relatively short half-life of 2 minutes, which makes it possible to contrast the neural activity in different experimental conditions only a few minutes apart. Second, the photons detected by the PET machine give a measure of the distribution of oxygen-15 across the brain, and this distribution shows a linear relationship to blood volume. The total amount of oxygen in a brain region is an indication of local neural activity because of the oversupply of oxygenated blood that follows the activity after it has occurred (see Section 4.1.1).

A typical PET experiment would include a relatively low number of conditions, with 4–8 as typical numbers. The conditions would typically be tested in blocks of 1–2 minutes, with often only two blocks per condition. In between blocks, there would be a short waiting period, during which a new injection would be performed.

The resulting dataset is a collection of volumetric brain images per participant, with their total number being equal to the number of conditions times the number of blocks per condition. In the next chapters, we introduce the image-processing and statistical methods needed to analyze such datasets. Given that a PET dataset is typically simpler than an fMRI dataset, with the latter containing many hundreds of images per participant, the relevant processing steps tend to be fewer for PET compared with fMRI.

Compared with fMRI, PET imaging has benefits and drawbacks as a measure of neural activity. An important benefit of PET is its ability to measure blood volume quantitatively. When the blood volume in a particular voxel increases by a factor of 2, so will the PET signal in that voxel. In contrast, the signal measured by a BOLD fMRI sequence depends on many factors and shows no simple relationship to blood volume. With PET imaging, we deal with less unknown parameters in our equations when we try to relate the measured signal to neural activity.

Positron emission tomography imaging also has a few disadvantages compared with fMRI. First, PET requires the injection of radionuclides. We mentioned the practical implications, such as the need for a cyclotron and associated costs, but even more important are the health risks associated with radioactivity. There is no need to exaggerate the health risks, as they are limited: The injected dose is small, and the radioactivity decays very quickly because of the short half-life. Nevertheless, there are stringent restrictions on the number of scans a person can be involved in (e.g., one per year).

Second, PET imaging has a spatial resolution that is poorer than typical fMRI scans, closer to 1 cm. This difference is actually not necessarily as problematic as it seems, because PET neural activity studies typically require averaging across participants because of the low number of data points per participant. In between-subject studies, the actual fMRI resolution is also limited by the extensive spatial smoothing needed to compensate for anatomical variability. Given the poor spatial resolution of PET, it is typically combined with an anatomical MRI scan. During the data analysis, the PET scans are coregistered with the anatomical MRI, which is used for the normalization of all the images to a standard template space (see Chapter 6). In most studies, the PET scans and the MRI images are obtained by different machines, although a minority of institutes have access to a combined PET-MRI scanner.

Third, PET imaging has a poor temporal resolution on the order of minutes rather than seconds, which is related to the long duration of the blocked stimulus presentation and the time in between blocks.

4.3.3 Unique Contributions of PET

The use of PET to measure neural activity has a historical importance and provides the most clear-cut connection to brain imaging methods such as fMRI and electroencephalography (EEG), but it is not the most common application of PET. In nuclear medicine, PET is most often used to measure metabolism in a variety of tissues. Given that glucose is the molecule that is most closely related to metabolism, these studies attach the tracer to glucose. A common radionuclide in this context is fluorine-18, which has a half-life of 110 minutes. It is not a drawback that fluorine's half-life is longer than that of oxygen-15 because these studies are not interested in temporal resolution. The compound formed by fluorine-18 and glucose is known as fluorodeoxyglucose (FDG).

Positron emission tomography imaging of metabolism is important for the diagnosis of cancer. In addition, metabolism has been shown to be related to several brain diseases. For example, hypometabolism in the temporoparietal region is an indication of neural degeneration in the context of Alzheimer's disease and mild cognitive impairment (Mosconi et al., 2008).

Imaging with other compounds might have the potential of providing an even more direct picture of the pathological process underlying Alzheimer's disease. For example, several compounds, including one known as the ^{11}C Pittsburgh compound B PET, might serve as a biomarker for the beta-amyloid deposits that characterize the disease (Johnson et al., 2013).

Finally, PET imaging has the potential to target specific neurotransmitter systems by attaching the tracer to a molecule of which the concentration is related to the activity of one specific neurotransmitter. Studies have focused on various systems, but for now the enterprise seems to be most promising for dopamine, measured through the compound 6-[18F]-fluoro-L-DOPA (Volkow et al., 1996).

4.4 Functional Near-Infrared Spectroscopy (fNIRS)

Functional near-infrared spectroscopy (fNIRS) is at first deceptively simple. It involves a machine that is much less massive and much cheaper than an MRI or PET. This machine shines a light on the skull and measures the light's reflection. This reflectance provides information about activity in the brain. Measuring brain activity by shining a light on the skull—it almost sounds too good to be true! Nevertheless, this is actually a correct (albeit simplistic) description of what happens.

In more scientific terms, light is directed to the skull by a set of small photo transmitters or emitters. The subject wears a head cap that contains many such photo transmitters as well as photo receivers or detectors (Fig. 4.6A). The reflectance of the light is picked up by the detectors (Fig. 4.6B). Of particular interest is the light at the near-infrared (NIR) range of the spectrum, more specifically 700–900 nanometers. The skin, tissue, and bone are largely transparent to light of this wavelength, which enables the light and its reflection to travel through these structures.

In contrast, hemoglobin and deoxyhemoglobin are strong absorbers of light in this part of the spectrum. These two molecules have a different profile of reflectance in the NIR range (Fig. 4.6C). When the concentration of these two molecules changes, so will the reflectance of light for different parts of the NIR range. It is important to note the complexity of the profiles and what this means for how we expect the absorbed light to change. A different ratio of oxy- and deoxyhemoglobin

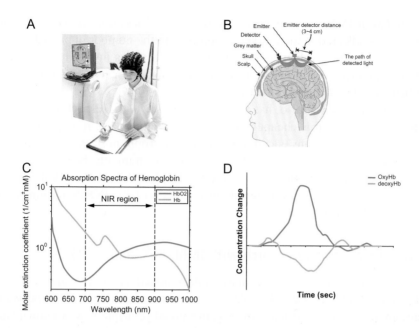

Figure 4.6 The setup and measurement of functional near-infrared spectroscopy. (A) An fNIRS machine with a subject wearing a head cap. (B) Illustration of the principle of light emission and detection used in fNIRS (from Naseer and Hong, 2015). (C) The absorption spectra of oxy- and deoxyhemogloblin (from Wikipedia). (D) The change in the concentration of oxy- and deoxyhemoglobin after a short burst of neural activity. (reproduced with permission from Gervain et al., 2011)

will not result in an overall increase in the reflected light. Instead, we will see a shift in the distribution of this reflected light across the near-infrared spectrum.

We have explained in the context of BOLD fMRI that neural activity is associated with a series of hemodynamic events that will indeed change the concentration of these molecules. As a consequence, the reflectance in the NIR range is related to neural activity. In fact, it can be said that fNIRS picks up the same BOLD contrast that is the basis of fMRI. The resulting measurement will have much of the same characteristics as the HRF found with BOLD fMRI, as illustrated in Figure 4.6D (see also Gervain et al., 2011). There is an initial increase of deoxyhemoglobin relative to oxyhemoglobin, similar to the initial dip mentioned earlier. It is followed by a large increase in oxyhemoglobin and decrease in deoxyhemoglobin with a delay of at least 4 seconds. This is followed by a smaller negative overshoot with more deoxyhemoglobin.

The method has its limits, though, compared with fMRI. A first important problem is that the bone scatters the light, that is transmitted and reflected. The reflected light that is received is spatially smoothed by this scatter and will not provide a fine spatial localization of the source of neural activity. Second, fNIRS can only measure superficial activity and will not pick up signals from within the sulci or from deeper structures. These two limitations put fNIRS at a major disadvantage compared with fMRI: poorer spatial resolution and less uniform coverage of the brain. This is reflected in the marked differences in the number of published papers using the two methods. Depending on your search terms inserted in online databases, the numbers seem to be at least 20 times smaller for fNIRS in relevant fields such behavioral and cognitive neuroscience.

Nevertheless, fNIRS also has some advantages with respect to fMRI. The machine is portable, it is cheaper than an MRI scanner, and it is less intrusive to subjects (e.g., no problems encountered with claustrophobia). In addition, some of the drawbacks of fNIRS are alleviated in research with infants, because they have a smaller head (most structures are not very deep) and a thinner skull (less light scatter) – all the more reason to test infants with a portable fNIRS machine and not in a noisy MRI scanner.

4.5 A Comparison of Research with fMRI, PET, and fNIRS

At this point, it is relevant to give an example of actual data obtained with the three methods on a similar research topic. As a case in point, we turn to the study of retinotopy in the visual cortex. This organizational principle is well known, and as such it is an ideal test case to test the spatial resolution of different methods and make comparisons (also see Fig. 3.3).

Retinotopy refers to the systematic mapping of the visual field on to the cortical surface. Neurons that are nearby in the cortex have similar receptive fields. This principle holds across all of the primary visual cortex, and again in many visual areas around it. The mapping works as follows: First, each hemisphere represents half of the receptive field, left or right from the point of fixation. The position in this hemifield is characterized by two parameters. First, there is eccentricity, which goes from foveal (the center of gaze) to peripheral. The second parameter is the visual angle, which goes in a semicircle from below over horizontal to above the point of fixation. The visual field is mapped in the primary visual cortex in such a way that the most foveal positions (the center of the gaze) are represented in the occipital pole. The more peripheral the position in the visual field, the more anterior we end up in the retinotopic map along the calcarine sulcus (medial occipital cortex). This mapping is exactly the same in primary visual cortex and in the surrounding areas. As a consequence, it does not matter which area in the medial occipital cortex you are recording from, because you will always see the same shift of cortical activity as a function of eccentricity. Figure 4.7A (left) illustrates this eccentricity mapping as found with fMRI.

The mapping of the visual angle is more complicated. In the primary visual cortex, activity starts ventrally in the cortex for visual positions far above the point of fixation, and then gradually moves up dorsally, with the fundus of the calcarine sulcus representing the horizontal meridian (this is the horizontal line that intersects with the point of fixation). In the cortical area surrounding the primary visual cortex, referred to as the second visual area (V2), the mapping of the visual angle

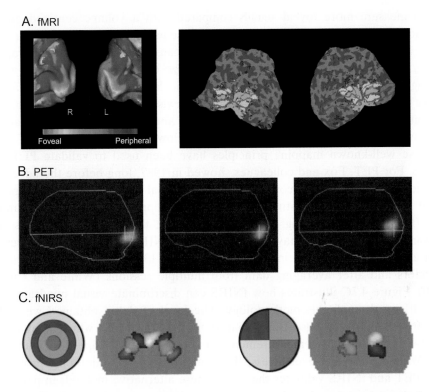

Figure 4.7 The measurement of cortical retinotopy with the three hemodynamic imaging methods.
(A) fMRI allows visualization of large-scale gradients, such as the mapping of the gradient from foveal to peripheral activation (*left*; image adapted with permission from Goesaert and Op de Beeck, 2010), as well as the finer alternation between the representation of the horizontal (blue) and vertical (yellow) meridian (*right*). (B) PET is able to uncover the shift of activity when moving from foveal (*left*), to parafoveal (*middle*), to peripheral (*right*) parts of the visual field (reproduced with permission from Fox et al., 1987). (C) Results from a single subject illustrate that fNIRS can also pick up the gradient of foveal-to-peripheral activation (*left*) and the four quadrants of the visual field.
(reproduced with permission from White and Culver, 2010)

reverses, starting with the higher-up visual position at the border of V1 and then moving to lower positions the more the cortical position moves away from V1. This is illustrated in the right panel of Figure 4.7A, which shows the representation of the vertical meridian (in yellow) that marks the border between V1 and V2 and the horizontal meridian (in blue) that runs along the depths of the calcarine sulcus. The mirror-image organization for the visual angle makes it very easy to use the vertical and horizontal meridians to delineate the borders between visual areas.

Functional MRI has sufficient spatial resolution to uncover the mapping of both parameters in a fair amount of detail. Figure 4.7A illustrates why a decrease in spatial resolution will not have a major impact on the measurement of eccentricity. A cubic centimeter volume centered at the most posterior tip of the calcarine sulcus would measure more foveal signals compared with a volume centered on the anterior half of the sulcus. In contrast, a decrease in spatial resolution will strongly harm the measurement of the visual angle, because it changes relatively rapidly across visual areas. A volumetric unit with a size of one cubic centimeter would average signals from all visual angles in a particular quadrant, such as all angles above the horizontal meridian. One aspect of the visual angle is clear, even at lower resolutions: The lower visual field is represented above the calcarine sulcus (also in V2), and the upper visual field is represented below the sulcus.

These well-known mapping principles have been used to validate PET and fNIRS. For PET, Fox and colleagues showed in 1987, long before the advent of functional MRI, that PET could discriminate foveal from parafoveal and parafoveal from very eccentric stimulation, as well as upper and lower field stimulation (Fox et al., 1987) (Fig. 4.7B). At that time, this was a tremendous step forward. Similar attempts have been made with fNIRS, which proved successful with a high-density system including distances of 13 mm between emitters and detectors and after averaging data from multiple sessions (White and Culver, 2010). Figure 4.7C illustrates how fNIRS can discriminate visual quadrants and eccentricity through this methodology. The level of detail obtained with PET and fNIRS is less precise than what is typical for fMRI, which allows very precise and quantitative measurements of receptive field properties (Dumoulin and Wandell, 2008). Nevertheless, the demonstration of retinotopic properties with PET and fNIRS validates the use of these alternative methods in particular niche applications.

Summary

- The hemodynamic response after a short burst of neural activity has a characteristic temporal profile that contains several components which relate to a combination of physiological processes.
- The sensitivity of hemodynamic imaging methods to each of these processes varies between imaging methods, and within a method it can further depend on imaging parameters.
- Functional magnetic resonance imaging is the most frequently used hemodynamic imaging method and is the noninvasive imaging method with the highest spatial resolution and a temporal sampling of seconds.
- Positron emission tomography measures the concentration of radioactive particles, which can be used to measure the hemodynamic response to neural activity at a reasonable spatial resolution and a low temporal sampling of one measurement per minute.
- Functional near-infrared spectroscopy measures the reflection of light and how it changes by blood oxygenation and serves its purpose as a hemodynamic imaging technique in niche applications such as imaging in infants.

Review Questions

1. Describe the components of the hemodynamic response function and the extent to which they can be measured by fMRI at different magnetic field strengths.
2. You work in a lab that has access to fMRI as well as fNIRS. What would you consider when choosing between these methods for a project that involves the analysis of retinotopic organization in ten-year-old children?
3. You have a hypothesis that the hemodynamic response function in medial temporal structures has a longer delay than in the parietal cortex. Which hemodynamic imaging method would you apply to test the hypothesis, and which imaging parameters might be important to pay attention to?

Further Reading

Huettel, S.A., Song, A.W. & McCarthy, G. (2004). *Functional Magnetic Resonance Imaging*. Sunderland, MA: Sinauer. (Chapters 6–7 contain extensive explanation of neural hemodynamics and the BOLD contrast.)

Toga, A.W. & Mazziotta, J. C (Eds.). (2002). *Brain Mapping: The Methods*. New York: Elsevier. (This book provides an in-depth coverage of many brain imaging methods; particularly useful are chapter 6 on fNIRS and chapter 18 on PET.)

CHAPTER FIVE

Designing a Hemodynamic Imaging Experiment

Learning Objectives

- Understanding the difficulties that can be encountered when designing and implementing an imaging experiment
- Understanding the subtraction logic as a fundamental building block in many experimental designs
- Understanding how the evolution over time of the hemodynamic response function constrains experimental design
- Understanding the difference between a block design and an event-related design, as well as the variations of these designs
- Acquiring the necessary knowledge to make informed decisions about which design might be most appropriate in a particular experimental context

STOP! Before you invest any more time learning about methods such as fMRI and PET, you need to be fully aware of what you are getting yourself into. If your end goal is to read imaging papers and to understand them, then the investment is reasonable – you read this book and then off you go! However, if you feel that you are starting to have an appetite for doing such research yourself, then you should be fully aware of what this means: hard work. We can back up this claim with some numbers, based on personal experience tutoring students and interns.

Suppose you are a master's degree student with a general theoretical background in psychology, including courses in neuroscience and statistics. You start with an internship of six months, and the goal is to complete your own experiment from scratch: formulating the research question, designing the study, writing the code for the experiment, acquiring and analyzing the data, and writing a report at the end. If the experiment is a behavioral study involving 1–2 hours of testing of 20–40 participants, then you will probably succeed in completing a full study. Moreover, you might even do a series of several experiments.

If you are even more adventurous and you aim to carry out an fMRI study, then your life as an intern would be very different. You will need to learn much more, and reading this book is one way to acquire at least part of this knowledge. Each step in the scientific process will take longer compared with a behavioral study. The data acquisition will be much more of a hassle per participant. Nothing compares to the data analysis, however, which could easily take you days per participant just to prepare the data. The first few subjects might take you a week or more per subject. In a behavioral experiment, in contrast, you might only need a few minutes to put the numbers in an Excel spreadsheet, not days or weeks. Twenty functional magnetic resonance imaging (fMRI) participants and an average of three days of pre-analysis per participant, and you are already busy for three months just on that small part of the whole enterprise. Needless to say, we have rarely encountered an intern who was able to complete a full study, from inception to a manuscript, in half a year. Luckily, an experienced researcher can proceed much faster, but even then the amount of required time, expertise, and technical resources is not to be underestimated.

Given this investment, it is crucial to make sure that the study you start with is worth the effort. This chapter provides important knowledge about what needs to be considered in order to design and implement a hemodynamic neuroimaging experiment of sufficient quality. It introduces and then discusses the experimental subtraction logic that is the basis for many experiments. Furthermore, we describe the most frequent designs that are appropriate for hemodynamic imaging. In the end, we also cover a few important difficulties and considerations that might be encountered when the chosen design is implemented in an actual experiment.

5.1 Think Before You Start an Experiment

Just because researchers have expensive MRI equipment at their disposal does not mean that any fMRI study they carry out is guaranteed to represent good and high-quality science. It is still up to the scientist to formulate relevant hypotheses and design a study in such a way that the data can be interpreted as providing evidence for or against some hypothesis. When it comes to good experimental design, *the expensive machines do not think for you.* They allow us to pick up the signal from brains at work, but they do not have the brains to know what these signals mean. Nor will the experimenters know when they have not thought carefully about the design of the study.

As do many scientific studies in general, there are also far too many brain imaging studies that lack scientific rigor. This situation is serious enough to elicit skeptical comments from some of the pioneers of cognitive neuroscience, people who were overall very positive about the potential of brain imaging.[1] Stephen Kosslyn, who started using PET and fMRI to address old questions about whether imagery involves image-like or propositional representations, wrote:

Attending a poster session at a recent meeting, I was reminded of the old adage "To the man who has only a hammer, the whole world looks like a nail." In this case, however, instead of a hammer we had a magnetic resonance imaging (MRI) machine and instead of nails we had a study. Many of the studies summarized in the posters did not seem to be designed to answer questions about the functioning of the brain; neither did they seem to bear on specific questions about the roles of particular brain regions. Rather, they could best be described as "exploratory." People were asked to engage in some task while the activity in their brains was monitored, and this activity was then interpreted post hoc. (Kosslyn, 1999)

Kosslyn goes on to acknowledge that this strategy may sometimes pay off. Indeed, when a new technique becomes available, it is already of high value just to show that it works. In early stages, validating the methodological advance might be more important than the scientific questions that could ultimately be answered with the novel technology. However, in the case of noninvasive human brain imaging, there has been a tremendous boom in the number of studies. Many of those studies could indeed be summed up: "Now that we have this machine ready, let's put somebody in the scanner with this or that old paradigm and see what happens."

In this book, which is focused on the methods we can use to noninvasively measure signals from the human brain, we will not go into detail about individual theories and hypotheses that could be tested by a good study. Nevertheless, theories are of the utmost importance. Someone who only knows about the methods could be of high value to further develop the methods, but this person will not be able to design a study with high theoretical relevance. If you want to use fMRI to advance knowledge about how mental processes are implemented in the brain, then you do not need to know only about how fMRI works; you also need to be a specialist in the psychological theories of mental functioning. Scientists such as Stephen Kosslyn are role models in this respect.

5.2 Which Conditions to Include: The Subtraction Method

5.2.1 The Subtraction Method

Suppose a scientist is interested in how people process visual images with a highly disturbing content, such as photographs of soldiers in combat and dead bodies. He/she puts participants in an MRI scanner and lets them watch a series of such photographs in one condition and a blank screen in another condition. Afterward the scientist compares the fMRI signal in the two conditions to find out which brain regions are more activated by the disturbing images than by the blank screen. Take a moment to think about how you would interpret the resulting brain activity.

This is an example of a lousy fMRI study. Note that the problem is not that the scientist would fail to find brain activity. In fact, there would probably be a difference in activity in most of the brain. However, the experiment is not designed to inform the researcher about why there is activation in the different regions. The problem is that the two conditions differ in so many respects that it is unclear which of them would underlie which of the many clusters of activity. One does not need to be a trained cognitive scientist to make a long list of differences: The images will activate the visual system while the blank screen will not; memory representations will be retrieved by the images, not by the blank screen; various emotions will be triggered by the images, but not by the blank screen, to just name a few differences.

What the scientist did in this experiment was make a direct comparison or subtraction of two conditions. This is referred to as the **subtraction method**. To be able to interpret brain activity in such a subtraction in terms of a particular mental process, the experiment has to be designed in such a way that the two conditions differ with respect to only one target mental process. The subtraction method was first used by Franciscus Donders in 1868 using differences in reaction time as the dependent measure (Donders, 1969): The difference in reaction time between two conditions was used as an indication for the time needed to complete the mental process in which the two conditions differed. This reaction time method is known as mental chronometry (Jensen, 2006).

The subtraction method does not limit experiments to just two conditions. A straightforward extension is the inclusion of **a series of conditions**, all of which differ from one other condition in only one mental process. A schematic example is given in Figure 5.1. In this case, an experiment is illustrated that includes three different manipulations or factors. Each factor has two levels, one in which a mental process of interest is not present and one in which this mental process is present. In Figure 5.1A, each of the three mental processes adds a particular amount of time to the reaction time of participants. In statistical terms, there are three main effects in this three-factorial design. The time spent on each of the three processes can be estimated by taking a condition in which this process is present and subtracting the condition in which this process is absent; all other factors are equal.

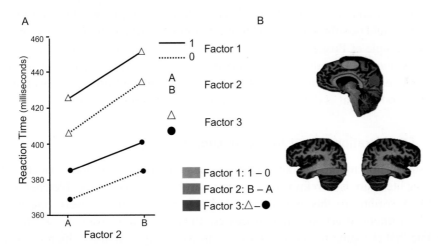

Figure 5.1 The subtraction logic as applied in mental chronometry and brain imaging. We illustrate a design with three factors. (A) The effect of each factor on reaction time. In this case, each factor has a main effect on reaction time. The main effect means that there is an increase in reaction time when one of the factors is changed, from 0 to 1, from A to B, or from circle to triangle, independently of the level of the other two factors. The increase in reaction time gives an indication of the time it takes to execute the process that is manipulated by each factor. (B) A subtraction of the imaging signal measured in the two levels of a factor is taken as an indication of where in the brain the process is localized.

   This schematic example refers to an actual study discussed by Posner (2005). In this experiment, the researchers presented numbers to participants who had to indicate for each number whether it was larger or smaller than five. Eight conditions were generated by manipulating three factors, each with two levels: the notation of the numbers (digits or spelled-out numbers), the distance between the number and five (close or far away), and the responding hand (left or right). Average response time was shortest when the number was shown as a digit, it was far away from five, and the participants responded with the right hand. Neuropsychological theories explain this result using the hypotheses that reading a digit occurs faster than reading a spelled-out number (encoding stage), that it is easier to decide that the number is below or above five when it is far away from five (comparison stage), and that responding is faster with the dominant hand (response stage). Each of these manipulations affects a different stage, and the effects are additive. This is very clear from the reaction time plot, which shows three main effects and no interactions. For example, the more time that it takes to process a spelled-out number compared with a digit can be derived by subtracting the two conditions and would be estimated to be close to 15 ms.

   The same subtraction logic can be used when participants perform such experiments in a scanner. In this case, we do not subtract reaction times but maps of brain activity. For each main effect in the reaction time plot, a subtraction of all the involved conditions can be performed. A schematic illustration is provided in Figure 5.1B. To find the brain regions related to the mental process manipulated through the second factor, the fMRI signal in all the conditions in which this process is absent would be subtracted from all the conditions in which this process is present. In the example of Posner (2005), this could be all conditions involving spelled-out numbers minus all conditions involving digits. This contrast will inform us about where the encoding of the number stimuli happens in the brain, or at least the part of the encoding that is different between spelled-out numbers and digits.

5.2.2 Considerations about the Subtraction Method

The subtraction method makes the crucial **assumption of additivity**, which in the imaging literature is also known as "pure insertion" (Friston, Price, Fletcher, et al., 1996). According to this assumption, it is possible to add, or insert, one mental process without affecting other processes. In the concrete example, we have to assume that changing something in the comparison stage will not influence processing in the encoding stage. If the assumption is not correct, then any brain activity (or reaction time difference) between conditions designed to target the comparison stage would be confounded by the unwanted influence in the encoding stage.

   The empirical data can already provide some indication about whether or not this assumption of additivity is valid. Suppose that the reaction time data in Figure 5.1 would show not only main effects but also interactions. This would suggest that the effect of manipulating one mental process depends on the presence of another mental process. Such an interaction effect would indicate that the effects of the different factors are not additive. For example, the extra processing involved for encoding a spelled-out number compared with a digit might be more or less pronounced depending on whether the comparison process proceeds rapidly or not. When the experiment includes the appropriate control conditions and when interaction effects are tested explicitly, then the assumption of additivity can be put to the test and statistical interpretations can be adapted accordingly. Testing such interactions can also be done at the level of brain activity, following a similar logic as for reaction time data.

Designing the perfect experiment is not straightforward and may even be impossible. Researchers have to deal with imperfect and incomplete knowledge about the brain and the mind. Science makes progress in small incremental steps, and, crucially, *often what is considered as one mental process at one point in history is subdivided further as science progresses*. We can take "attention" as an example. "Attention" is an umbrella term for many different processes. There is the classical distinction between arousal, distributed attention, and selective attention, and between exogenous (stimulus-driven) and endogenous attention. Cognitive psychologist Michael Posner and others have further divided selective attention in subprocesses based on neuropsychological and neuroimaging evidence (Gazzaniga, 1995). To allow the focus of attention shift from one item to another, attention first has to be disengaged from the current focus, then it has to shift, and finally it has to be engaged on the new item. Needless to say, only a cognitive scientist who has a very sophisticated knowledge of psychological theories of attention can design an experiment that is relevant to advance the current state of knowledge about attention. Even then, what current theories assume to be one process might be further divided later on.

The difficulties with designing perfect experiments and limitations of the current state of the art do not relieve scientists from the obligation to try to strive in the direction of the ideal scientific experiment as much as possible. Too often, studies are published in which conditions differ in many different aspects and yet the authors jump to conclusions about what the results reveal. Invalid conclusions are often based on a particular way of making inferences ("reverse inference"; see the section on statistical inference in Chapter 7), which is the only available fallback option when a study was not designed properly. It is important to note that in such cases it is not the technique itself nor the more general neuroscientific approach to mental functions that is to blame for the interpretational problems, but the inappropriate use by scientists who have not designed their experiments properly. The scientist is to blame, not the imaging method.

It is very common, and not as much of a problem, for scientists to compare conditions that do not satisfy the "one-process-difference" assumption as a first *exploratory analysis*. To return to the experiment with the disturbing pictures of soldiers and bodies, the contrast of this condition with a blank screen condition would be very much acceptable as a means of getting a first exploratory view on the whole system of brain regions involved when processing the pictures. However, this should be only a first step, without any grand conclusions drawn from it. The experiment should include further conditions that allow one to determine which mental processes are associated with each of the many different peaks of activity found in the exploratory contrast. A related approach is the use of *functional localizer* contrasts, which are used to localize brain regions of interest. Sometimes this localizer contrast itself involves conditions that are again more different from each other than the conditions in the actual experiment of interest.

Finally, the subtraction method is typically introduced as a way to manipulate mental functions in a categorical or all-or-none fashion: The function is either involved or not involved, and conditions are pair-wise subtracted. However, this most simple case can be extended toward so-called *parametric designs*, in which the degree of involvement is manipulated systematically in a parametric manner. For example, instead of having one condition that involves selective attention and another that does not, selective attention could be manipulated in degrees.

Now that we have given an overview of all these important considerations, it would be a good exercise to go back to the researcher interested in delineating and localizing the different mental processes involved when disturbing pictures are processed and think about how you would approach this general question: Which conditions would be included in your experiment?

5.3 How to Present the Conditions: The Block Design

5.3.1 The Block Design and the Hemodynamic Response Function

Once we have decided about which hypotheses to investigate and which experimental conditions are needed, we face the question of how to present those conditions. It is useful to first see how we would do this in the case of a simple behavioral experiment, then contrast the procedure with what we would do for an fMRI experiment, and finally discuss how this would be different with the other hemodynamic imaging methods.

Consider the abstract case of an experiment with conditions A and B. One trial of each condition takes a few seconds. In which order will we show the conditions? In some cases, when the two conditions are difficult to switch, researchers might opt to present the conditions in a blocked manner with several trials of condition A before a switch to condition B. Situations in which this might be necessary include, for example, experiments that involve switches in complicated task instructions, or two conditions that are different in terms of the room in which the participants are seated. However, in most experiments, the researchers prefer a different approach and use a (pseudo-)random trial order so that subjects cannot predict which condition is coming next. This is the preferred approach followed in most behavioral experiments.

Using a random trial order is not a straightforward choice in the case of an fMRI experiment. In Chapter 4 we discussed the HRF (hemodynamic response function).

Even if the trial itself and all neural activity associated with it takes only 2 seconds, then the effect of this trial on the hemodynamic signal is "smeared" in time: The peak of the HRF is delayed with 6 seconds, and its total duration is more than 12 seconds from onset to the point at which it has gone back to baseline. If a researcher would let a trial of 2 seconds (s) of condition A be followed immediately by a trial of condition B, then the blood-oxygenation-level dependent (BOLD) signal changes related to condition B would start even before the signal changes related to the previous trial of condition A have reached their peak.

This problem is illustrated in Figure 5.2 for the simplest design possible: trials of one active condition interleaved with a baseline. Each continuous blue line shows a simulated (idealized, non-noisy) BOLD response related to the trials of the condition that are presented each time there is a vertical red tick mark on top. To avoid the problem of overlapping HRFs when trials come too close in time, researchers could opt to space the trials with as much time as is needed to let the HRF of the previous trial return to baseline. In Figure 5.2A, the trials are spaced by 16 s (interstimulus interval [ISI]), which is indeed sufficient to achieve this goal.

It is obvious that this design is not very efficient. In a behavioral experiment, participants could complete many more trials in the same time window. Also, we would expect, given that the HRF is additive, that one stimulus would elicit fewer changes in the BOLD signal compared with a design in which five times as many stimuli are presented.

Nevertheless, it is not an option just to present stimuli with a short ISI of fixed duration. Figure 5.2B shows what the modeled BOLD response would look like. This signal starts with a strong gradual signal increase, even stronger than that in Figure 5.2A because the HRF of the second trial adds to the HRF of the first trial. Then the signal reaches an asymptotic level with only very minor fluctuations related to when the condition is present and when it is not. The very large ups and downs that were visible with ISI = 16 s have been reduced strongly at ISI = 2 s.

To solve this issue, researchers often decide to present trials in a blocked manner and alternate blocks of different conditions, commonly referred to as a **block design**. Within blocks, the HRFs associated with individual trials add together to generate a strong cumulative signal. When a block of another condition starts, in the simplest case a block of baseline, the signal related to the first block goes down, even all the way to baseline if block length is long enough. Figure 5.2C illustrates the resulting modeled BOLD signal. The condition-related ups and downs in the signal are even larger than in the sparse design shown in Figure 5.2A. The block alternation is perfectly visible in the BOLD response.

The block design is a *very efficient* design. Participants can be subjected to a constant train of trials, and there is no need to wait a long time between individual trials. The block design also has a *high power and sensitivity to detect changes in the BOLD signal* because the differences in signal between conditions are amplified compared with a slower and sparser design, and even more with respect to a condition order in which trials of different conditions alternate.

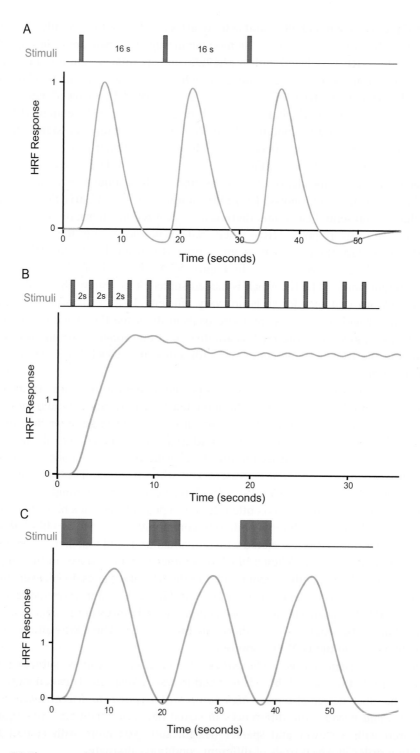

Figure 5.2 The expected hemodynamic signal changes related to different trial sequences. (A) Slow event-related design. (B) Fast event-related design with alternation of stimulus trials and null events. (C) Block design.

Nevertheless, the block design also has several drawbacks. First, participants can predict the condition to which the next trial will belong. If for any reason subjects tend to "prepare" themselves differently for different conditions (e.g., assign attention elsewhere), then the block design provides ample opportunity to do so. This predictability and associated preparatory effects increase the odds that unwanted cognitive processes confound that one mental function that the researchers had set out to isolate by contrasting two conditions. Second, the predictability might also make the task more boring for the participants. Third, the block-wise presentation might be incompatible with addressing some experimental questions (e.g., trial-to-trial fluctuations in performance). Fourth, with a block design it is *impossible to estimate the single-trial response function*, that is, which effect was elicited by a single trial. This (modeled) single-trial response is very nicely visible in Figure 5.2A, but in Figure 5.2C we only recover the response to the block of trials as a whole. Going from the block response back to a single-trial response is possible if one makes assumptions about the exact shape and additivity of the HRF, but researchers interested in single-stimulus response functions prefer not to make such assumptions. Indeed, even though the HRF tends to have the same general characteristics overall (delayed in time, temporally smoothed), its exact form can differ between regions and participants (Aguirre et al., 1998).

All hemodynamic imaging methods provide data that are temporally filtered through a hemodynamic imaging method. Nevertheless, the choice of design is not exactly the same for the individual methods. For fMRI and functional near-infrared spectroscopy (fNIRS) we have a freedom of choice between using a block design or not, and the same arguments will be in play in both cases (efficiency, power, cognitive factors and predictability, estimation). The situation is different for positron emission tomography (PET). In PET, we cumulate the signal across longer periods of time after the injection of a tracer. During all this time, only one condition can be presented, resulting in a design with long blocks. The number of long blocks will also be low, because each block has to be preceded by a tracer injection. A design with long blocks, a relatively low number of conditions, and a low number of blocks per condition is the only possible design for a PET task activation study.

5.3.2 The Block Design in Practice in fMRI and fNIRS

In practice, there is a large variability in the scientific literature in terms of the exact temporal succession of trials and blocks in a block design. Over time, different laboratories have converged toward very different practices within the very large space of possibilities that remains after considering the restrictions mentioned above. For example, *block length* has to be long enough, but how long? In the literature, the length ranges from "short-block" designs with blocks of 6–12 s, "intermediate-block" designs with blocks of 12–21 s, and "long-block" designs with blocks up to 30 s and more.

When comparing block length between studies, it is important to consider how blocks from different conditions follow each other. Some labs prefer to have a period of "rest" in between successive blocks from different conditions. These rest intervals allow the signal to return to baseline. Figure 5.2C is an example of such a condition/rest alternation. This *rest interval* effectively increases the onset asynchrony of successive blocks with the time of the rest interval. The fluctuations in signal, therefore, would be larger than they would be when blocks of different conditions succeed each other immediately. Which block organization to use is subject to the same trade-off as when comparing a block design with a very sparse design: The rest breaks increase the signal changes, but they allow for less activation of the brain and fewer presentations of the conditions of interest. If one is interested in estimating the response to a block of trials, then the rest breaks are essential. Otherwise, it is often a matter of preference and habit.

In many studies, block length is constant, but in some other studies block length is varied from block to block. In those cases, the power of the block design is probably close to the power of a block design with a constant block length equal to the average of the varying block length. Nevertheless, the variation in block length can be useful in several contexts, for example, in cases where the researchers want to make the alternation from one block to the other unpredictable.

Even when working with blocks, researchers try not to have the different conditions come in a fixed order. For example, with four conditions, the order [1 2 3 4] would not be the only one used. This is all the more important when blocks from different conditions follow each other without a rest break in between. Counterbalancing condition order avoids the situation in which the signal measured in one particular condition A could be biased by the fact that this condition is always or predominantly preceded by different conditions than those preceding condition B. Most studies make sure that this counterbalancing is as perfect as possible for the immediately preceding condition, so-called **one-back counterbalancing**.

The number of blocks is another point to consider. The fMRI signal is noisy, and thus conditions have to be repeated to increase the signal-to-noise ratio in the data. Most of the time, an fMRI experiment will require tens of minutes or even more than an hour of testing to acquire enough data. It is not optimal to acquire data for that long, without pause, using a pulse sequence that runs continuously. Participants cannot maintain concentration on a task without sometimes taking a break. In behavioral experiments, breaks are included to allow subjects to relax. The same procedure is followed in fMRI studies, and data acquisition is stopped every 5–10 minutes. Another benefit of splitting data collection into individual runs relates to the frequent minor problems that might occur during data acquisition (e.g., the subject has to sneeze). By dividing the data into smaller bits and pieces, it is easier to throw away one piece of data, if necessary, without any effect on the other images acquired in other runs. A period of continuous data acquisition is often referred to as a "run" or a "time series." There is a practical limit to how short such runs can be. For the data analysis, it is advisable to have each condition appear in each run, if possible for at least two blocks so that the average onset time of all conditions is as similar as possible (e.g., the first condition is also the last one).

Below is an example condition order for one run of an experiment that has been performed with slight variations by many labs. The experiment includes four conditions differing by which type of image was shown: (1) faces, (2) objects, (3) scenes, and (4) scrambled images (unrecognizable texture-like pictures). Condition 0 is a rest condition (no image shown; just a blank screen). Each block lasts 15 s, and rest breaks are not systematically included between successive stimulus blocks.

Condition order: [0 1 2 3 4 0 2 4 1 3 0 3 1 4 2 0 4 3 2 1 0]

This run includes 21 blocks, with a total duration of 315 s (6 minutes and 15 seconds). Four such runs provide 16 blocks per image condition, which is sufficient to find significant activation for contrasts with a relatively large effect size (such as faces – objects, see the following).

5.3.3 A Few Examples of Classical Studies Using a Block Design

In this section, we illustrate the typical results obtained in a block design. The example studies are also an example of the iterative refinement of the contrasts that are included in successive studies.

In 1995, Malach and colleagues reported an experiment that included a range of conditions divided in two groups differing in whether or not the presented images included an object (Malach et al., 1995). The object conditions included common objects (teddy bear, car, . . .), abstract sculptures, and faces. The non-object conditions included texture patterns and gratings. The authors found a relatively large region in the lateral occipital cortex that responds more strongly to all of the object conditions than to the non-object conditions. This region is commonly referred to as the "lateral occipital complex" (LOC).

Figure 5.3 illustrates the fMRI signal (here expressed in normalized units on the Y-axis) measured in the LOC (red line) and primary visual cortex (blue line) for each of these conditions. Non-shaded areas represent resting periods with a blank screen (no images presented). Purple areas include all blocks of object conditions, and dark gray areas all blocks of non-object conditions. The LOC shows a higher signal each time a block of object images is presented compared with when non-object images are presented.

The different object condition blocks are relevant to exclude potential confounds. The condition with the abstract sculptures is particularly important. These abstract sculptures do not activate strong semantic associations, making it unlikely that the LOC activity would be related to semantic processing.

This object-related activation was also demonstrated with PET by (Kanwisher, Woods, Jacoboni, et al., 1997). Illustrating the different design choices for PET, the experiment included in total 12 blocks of 60 seconds each, including 4 blocks of 3 conditions: familiar objects, unfamiliar objects, and scrambled images.

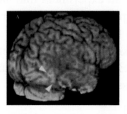

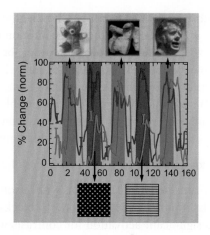

——— Lateral occipital complex
——— Primary visual cortex

Figure 5.3 The localization of object-selective brain regions using a block fMRI experiment. The brain image shows the object-selective lateral occipital complex (LOC) in red, close to the motion-selective middle temporal area in green. The hemodynamic signal changes in the LOC (red line) and in the primary visual cortex (blue line) are shown for a no-stimulus baseline (light gray bars), for several object conditions (purple bars), and for several texture conditions (dark gray bars).
Images reproduced with permission from Malach et al., 1995. Copyright (1997) National Academy of Sciences

Later on, researchers wondered whether all regions would, as the LOC does, respond the same to faces and other objects. One of the arguments to expect in potential differences is the occurrence of neuropsychological patients who cannot recognize faces, although they have no problems with other objects. This syndrome is known as prosopagnosia. The most famous demonstration of face-selective regions in the human brain is the 1997 study conducted by Nancy Kanwisher and colleagues (Kanwisher, McDermott and Chun, 1997). They found a region in the ventral occipitotemporal cortex, more specifically in the fusiform gyrus, which shows a higher signal when faces are presented compared with when other object images are shown. This region is known as the fusiform face area (FFA). The basic finding is illustrated in Figure 5.4. The brain slice shows the significantly activated voxels in the contrast of faces minus objects. The outline of the FFA is shown with a green line. The time course plot on the right shows the signal changes in the FFA voxels, with an increased signal during the face blocks.

The contrast between objects and non-objects was a very important first step, in particular from a neuroscience perspective, but the distinction could be criticized as being very nonspecific. Few psychological experiments compare objects and non-object texture images. The contrast between faces and other objects is much more relevant, and neuropsychological and other studies often contrast object processing with face processing. Nevertheless, faces and objects also differ in many respects. Since 1997, many studies have tried to identify which mental process is responsible for the differential response to faces and objects in regions such as the FFA. Potential candidates are category membership, visual shape properties, and holistic

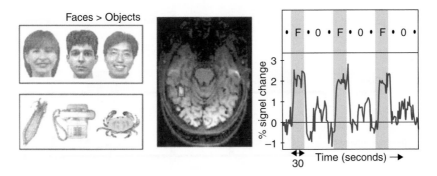

Figure 5.4 The localization of face-selective brain regions using a block fMRI experiment comparing blocks of successively presented face images with blocks of non-face images. The signal in the localized region (within green outline) is shown for three conditions: fixation baseline (denoted by a dot), face blocks (F), and object blocks (O).
Reproduced with permission from Kanwisher, McDermott and Chun, 1997

processing (Bracci and Op de Beeck, 2016; Haxby et al., 2000; Tarr and Gauthier, 2000). This process of further refining our understanding of the functional specialization of these regions continues today (Bracci et al., 2017).

5.4 The Event-Related Design

Despite the power of the block design, its drawbacks have motivated many scientists to search for alternative designs. In addition to the block design, we have already referred to one alternative in which a very long ISI is used. This design is often referred to as the **slow event-related design**. When the experiment includes two conditions, it might look like Figure 5.5B. The red and blue bars refer to the two conditions in a two-condition experiment. A slow event-related design might have a fixed long ISI as in the figure, or an ISI that is long on average and varies from trial to trial. The technical term for such interval variation is **jitter**.

Based on Figure 5.2B, which was used to introduce the block design, it can already be observed that simply alternating the two conditions without an ISI of many seconds might not work. Such an **alternating event-related design** has only been used for illustrative purposes, such as in the study shown in Figure 5.6 (Bandettini and Cox, 2000). These researchers presented a visual stimulus for 2 seconds and manipulated the ISI. With long ISIs of 10–12 seconds, the alternation of the stimulus is visible in the raw fMRI signal in Figure 5.6A (see time courses on the left for those conditions). For very short ISIs of only two to four seconds, this modulation has disappeared.

Instead of plotting the continuous signal, it is also possible to extract intervals from the signal belonging to different trials, plot all these intervals on the same scale with 0 = stimulus onset, and then average all the intervals. This gives an

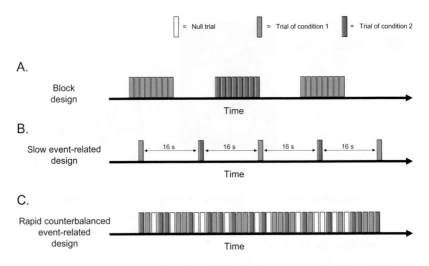

Figure 5.5 Different fMRI designs: (A) block, (B) slow event-related, and (C) rapid event-related.

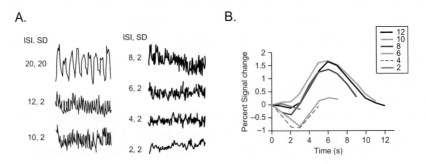

Figure 5.6 Hemodynamic signal variation in visual cortex when stimulus trials (SD: stimulus duration) alternate with no-stimulus trials at a range of fixed interstimulus intervals (ISI). (A) Raw time series. (B) Cycle-averaged time series, with time zero = stimulus onset.
Figure based (with permission) on Bandettini and Cox, 2000

event-related response. We will encounter this type of analysis again in the context of electrophysiological imaging (see Chapter 11). With the longer ISIs in Figure 5.6, the event-related response looks very much like a typical HRF (Fig. 5.6B). Indeed, a slow event-related design is ideal for estimating the response function. For ISIs below 8 s, there is no clear event-related response present. All of this seems to be in favor of using a slow event-related design. This leaves us with all the drawbacks of this design, including its low efficiency and the consideration that it is pretty boring for participants.

For those reasons, researchers regularly resort to another design, the **rapid counterbalanced event-related design**. Here the trials of the different conditions are presented in rapid succession, possibly without any further ISI than the trial

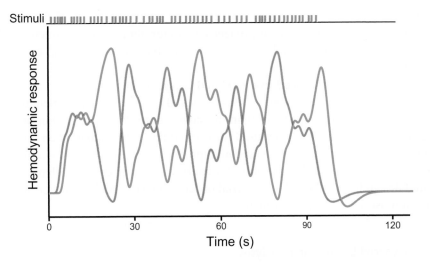

Figure 5.7 The modulation of the hemodynamic signal in a rapid counterbalanced event-related design. The top row depicts the timing of the trials of two conditions. The expected hemodynamic responses for the two conditions are shown below, as computed by convolving the two trial time series with the HRF.

duration. Thus, the next stimulus or trial might start when the previous one ended. Importantly, the conditions are not alternating in a fixed order, but the order is more random. A condition can follow itself, while at other times there might be a relatively high number of trials in between two occurrences of a particular condition. The order is counterbalanced so that each condition follows each condition an equal number of times. An example sequence is given in Figure 5.5C, where trials of two conditions are presented in rapid succession, intermixed with trials or "null events" of a baseline condition.

Such a fast event-related design has been shown to provide enough sensitivity to pick up significant differences between conditions, even with trials as short as 2 seconds (Buckner, 1998; Dale and Buckner, 1997). How can this counterbalanced design work given that the alternating design fails to show a clear signal? This is explained in Figure 5.7. This figure shows the modeled BOLD signal for two conditions in orange and blue. The occurrence of trials of these two conditions is shown by the time stamps on top. When we follow the orange signal, we see that it starts rising after the blue signal, but then the orange signal reaches a very high peak, while the blue signal goes down to zero. This peak in a difference of signal occurs after a series of trials of the orange condition. At this point in time, there is a large contrast between the two conditions, much more than ever happens in the alternating design. Such a contrast is seen each time a particular condition occurs frequently in a relatively short period of time. In a random sequence, such frequency peaks happen regularly, and they are responsible for why this design provides a useful signal.

The order of conditions in this design is typically not a fully random sequence. It has to be counterbalanced, and among different counterbalanced sequences some are better than others (*more efficient*) in terms of the strength of the resulting contrast. There are different approaches to determining these sequences. Two examples are the method used by the freely available function optseq2 and genetic algorithms.

The rapid counterbalanced event-related design is in many ways a reasonable compromise. It has an intermediate sensitivity and power, much more than the rapid alternating design, and also more than the slow event-related design, but much less than the block design. It can be used for estimation, in particular when one of the counterbalanced conditions is a rest condition. Nevertheless, the slow event-related design is still better for that purpose. Of course, the rapid counterbalanced event-related design has the benefit of the trial order being very similar to what would be done in most behavioral experiments.

More Advanced Designs and Analyses

The distinction between block and event-related designs is useful in introducing the relevant issues and concepts such as sensitivity and efficiency. In practice, this distinction is much more fuzzy because often researchers opt to use intermediate approaches. For example, sometimes the block length in a block design becomes as short as 4–6 seconds, closer to the timing of the classic event-related design than to the block length in the stereotypical block design (see also Section 5.3.2). Furthermore, over the years many different designs and extensions have been developed and used. Two of these designs are discussed in Chapter 8, which covers advanced statistical analyses, because the designs are inherently connected to particular approaches of data analysis. A first example is the condition-rich event-related design in which many tens of conditions are included instead of the traditional design with only a few conditions. This gives fewer trials per condition and thus a lower signal-to-noise ratio per voxel, which is compensated for by a specific analysis approach that combines the signal across voxels: multi-voxel pattern analysis. A second example is the fMRI adaptation design in which each event (or block) includes at least two stimuli and the researchers manipulate whether these two stimuli are the same or different.

5.5 The Baseline or Rest Condition

5.5.1 The Role of a Baseline in Task-Based fMRI

The willingness to satisfy the assumptions of the subtraction method could lead to the choice to optimize all conditions in an experiment to be as similar as possible, differing from at least one other condition in only one cognitive process. Taken to its extreme, this approach could cause different studies to have no condition in common. The drawback is obvious: It would be very difficult to compare the results from different studies.

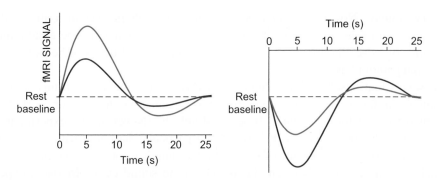

Figure 5.8 The importance of a resting baseline to disambiguate more activation from less deactivation. The hemodynamic response (fMRI signal) is shown for two conditions. The red condition is associated with higher signal values compared with the blue condition in both plots. The signal level is expressed relative to the signal in a resting baseline.
Figure inspired by Jody Culham

Furthermore, in this approach it might be hard for researchers to interpret the differences in activity between the experimental conditions. Consider the two plots in Figure 5.8. In both cases, there is one condition with a higher signal compared with the other condition. With just those two conditions in the experiment, a contrast of them would only show the differences among them. It would not inform us about whether the higher condition is more activated (left plot) or less deactivated (right plot).

The comparison of results from different experiments and the interpretation of the results from contrasts are much easier when each experiment includes a baseline that is as similar as possible between experiments and, as such, is the agreed null condition or baseline for all researchers. Such a baseline differentiates between differences in activation (left plot) and differences in deactivation (right plot).

When present, the baseline condition is often used to calculate fMRI *responses* instead of the raw fMRI signal. In the case of the study of Kanwisher, McDermott and Chun (1997), the Y-axis in the time course plot is labeled "% signal change" (Fig. 5.4). This index is used regularly. It refers to the signal change in comparison to a baseline condition, which in visual studies is often a blank screen with a fixation spot. The percent signal change is defined as:

$$100 \times (\text{signal}(t) - \text{baseline})/\text{baseline}$$

(Here signal (*t*) is the signal measured at each time point *t* and baseline is the signal averaged across all the baseline blocks.)

While the raw BOLD-related fMRI signal value in MRI images often takes high values such as 600–900, this overall value is now subtracted away. The modulations due to differences in blood oxygenation are relatively small in relation to this overall value. A modulation in terms of percent signal change of 2–3%, as seen in the plot, is very common. Now you understand why some researchers voice the criticism that human brain imaging is all about small percentages of signal change among huge amounts of noise, like looking for a needle in a haystack. Luckily, it helps to know something about hay.

It seems that baselines have emerged in fMRI experiments in an unsystematic manner. As far as we know, there has never been a conference or workgroup devoted to what the "standard" baseline should be. Nevertheless, experimenters have primarily converged on the use of one particular baseline, with only minor deviations. For many domains of study, the baseline is a total rest baseline during which no sensory input is given (blank screen; no sound cues). In visual experiments, in which subjects are often asked to focus on a fixation spot while stimuli are presented, the baseline is principally a fixation condition during which this fixation spot is shown without any other stimuli.

How the baseline is intermingled with the experimental conditions can be approached in a variety of ways. It can be treated as yet another experimental condition (same number of trials; part of counterbalancing); in event-related designs, it is often part of the counterbalancing but more frequent than the other conditions; sometimes it is not part of counterbalancing and even less frequent than the other conditions (e.g., only at the start and at the end of each run); and sometimes each block of an experimental condition is followed by a block of the baseline condition.

5.5.2 Regions Activated during a Resting Baseline

For quite some time, researchers included a rest condition as a baseline without being particularly interested in what was going on during this condition. In the previous decade, we saw a surge of studies being devoted to what the brain does during rest (Raichle and Snyder, 2007). There are many brain regions active during rest. More intriguingly, there are many brain regions that are more active during rest than during the performance of an active task. The activated and deactivated regions in three example datasets are shown in Figure 5.9. In each case, the color map represents a t-contrast between an active task condition and a passive baseline. Yellow/red colors indicate more activation in the task condition, blue refers to more activation in the passive baseline. The tasks are very different: (Fig. 5.9A) Subtracting two numbers and determining whether the outcome is odd or even (Bulthe, De Smedt and Op de Beeck, 2014); (Fig. 5.9B) determining when a repetition occurs in a series of images of everyday objects; (Fig. 5.9C) determining when a repetition occurs in a series of texture patterns. Despite the obvious differences between these task contexts from the perspective of a cognitive scientist, the three tasks essentially activate the same set of regions, in particular, visual regions in the occipital cortex, regions around the intraparietal sulcus, and the lateral prefrontal cortex. Of course, there are minor differences which can be picked up. The data in Figure 5.9B and C were obtained

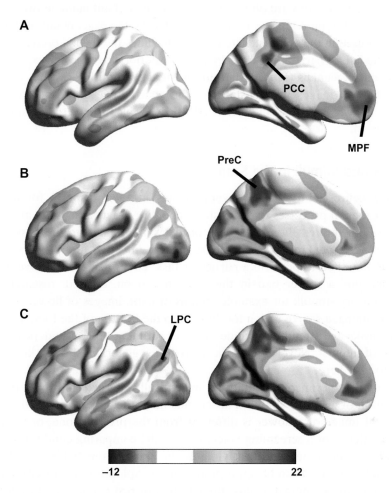

Figure 5.9 fMRI activation in a contrast of an active task minus a passive no-stimulus baseline.
The baseline involved passive viewing of a blank screen with a fixation dot. The active tasks are (A)
number subtraction task (16 subjects), (B) one-back repetition detection with object images (20 subjects),
(C) one-back repetition detection with texture patterns (20 subjects). The color maps represent *t*-values
from a second-level random-effects analysis. Visualizations generated by BrainNet Viewer.

from the same set of 20 subjects. A direct contrast of these two active tasks
reveals a stronger activation of the lateral occipital cortex in the task with
everyday objects, similar to the aforementioned object-selective responses first
reported by Malach et al. (1995). However, no matter how important these
differences are, we should not forget that they are added to a general activation
pattern which is largely shared.

We now turn to brain regions that are more activated in the resting baseline.
There is typically a whole set of regions that are *more* active during the resting

condition. These regions are often referred to as the **default mode network**. Again, this network of brain regions is found irrespective of the exact details of the active task that is used in the contrast. The network includes the medial prefrontal cortex (MPF), the lateral parietal cortex (LPC), the posterior cingulate cortex (PCC), and the adjacent precuneus (PreC). The interest in activity during rest has resulted in the practice of doing a resting-state scan in which subjects are not performing any task, known as resting-state fMRI (RS-fMRI, which is covered in more detail in Chapter 8).

5.6 Task and Stimuli in the Scanner

Cognitive neuroscientists have several means at their disposal for activating particular mental processes of interest. Some more practical matters are covered in Box 5.1. In the text here, we focus on decisions related to the design of the study. Broadly speaking, we can separate them into two groups. First, participants can be asked to perform a particular task: count backward, move an index finger, imagine a flower bed in the sun, and so on. Second, researchers can present sensory stimuli: for example, beams of light, images of flowers, a human voice screaming, a stroke with a toothbrush to the bottom of the foot. The choice of which tasks and stimuli to include in the experiment obviously depends on the question of interest. Nevertheless, there are a few generalized remarks and some advice to give here.

First of all, experimental conditions are typically characterized by a particular combination of task and stimuli. Participants might be asked to indicate whether the current image of a flower is different from the previous one, or to rate the negative valence of a screaming voice. Obviously, comparing conditions that are different in both stimuli and task violates the assumptions behind the Donders subtraction method. It can be appropriate for an exploratory localizer contrast or for an exploratory contrast against the baseline or rest condition, but not for the contrasts of interest. For a contrast of interest, one should either change the stimuli and keep the task the same or manipulate the task executed with the same sensory stimulation.

Second, the choice of task is important for all cognitive neuroscience experiments. A cognitive neuroscientist interested in task effects will opt for those tasks that are theoretically relevant, and here there might not be much difference between a typical behavioral experiment in the field and an imaging study. For example, a PET study on working memory will, of course, include a working memory task in the experimental design. However, the choice of task is less straightforward when a researcher is interested in stimulus effects and wants to compare different stimulus conditions while keeping the task the same. Here there are some particular questions about task effects that emerge in imaging and that are not typically asked in behavioral experiments. In behavioral experiments, researchers need to have participants perform a task that provides the wanted behavioral response. In an

Box 5.1 From the Design to Scanning

Once all the details about the design have been decided on, the ideas have to be brought in practice. There are several important steps to consider. First, the experiment has to be programmed. For this there is a wide range of software available, including software that is also commonly used for behavioral experiments: E-Prime, Presentation, MATLAB and Psychtoolbox, Python/PsychoPy, and many more. Apart from the many functions that are also needed for a behavioral study, the programming for an fMRI study might include a few extra elements such as the need to synchronize the imaging data acquisition with the behavioral/stimulus protocol by reading in the trigger signal from the scanner; presenting the stimuli through other means than standard plug-and-play hardware; and reading behavioral responses by hardware other than a standard keyboard. Given that most new researchers start scanning in a facility that is already used by other and more experienced researchers, getting started typically involves acquiring knowledge about local customs and about what is already available on site.

Second, at most universities obtaining ethical approval for an fMRI or PET study will necessitate a longer administrative procedure compared with a standard behavioral experiment. Participants in the experiments will also have to fill in more paperwork: not only an informed consent but also medical screening forms. For special populations (e.g., children), the scanning might be preceded by a practice session in a mock scanner or dummy scanner. A mock scanner looks like a real scanner, but there is no magnetic field and no working costs.

Third, the selection of participants is also subject to several considerations, such as safety issues (no metal in the body), handedness (often researchers opt to include only right-handers because left-handers might be more variable in brain organization), and gender (in the past, some labs used only male subjects, for several reasons, one being assumed gender differences in hemispheric asymmetry (Sommer et al., 2004)). The number of subjects needed depends on the expected effect size and the signal-to-noise ratio with which the effect is measured. This is not easy to determine in fMRI, which is one of the reasons why power analyses prior to performing a study are rarely performed and the desired number of participants is under debate (Kolossa and Kopp, 2018). Studies that depend on group-based statistics often include 12–20 participants per group, with recent studies more often using even larger sample sizes (also see Box 6.2 in Chapter 6). For within-subject designs, it is often advisable to have at least 16–20 participants. However, studies have been published that demonstrate very robust and replicable findings with as few as 3–5 participants. In these cases, effect size is so large or data collection per participant is so intensive that effects are strongly significant in each individual participant (Formisano et al., 2008; Kay et al., 2008).

Then there is the actual scan session. In most countries, legislation requires that scanning be performed or at least supervised by a certified radio-technician. Even attending the scan session requires training in safety. A good preparation is critical to let everything proceed smoothly. All equipment, software, imaging sequences, and design choices have to be tested and decided on in advance. Safety is the priority, and of course time is money: The scan might cost hundreds of euros per hour. Finally, the attending experimenter should keep a detailed logbook covering everything that has happened during scanning. Otherwise, the data might be useless. Indeed, imaging data as they come from the scanner typically do not contain any information on the stimuli and the task(s) that were presented. If the logbook does not tell the researcher which stimulus sequence was used in run 6, then the MRI data of run 6 are useless. Likewise, PET data will not tell us that the subject has fallen asleep in block 3 or reported feeling dizzy in block 5; only the logbook can.

imaging study, researchers do not necessarily need behavioral responses. Researchers can investigate brain activity triggered by the experimenter's design without the need for any overt behavioral response related to the process of interest. Thus, there is the possibility of including no task at all (passive perception of the presented stimuli), or, alternatively, to ask subjects to attend to stimulus features that are irrelevant to what the researchers are interested in. The latter type of task is often referred to as an "orthogonal task". For example, a researcher might be interested in the difference in activity between faces and other objects and ask the participants to press a button every time the fixation spot changes color.

However, it must be said that no matter how hard the researchers do their best to use the best task available, it is very hard to avoid the criticism that stimulus effects might be confounded by task effects or "attention"—sometimes to the understandable frustration of researchers. The following anecdote illustrates this feeling. One autumn in the mid-2000s, a pumpkin decorated in Halloween style appeared in the Kanwisher lab at the Massachusetts Institute of Technology where one of us was working at that time. The pumpkin sat on the sofa used for the weekly lab meeting and held a text balloon with "could this just be due to attention?" written on it. The question was never irrelevant.

Third, for stimulus presentation and response registration the scanner environment brings with it quite a number of pragmatic challenges. Among the hemodynamic imaging methods, fNIRS involves the fewest problems and fMRI the most. Concerning the latter, visual scientists prefer to present stimuli on well-calibrated monitors. For an fMRI experiment, they have to use goggles or project the stimuli on a screen in front of a subject's eyes. Stimulus control is a challenge with these devices, and for some psychophysical experiments it might not be sufficient when embarking on an fMRI experiment. Studies of auditory perception have to consider not only the quality of the audio presentation but also the interference of the noise of the scanner during data acquisition. Auditory experiments often apply a more sparse data acquisition, so that there are a few seconds of silence in between two successive volume acquisitions in order to present the auditory stimuli without interference. Studies of somatosensation and visuomotor coordination often need special equipment to stimulate subjects or for the performance of visually guided motor actions, and of course such equipment has to be nonmagnetic and certified for use in a strong magnetic field. The same goes for the equipment needed to record all sorts of behavioral responses, even for the simplest button presses. Controlling for the effect of eye movements is useful in constraining the interpretation of brain activation differences. However, using eye-tracking devices inside a scanner can be quite difficult, and the data acquired are typically far inferior to what can be obtained outside the scanner. Verbal responses are also used, but again researchers have to deal with interference from scanner noise and with the obvious risk for confounding head movements during speaking. Thus, whatever the field of study you are interested in, you can expect a marked difference in the methods and equipment used between an fMRI study and a behavioral study. Choosing to use fMRI often results in the need for pragmatic compromises.

Summary

- Designing and implementing a hemodynamic imaging experiment requires thorough planning to develop a proper design that allows for interpretable data. It also involves many administrative and technical hurdles.
- The design of many imaging studies involves the subtraction method, which requires an up-to-date knowledge of cognitive science and brings with it several assumptions.
- The block design is the most efficient design for hemodynamic imaging because of the temporal characteristics of the hemodynamic response function, but this design includes various cognitive confounds and a loss of the ability to estimate the neural response to stimulus and task events.
- The event-related design suffers from a lower efficiency, but is more related to typical behavioral designs and it allows for an estimation of the neural response to individual events.

Review Questions

1. Explain why a good application of the subtraction method 20 years ago might now be considered a poor design if the same study were to be implemented today.
2. Explain how the temporal characteristics of the hemodynamic response function constrain the experimental design in hemodynamic imaging.
3. Explain the benefits and disadvantages of the event-related design compared with the block design.
4. What do researchers have to consider when they chose the baseline condition in an fMRI experiment?

Further Reading

Designing experiments is rarely the topic of long texts. Instead, there are many excellent online resources that include slide presentations about experimental design. The following list contains a few examples:
www.fil.ion.ucl.ac.uk/spm/course/
imaging.mrc-cbu.cam.ac.uk/imaging/DesignEfficiency
www.fmri4newbies.com/tutorials/

Notes

1 This is one of several quotes put together by Jody Culham; see www.slideserve.com/webb/basics-of-experimental-design-for-fmri-block-designs.

CHAPTER SIX

Image Processing

Learning Objectives

- Understanding the complexity of neuroimaging analyses and how this complexity can be mastered
- Acquiring knowledge of the most important concepts and steps of image processing
- Being aware of the importance of performing quality control and of allowing external quality control (open science)

What can we infer from a brain imaging experiment? Some people are tempted to infer too much, whereas others maintain an unreasonable skepticism. The only two ways to answer the question is either to ask an expert (the easy way) or to become more knowledgeable yourself about data analysis and interpretation. The latter is what we try to achieve in this and the following two chapters.

Data analysis for hemodynamic imaging can be divided conceptually into three steps: preprocessing, statistical model fitting, and statistical inference (Fig. 6.1).

In this chapter, we focus on preprocessing; the other two steps are covered in Chapter 7. Preprocessing primarily involves image processing, which does not exist for the analysis of behavioral data. Here we introduce several important preprocessing steps: quality control, motion correction, coregistration, normalization, and spatial smoothing. Several of these steps are also involved in other types of brain imaging, so part of the acquired knowledge will be transferable to those methods.

Quality control is important throughout. It is covered in Boxes 6.1 and 6.2, which cover both the quality control at the technical level provided by the individual researcher, as well as quality control provided by the scientific community.

We focus more on functional magnetic resonance imaging (fMRI) than on positron emission tomography (PET) and functional near-infrared spectroscopy (fNIRS). This choice is in line with the relative user frequencies of the different methods. In addition, the analysis of fMRI data typically involves the most processing steps, of which a subset is also relevant for the other methods.

6.1 Software Packages

Many software tools are available for basic and more advanced data analyses. The choice might depend on many factors, the first being the researcher's knowledge level

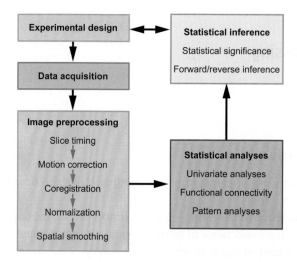

Figure 6.1 Overview of the major steps in the data analysis of an fMRI experiment. These steps include image processing, statistical analyses, and statistical inference. The two prior steps in the experimental process, experimental design and data acquisition, are also included, because valid statistical inference depends heavily on a proper experimental design – hence the bidirectional arrow on top.

and flexibility. The required flexibility typically increases the more the researcher knows. An inexperienced researcher might prefer a "click-this-or-that-button-for-option-1-or-2" package that can do everything from image processing to performing heavy statistical analyses, all in an effort to keep complexity and flexibility to a minimum. In contrast, an expert might be perfectly happily with a large collection of separate tools and functions from which to build a processing pipeline suited for the needs at hand. A second factor is a potential preference for operating system, which can be the choice of an individual researcher or of the university environment. Possible options are Microsoft Windows, Macintosh/Apple, and Linux. The most important factor is probably the researcher's background, such as the labs in which they have been trained, and the software being used by other nearby researchers.

Given the introductory nature of this book, we primarily discuss packages that are very useful for beginners, while at the same time allowing enough functionality and flexibility for expert users. Statistical Parametric Mapping (SPM) software is actually a toolbox running under MATLAB, a numerical package. SPM is free, but MATLAB is not. The package has several positive points. First, SPM allows for quite a lot of flexibility, while also having an intuitive user interface. Second, SPM runs under Microsoft Windows as well as under Mac and Linux. Third, MATLAB is used for many other purposes in many labs, including stimulus presentation, standard inferential statistics, and even creating figures, so students can get a lot out of using (and paying for) this one common software environment. Fourth, there are a large number of toolboxes available to implement a wide range of advanced analysis methods within the SPM environment.

Box 6.1 Preprocessing Step 0: Quality Control

Quality control should be a constant point of attention: during scanning, when copying data, and before starting the actual preprocessing. During later steps of the processing, appropriate checks should be done to make sure that everything has gone as planned. Many parts of the data analysis can be automated by scripts so that several steps run successively without the need of human intervention. Automatization is very efficient, but it results in a greater distance between the human experimenter and the data. For that reason, automatization should be used with care and can never fully replace human quality control.

As a starter, it is better to cut the analysis into smaller pieces and run it step by step. This is a good advice when you are a newcomer who is learning how to analyze imaging data, but also when you are the world's expert who is setting up a new innovative procedure. Automatization at a later stage is perfectly fine but should be followed up by systematic checks of the most critical points in the analysis stream to make sure that everything has been implemented as intended. These checks require some time, but detecting problems early avoids much larger time losses later on.

General problems with the images might already be detected during scanning itself. Box Figure 6.1 shows a few of the problems that might occur in (f)MRI. The physical mechanisms that lead to such artifacts were introduced in Chapter 2. However, it is not because the images look perfect during scanning that they will still remain so

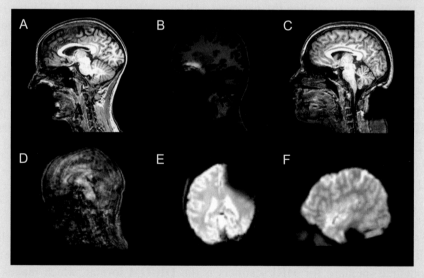

Box Figure 6.1 Obvious artifacts in MRI images. (A) Signal dropout in the mouth region due to dental wire. (B) Signal dropout in mouth region and artifact in frontal cortex due to dental implants. (C) Signal dropout due to hairclip. (D) T1-weighted image corrupted by subject motion.
(E) T2*-weighted image with signal dropout due to hairclip. (F) T2*-weighted image with signal dropout around the ear canals. In contrast to all other shown artifacts, this last artifact is always present in a T2*-weighted image.

when you start preprocessing. After scanning, the image files have to be copied and transferred to the server or workstation on which the analysis will be performed. It is good practice to check these files at their new location prior to starting the preprocessing. You can check the file names, file size (all runs of equal length should have data files of an equal size), and the number of files. You can open a subset of the files and inspect some time points to make sure that the data look as they should. These detailed suggestions are just a few illustrations of the strict and neurotic mindset that you need when working with imaging data.

Other free packages with a large user bases include the FMRIB Software Library (FSL) and the Analysis of Functional NeuroImages (AFNI) software. For those who are familiar with the increasingly popular Python programming language, there are additional options such as NiPy. These packages run most naturally under Linux, which is also available on Windows using a virtual machine.

These packages include not only the tools to analyze functional data from pre-processing to statistical analyses, but also features for the analysis of anatomical data, including surface-based analyses, and for data visualization. Some packages are more specifically focused on these aspects, such as FreeSurfer. Basic functionality for image visualization, as well as more advanced tools, can also be found on the nitrc.org webpage (including the packages MRIcro, MRIcroGL, and MRIcron).

Finally, there is a comprehensive commercial software package, BrainVoyager. It is user-friendly and comprehensive, but relatively expensive and less flexible in its use compared with the free packages.

For a relatively inexperienced user, it is advisable to opt for a software package that is used by one's closest colleagues. All software packages have email lists for discussion and problem solving, which can be helpful, but they can be a poor substitute for an experienced colleague who can help you out when needed. There is a Dutch saying that a good neighbor is more useful than a faraway friend, and this also applies to brain imagers.

6.2 Properties of the Images

The image files contain information about the image signal values as well as additional "header" information, such as some of the imaging parameters. A longtime standard for MRI scanners is the **DICOM** format, which makes the data structure relatively unintuitive because each slice corresponds to a separate file. For that reason, this format is typically converted to a different format. There was for a long time a lack of a real standard for the data format used for analyses. Different scanner companies used different output formats (such as PAR/REC by Philips), and many of the software packages had different native formats (e.g., img/hdr for SPM). Often, therefore, the data analysis had to begin with converting the images from one format to another. Software packages such as MRIcron included elaborate conversion tools.

During the past decade, a new standard emerged, **NIfTI** (file extension .nii). In NIfTI, there is only one file, because the header information is integrated with the data, and this is done per run. For functional imaging, the data in this file have four dimensions: three spatial – X (left-right), Y (posterior-anterior), and Z (inferior-superior) – and one temporal dimension.

The NIfTI format is also meant to solve long-term confusion about the direction of the X-dimension, which is the left-right orientation. For the other two spatial dimensions, it is easy to check the direction of the dimension in the images. However, brains are relatively symmetric on the left-right dimension, and the images cannot unambiguously inform us about what is left and what is right. Older image formats did not contain this information directly. Adding to the confusion, there were different conventions in different scientific disciplines. Neurologists prefer the arguably most logical approach to put left on the left and right on the right (neurological convention). Radiologists do the opposite, putting left on the right and right on the left (radiological convention), a convention dating from the period when radiologists worked with printed films.

The NIfTI format, when used properly, conveys the information about which direction is which. Nevertheless, to be absolutely sure, most MRI centers and laboratories explicitly test after major changes have occurred or been implemented (e.g., new type of scanner) whether what they think is left is indeed left. A proper way to do this is to tape a vitamin E capsule to one side of a subject's head and write down which side it is on. The capsule will be visible on the MRI images.

6.3 Preprocessing Step 1: Slice Timing

The sequences used in most blood-oxygenation-level dependent (BOLD) fMRI experiments acquire data slice by slice. The parameter settings of the sequence determine the exact timing of the slices and the order in which slices are acquired. Typical orders are descending, ascending, and interleaved (see Chapter 2).

The differences in timing can go up to almost the full duration of the repetition time (TR). The temporal resolution of BOLD fMRI is low, but still a time difference of 2–3 seconds might matter. Suppose that we take the start of a TR as the reference time zero, and a stimulus is presented at this time. In a slice that is acquired near time zero, we expect the peak of the hemodynamic response to occur about 6 seconds later. However, in a sequence with TR = 3 s there might be a slice that is acquired almost 3 seconds later. In that last slice, we expect the peak of the hemodynamic response to already occur 3 seconds after the acquisition of the slice, which is one sample time point earlier.

In this preprocessing step, we compensate for such differences in slice timing. In the example above, we could already get close to a full compensation by shifting the measured BOLD signal for the last slice with one time point. Thus, the signal for time point t is given to time point t - 1. Through this approach, the difference between the first and the last slice would be minimized. However, there are many different slices, and their timing evenly spans the full time interval between the first and the last slice. For this reason, slice timing correction involves more than just shifting time points, instead we need to interpolate the values between time points. Take, as an example, the slice that has been acquired in the middle of the TR. For a particular voxel the measured fMRI signal was 672 at time t - 1 and 676 at time t. We need to shift the signal by half a TR; in that case, the simplest interpolation function to determine the new value at time t - 1 is by taking the average between 672 and 676. Algorithms for correcting slice timing allow a choice between several interpolation functions.

In contrast to most other preprocessing steps, it is not unusual for fMRI analysis pipelines to omit the step of slice timing. Its benefits might in some experiments be minimal, for example, when the TR is very short and when using block designs (resulting in predictors that are more smoothed in time). In such cases, its benefits might not weigh as heavily as the possible negative effect that the interpolation would slightly increase the noise in the data.

6.4 Preprocessing Step 2: Motion Correction

Apart from fNIRS, in which the position of the sensors relative to the brain is constant, the head might move relative to the reference frame used during scanning. For example, an MRI operator decides at the start of the scan session which volume will be imaged and how the slices will be positioned. However, there are several reasons why *the exact position of the anatomy in this volume will vary from time point to time point.*

First, participants will move in the scanner. In a close to perfect participant, this movement might be very minimal, only about one-tenth of a millimeter. In such a case, running through the images as in a movie might not show any gross movements and you might only see changes due to physiological processes such as heart beat (flicker in large blood vessels). In other participants, the degree of motion could be relatively large. There are fast, abrupt movements, as well as slower changes, on the order of several millimeters. There are several ways to minimize the amount of motion. One of them is physical restraint of the participants. Today, most researchers work with putting padding and straps to restrain the head while still preserving comfort. Previously, it was more common to go for more invasive means of restraint such as a bite bar with a custom-made (for each participant) dental form. Another way to restrict motion is to instruct participants by stressing the need to remain still and giving feedback about their performance ("I noticed a few small movements in the previous scan; could you please try to avoid this as much as possible?").

A second source of changes in anatomical position are instabilities in the hardware of the scanner. For example, if a pulse sequence pushes the limits of the

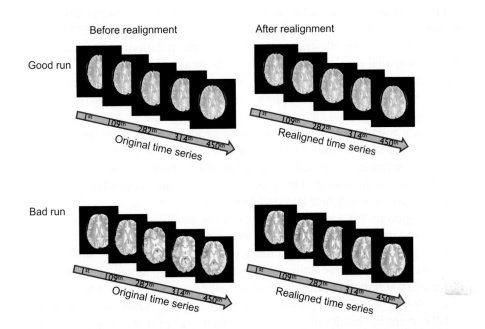

Before realignment   After realignment

Good run

1st 109th 282th 314th 450th
Original time series

1st 109th 282th 314th 450th
Realigned time series

Bad run

1st 109th 282th 314th 450th
Original time series

1st 109th 282th 314th 450th
Realigned time series

Figure 6.2 Example images before and after motion correction of a time series with little subject motion ("good run") and a time series with large amounts of motion ("bad run"). Motion correction was performed with the SPM toolbox.

hardware, then some of the gradient coils might increase slightly in temperature. This would change the magnetic field gradient induced and could shift the images slightly and very gradually during a run of continuous data acquisition.

It is impossible to completely avoid motion issues. For that reason, motion correction is always needed. Figure 6.2 shows images from a run with relatively small amounts of motion (top row), and another run with an amount of motion that is problematic. In most software packages, motion correction is accomplished by applying a **rigid transformation** to the images. A rigid transformation is a combination of three orthogonal translation directions and three orthogonal rotation directions. In the mathematical formulae that implement the motion correction, these six parameters are combined into a transformation matrix. First, the transformation matrix has to be *estimated*. One image is selected as the reference that is not transformed; sometimes the average of all untransformed images is taken as the reference. Then the transformation matrix is calculated for each image so that the distance with the reference image is minimized. Software packages often have multiple options for minimizing the cost function (mutual information, least squares, etc.).

Once the transformation parameters have been estimated, they have to be applied to the original images to obtain a transformed or resliced image (Fig. 6.3 on the right). **Reslicing** requires the choice of an interpolation function. As an example, if a set of voxels has values [2 4 5 3 2, ...] and they have to be shifted by one-third of a voxel, then the new values depend on the interpolation function. A simple linear interpolation would give as new values [2.67 4.33 4.33 2.67, ...]. This example immediately illustrates a problem of interpolation: It introduces a certain degree of spatial smoothing by flattening the peak values. The peak of 5 has been reduced in the interpolated values. Often researchers use more complex functions to avoid this problem, such as spline interpolation. These methods require more computing time.

This is a good time to note that software packages often allow the researcher not to reslice the images after each preprocessing step, but to combine all the transformation matrices computed in the different preprocessing steps and then do the reslicing in one final step. This procedure avoids the accumulation of noise and rounding errors across multiple reslicing steps.

It is important for a researcher to check the motion-correction parameters. The three translation parameters from the two example runs in Figure 6.2 are displayed in Figure 6.3. The top row illustrates a relatively stable run with little motion, the bottom row a very unstable run. With voxels of only 2–3 mm in size, the second case requires a translation of the data by more than one voxel in some time points. Such a large amount of motion is particularly problematic if it is relatively abrupt, because it will corrupt the history of excitation of voxels and probably also the images if the motion occurs during the acquisition of a volume. One way to summarize the amount of rapid motion is by computing how much the translation of each time point differs relative to the translation in the previous time point by calculating the Euclidean distance across the three translation parameters (Fig. 6.3, right). This

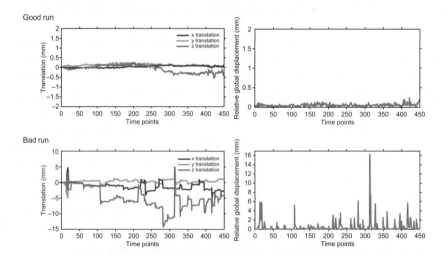

Figure 6.3 Motion-correction parameters in the case of small (top row) and large (bottom row) amounts of subject motion. The data represent the same two time series shown in Figure 6.2. The graphs on the left show the three translation parameters, the graphs on the right show the global displacement (Euclidean distance) in each time point relative to the previous time point.

"relative translation" index shows that all relative translations remain within the limit of one voxel in the top row but not in the second row.

There are several good arguments for not using data that require extensive motion correction. First, some movements cannot be corrected for. A subject's movement will happen at a relatively random time with respect to the pulse sequence. When a subject has moved abruptly in the middle of the acquisition of a volume, then all the slices acquired after the movement are shifted compared with the slices acquired earlier. For example, with an interleaved slice order, all odd slices might be shifted compared with the even slices. Motion-correction methods through rigid transformations cannot solve such a shift within the volume.

Second, the movement might mess up the image quality because of instabilities in the fMRI signal. The movement could transiently alter the magnetic field and its inhomogeneities, as well as the history of excitation that nuclei have experienced. Such instabilities might take many seconds to stabilize again, much longer than the actual movement.

Third, it would be a problem if the amount or type of motion were confounded with the occurrence of specific conditions in the experimental paradigm. For example, in an experiment where one condition requires participants to make a complex motor response and another condition does not, it is possible that the complex motor response would be associated with a small change in head position. In that case, it would be hard to dissociate neural activity from motion artifacts. The resulting "brain activity" might look suspiciously like what would be expected if the images in one condition were translated and/or rotated compared with another condition, for example, with positive activity at the outer edge of one side of the brain combined with negative activity at the opposite outer edge.

6.5 Preprocessing Step 3: Coregistration

Even when researchers are interested in functional imaging, they also perform a structural, anatomical scan. They do so for several reasons. First, typically the functional images are not sufficient to support a good localization of the measured effects, because they have a relatively poor spatial resolution. Second, the constraints on the timing for data acquisition often force researchers to scan an incomplete volume, which, combined with the poor spatial resolution, might not give a good indication of functional localization.

The coregistration step brings different image modalities, such as a functional scan and an anatomical volume, into one and the same spatial coordinate frame. We looked at image alignment earlier when discussing motion correction, but the problem is more complicated for coregistration because the images represent different modalities. For the most part, the matrix size is different, with a larger field of view and a higher resolution in anatomical scans. The different modalities might each exhibit specific geometric distortions of the images. For MRI, the dependence on different contrast parameters (e.g., T1 and T2 weighting for, respectively,

Anatomy:

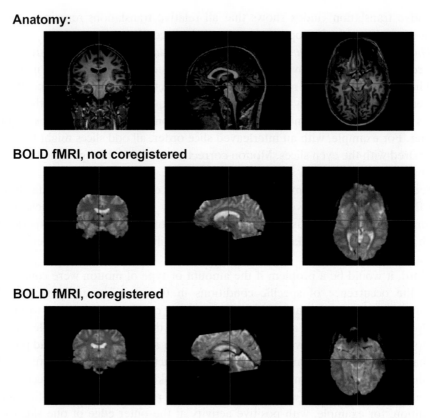

BOLD fMRI, not coregistered

BOLD fMRI, coregistered

Figure 6.4 Example of the input images for coregistration between a T1-weighted anatomical scan (*top row*) and T2*-weighted functional MRI scan (*middle row*). The latter is also shown after coregistration (*bottom row*). Coregistration was performed with the SPM toolbox.

structural and functional imaging), might mean that what is whiter in one image would in fact be darker in another image. There are also clear differences between a PET scan and a structural MRI. For all those reasons, neither calculating a simple cost function, such as a distance or correlation metric between the two volumes, nor a simple rigid transformation to align the two modalities would be sufficient. Coregistration methods use complex cost functions such as mutual information and possibly also transformations with more degrees of freedom than a simple rigid transformation.

Figure 6.4 illustrates typical input data for coregistration, with a structural MRI image on top and a functional MRI volume below. In this case, a translation of one of the two images along the vertical (Z) direction along with a slight anterior-posterior shift and a small rotation are necessary to coregister the two images.

The researcher has to decide which image is to be the reference to remain unchanged and which image is to be transformed. Both choices have their followers. It is most natural to take the anatomical image as the reference, because it contains the most spatial information and has the largest field of view. However, this will result in one extra transformation being applied to the functional images, and for that reason it is not uncommon to use the functional images as reference. There are many functional images in one dataset, primarily the one used for coregistration is the same image that was taken as reference for motion correction, after which the spatial transformation is applied to all other images.

6.6 Preprocessing Step 4: Normalization

Normalization refers to the procedure used to bring all the data from the different subjects into one common spatial reference space. Most of the time, the normalization parameters are calculated using structural images, although normalization might also be relatively successful with functional images of high enough resolution and field of view. Given this reliance on structural images, we introduced the different approaches to spatial normalization in Section 3.1.2. There, the reader learned about important concepts such as volume- and surface-based normalization, segmentation, and population templates and atlases.

Here we describe normalization as a step within a standard analysis stream prior to the actual statistical processing. In many cases, researchers wish to combine data across participants and use this combination explicitly in their analyses. Before doing so, it is necessary to normalize the data of each individual to a template reference frame. As a result, the statistical analyses of functional effects are based on normalized data. Note that normalization entails more than a simple rigid transformation as was done for motion correction, because neuroanatomy differs among people. However, researchers can also choose to perform statistical analyses on non-normalized functional data that remain in the native subject space. After statistical analysis, researchers can then opt to normalize the data or not. As long as spatial coordinates do not need to be combined across participants (single-subject analyses), a study can be completed without using any normalization.

Once the normalization parameters have been estimated, they can be applied to the anatomical image (a new image is resliced/written) as well as to all functional images that have been coregistered with this anatomical image. This step should be followed by a visual inspection of the normalized anatomy together with the template and (a subset of) the normalized functional images to assure that normalization has been successful. Again, investing a few minutes in this quality control can save many hours of wasted time later on.

6.7 Preprocessing Step 5: Spatial Smoothing

As a last step in the preprocessing of fMRI images, researchers often resort to spatial smoothing. This is a way of blurring the images, which in image processing

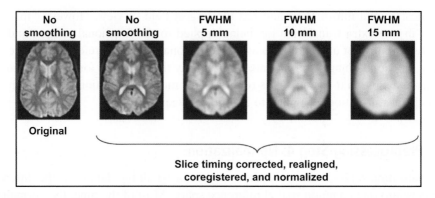

Figure 6.5 Functional MRI images at various levels of smoothing. Spatial smoothing was performed with the SPM toolbox.

terminology corresponds to a low-pass filtering of the images. Modulations at high spatial frequencies (fine details) are attenuated at the benefit of contrast at lower spatial frequencies. There are multiple filtering kernels in use. By far the most common is a **Gaussian filter**. The amount of filtering by a Gaussian kernel is summarized by the width of this function, in which its height is at half of its maximum, the so-called **full width at half maximum (FWHM)**. Figure 6.5 illustrates the effect of spatial smoothing on fMRI images.

Why would researchers want to reduce the higher spatial frequencies in their signals? Researchers would be expected to try to optimize the spatial resolution of their data, and spatial smoothing seems to go against this goal. To explain the use of spatial smoothing, we have to understand that spatial resolution is a function not only of the highest spatial frequency that we can measure. In addition to voxel size, spatial resolution is also limited by the signal-to-noise ratio at different spatial frequencies. If the higher spatial frequencies chiefly represent noise and very little signal, then the researcher is better off removing these higher spatial frequencies.

With fMRI images, we know the signal is spatially smoothed anyway, because we measure hemodynamic correlates of neural activity. At the same time, fMRI images contain quite a lot of noise at the individual voxel level, which is a high spatial frequency relative to the spatial resolution of the image. As a consequence, the overall signal-to-noise ratio can be improved by spatial smoothing, which strengthens the lower spatial frequencies that represent the signal at the expense of the higher spatial frequencies that are primarily dominated by noise (Friston et al., 1995). This is the advice of the **Matched Filter Theorem**: It is best to filter the data with a filter kernel that has the same amplitude spectrum as the signal that the researcher wants to measure among noise with a different amplitude spectrum.

Following these arguments, many fMRI studies include a level of *smoothing by about twice the voxel size*. Studies that aim to combine data across subjects tend to

Box 6.2 External Quality Control through Transparency and Reproducibility

Science in general is under increased scrutiny because of reports of questionable research practices and a relatively low rate of reproducibility. This is particularly true for fields in which statistics play a big role, effect sizes are small, and a tendency exists to have many different research groups investigating many different hypotheses. The targeted domains include biomedical and behavioral sciences, and human brain imaging is right in the middle. Poldrack and colleagues (2017) have illustrated a number of problems specific to research with fMRI, and they have proposed solutions that have relevance for brain imaging and neuroscience in general. First, on average human neuroimaging studies lack sufficient statistical power, with a number of subjects that is too low given the typical effect size that is observed and to be expected. Insufficient power increases the possibility of false negatives, decreases the trustworthiness of effect size estimates in studies with positive effects, and increases the potential impact of questionable research practices. Here it is important to determine the necessary number of participants a priori, taking into account expected and meaningful effect sizes, ideally through a power analysis.

Second, there is a large degree of flexibility and possibility for exploration in the analysis of functional imaging data. The number of choices in which analyses steps to run and which parameter options to go for is enormous. Each of these choices might impact the results, and together they can have a huge influence on the final results (Carp, 2012). In the worst case, some of the choices have been influenced by knowing about the results obtained with these choices, in which case the analyses become partially circular (see further in Chapter 8). The tightest safeguard against the latter problem is a formal preregistration of the complete analysis stream and the a priori hypotheses.

Another important practice is to make methods sections as complete and transparent as possible. A fully transparent methods section, in which the research process is detailed in all its aspects (e.g., exactly how the choice for each parameter was decided; how exactly the data were looked at in each and every step of the process), would in its asymptote be very similar in informational content as in a preregistered study. However, there is probably not any non-preregistered study that reaches this asymptotic level. Such incomplete study reporting is a third major problem in the current literature.

Because of such problems, neuroimaging research is less replicable than it should be. In addition to solving the individual problems, we need solutions that target replicability directly, such as more replication efforts, more focus on meta-analytic approaches and innovative tools to do so (e.g., www.neurosynth.org; see Yarkoni et al., 2011), and more data sharing as a way to promote replicability. Data sharing also helps to increase sample size. Large databases and repositories have been constructed to which many labs have uploaded their data. Some of these initiatives are aimed at specific niches, such as databases of resting-state fMRI (see Chapter 8) in ADHD (ADHD-200) and autism (ABIDE). Another promising approach is the start of large imaging consortia that focus on the collection of standardized data of a wide variety of measures such as multiple imaging modalities and a range of behavioral tasks. Setting up such a collaboration typically also involves the development of standardized imaging and analysis protocols and making the data openly available. Example consortia include the Human Connectome Project and, specifically for Alzheimer's, the Alzheimer's Disease Neuroimaging Initiative (ADNI).

To be clear, no one claims that most neuroimaging results are bogus; in fact, many key findings have been documented over and over again. There is no need to become depressed or cynical about progress in this field. Impressive textbooks can be filled with findings that have been replicated convincingly. Nevertheless, if you take the positive findings of a randomly chosen neuroimaging paper and try to replicate them, your chance of success would likely be lower than it should be.

include an even larger smoothing level to compensate for the inter-individual differences in anatomy (Mikl et al., 2008).

Aside from these signal-processing considerations, there are also statistical arguments in favor of spatial smoothing. Some of the statistical approaches applied to imaging data, such as statistical parametric mapping, make assumptions about the data. These assumptions sound familiar to most scientists who have taken a course on parametric statistics, such as the assumption that errors are distributed according to a normal/Gaussian distribution. It has been shown that spatial smoothing with a Gaussian kernel makes it more likely that similar assumptions hold (Worsley et al., 1996), and this can be an additional argument for performing (sufficient) spatial smoothing.

Summary

- Data analysis starts with image processing, including slice timing, motion correction, coregistration, normalization, and spatial smoothing.
- During all steps, it is important to perform quality control and consider whether the appropriate parameter settings are being used.
- Each step can influence the end result, necessitating transparency about which parameters have been used and why.

Review Questions

1. Describe motion correction and explain why this step is important and how inaccuracies in this step might affect the outcome of an fMRI analysis.
2. Explain why fMRI researchers spatially smooth their data as well as the factors that might be taken into account to decide on the most appropriate level of smoothing.

3. Two researchers, Hillary and Donald, analyze the same dataset. They use exactly the same script and parameter settings for the statistical analysis, but they work independently for the image preprocessing that includes the steps of motion correction, coregistration, normalization, and smoothing (different script, different parameters). After the statistical analysis, both find one cluster of significantly activated voxels. However, Donald's cluster is larger than Hillary's, and it is shifted one centimeter to the right. Explain for each preprocessing step whether and how it might contribute to these differences.

Further Reading

Poldrack, R. A., Baker, C. I., Durnez, J., et al. (2017). Scanning the horizon: towards transparent and reproducible neuroimaging research. *Nature Reviews Neuroscience*, **18**(2), 115–126. (This article describes the actions that can be taken to increase the transparency and reproducibility of human neuroimaging research.)

Poldrack, R. A., Mumford, J. A. & Nichols, T. E. (2011). *Handbook of Functional MRI Data Analysis*. Cambridge: Cambridge University Press. (This book provides a more in-depth and very concrete explanation of the important concepts and steps involved when analyzing fMRI data.)

Some of the online resources mentioned in this chapter:

www.humanconnectomeproject.org

www.neurosynth.org

CHAPTER SEVEN

Basic Statistical Analyses

Learning Objectives

- Learning how to compile an appropriate general linear model
- Understanding the application of basic statistical tests in the context of neuroimaging research
- Understanding the need to correct for multiple comparisons and the main approaches for doing so
- Learning about the many ways in which a statistical inference might go wrong

Here we describe the core of the statistical analysis of hemodynamic imaging data. Following on the introduction in preprocessing in the previous chapter, we introduce the next two components of the analysis stream: statistical model fitting, and statistical inference.

Model fitting and inference are common to analyses of many types of data, including behavioral data, but the types of models and statistics tend to be much more complicated in the case of neuroimaging data. From this perspective, referring to it as "basic" neuroimaging statistical analysis does not do justice to the complexity of what we cover in this chapter.

7.1 Statistical Analyses: The General Linear Model

7.1.1 Simple Linear Regression

To start with a simple example, suppose you do a behavioral experiment in which you test how fast a person can react to a burst of noise. You test this reaction time 100 times over the course of 1 hour. Sometimes there is a distracting event happening outside the testing room that involves a varying number of people. You have the hypothesis that the reaction time might be prolonged by this distracting event, with reaction times becoming slower as more people are involved.

To test such a hypothesis, the researcher could quantify the relationship between the occurrence of the distracting event and the reaction time. The easiest approach would be to test for a linear relationship by computing the correlation between the occurrence of the event and number of people involved and the reaction time. A similar way to express the potential dependence of reaction time on the distracting event is to compute how much the reaction time increases for each person added to the distracting event. This gives us the formula for a simple linear regression, as follows:

$$Y = \beta_0 + X_1\beta_1 + \varepsilon$$

$$Y = [y_1 y_2 \ldots y_n]' \quad X_1 = [x_1 x_2 \ldots x_n]'$$

n = number of time points in the (in)dependent variable

In this formula, X_1 and Y are vectors (series of numbers). The superscript T signals that the vector is a column of numbers (without the superscript, the vector forms a row). The independent variable, X_1, contains the number of people at the n points of time at which the reaction time was measured (with the number being zero if no distracting event occurred). The dependent variable, Y, contains the actual reaction times measured at these time points. The other characters represent single-number parameters that capture the relationship between X_1 and Y. The constant to be added to X_1 to account for the difference in average value between the two vectors is represented by β_0. The aforementioned dependence of reaction time on the elapsed time is represented by β_1. The variation in reaction time that is not captured by the beta parameters β is represented by ε.

The same simple regression formula is used in the context of functional magnetic resonance imaging (fMRI) analyses. Now Y is the measured fMRI signal at a series of time points. The independent variable is again X_1, which could represent the presence or absence of a particular experimental condition. A simple example would be the number of visual stimuli shown on a projection screen.

7.1.2 Multiple Linear Regression

After finding that reaction time increases as a function of the number of people in the event, you think about a second variable that might influence reaction time. In some sessions, the participant has been drinking coffee before the experiment, with the amount ranging from 1 to 3 cups. You predict that reaction time will speed up linearly with the number of cups. To test the relationship between a dependent variable and multiple independent variables, we perform a multiple regression analysis.

In multiple regression, we use the same basic formula but now with multiple independent variables:

$$Y = \beta_0 + X\beta + \varepsilon$$

$$Y = [y_1 y_2 \ldots y_n]' \quad X = [X_1 X_2 \ldots X_p], \text{with } X_p = [x_{1p} x_{2p} \ldots x_{np}]'$$

$$\beta = [\beta_1 \beta_2 \ldots \beta_p]'$$

n = number of time points in the (in)dependent variable

p = number of independent variables (predictors)

Here **X** is a matrix in which each column corresponds to the values of one independent variable. All these vectors/columns together form the matrix. Each independent variable has one associated β parameter. The variation in **Y** that is not captured by all the independent variables is represented in the error term ε.

7.1.3 The General Linear Model Applied to fMRI Data

The multiple regression model as applied to fMRI data is typically referred to as the general linear model (GLM). With fMRI data, each vector has as many data points as the number of scans included. The matrix **Y** contains the fMRI signal at each time point (blood-oxygenation-level dependent [BOLD] time series). The matrix **X** contains all independent variables that the researchers want to include and is referred to as the "design matrix." This general linear model is visualized in Figure 7.1.

The independent variables in the design matrix can be classified in two groups. First, we have the experimental conditions that the researcher is interested in, the **regressors of interest**. Each regressor of interest is typically associated with one experimental condition, and there are at least as many regressors of interest as there are experimental conditions in the experiment. Second, we have other variables that we might expect to predict part of the variation in the fMRI signal, but that are not

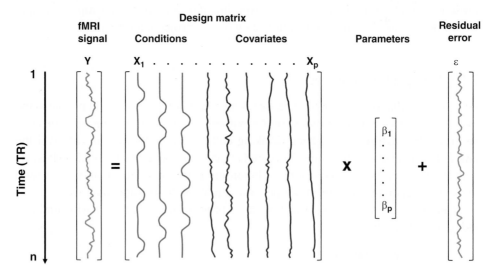

Figure 7.1 Visualization of the general linear model as applied to real fMRI data. The dependent variable Y is the signal of one random voxel in one time series of $n = 75$ time points with a repetition time (TR) of 3 seconds (s). The experimental design contains 3 conditions, which were each presented for 4 blocks of 15 s each. The six motion-correction parameters (translations and rotations) are included as covariates. As a consequence, $p = 9$.
Figure inspired by Monti, 2011

of primary interest to the researcher. These variables are referred to as **covariates** or **nuisance regressors**.

The GLM is applied to the data of individual voxels. Often a selection is made prior to implementing the model to avoid performing all the heavy computations to data of which it is clear that they are not relevant. For example, voxels that are outside the brain have no relevance. Still, the analyses might include computing hundreds of thousands of individual GLMs. This approach of analyzing each voxel separately is sometimes referred to as a univariate or voxel-wise analysis.

The actual regressors do not simply correspond to the exact timing of experimental conditions or other events but already include what we know about the measured hemodynamic signal and its dynamics through the hemodynamic response function. This knowledge is already used during the construction of the design matrix by convolving the original regressor that indicates the time of occurrence of particular events with the hemodynamic response function. As a consequence of this **convolution with the hemodynamic response function** (HRF), even when the original regressor was a series of 0 (condition not present) and 1 (condition presented), the actual regressor in the design matrix would be a continuous variable with the peak occurring about 6 seconds after the occurrence of each 1.

The convolution with the default HRF is a standard approach, and the majority of research studies would not go further than this. However, more complex approaches exist. Typically, these approaches provide more than one regressor per condition, resulting in a model that is more complex and uses more degrees of freedom. This extended model allows more flexibility to account for differences in the timing and the shape of the HRF between different brain regions. One example is the addition of the time derivative of the convolved regressor.

For more complex approaches, the need to include additional variables is a potential disadvantage. The same is true for the nuisance regressors. They are helpful only if they explain at least some variation in the dependent variable. All variation that is predicted by the design matrix is subtracted from the remaining error term. The size of this error term is important, because it has an important role later on to determine significance of effects (the betas in the GLM). The smaller the error term, the easier a beta of a particular size might become significant. Possible candidates to be included as nuisance regressors include movement of the subject as determined through the motion-correction preprocessing step, the reaction time of behavioral responses, eye movement data, and physiological parameters such as heart rate and respiration.

7.1.4 Data Cleaning prior to Applying the GLM

Prior to applying a GLM, we can also remove noise from the signal before the GLM model is applied. Of course, this will be done only for factors that are of absolutely no interest to the researcher. Most software packages include a **high-pass filtering** step in which very slow drifts in the signal are filtered out. In many experiments, it can be decided a priori that these very low frequencies can only contain noise. The most optimal cutoff value for the filter depends on the experimental design.

Let us consider a specific design as an example. The design contains a continuous alternation of two experimental conditions A and B and a resting baseline R, with an order A R B R A R B R, with each block taking about 15 seconds. In this design, we know that a signal variation with a frequency slower than 1 cycle per 2 minutes would not be related to our experimental manipulations, as conditions A and B follow each other much more rapidly (we already have a second occurrence of A 1 minute after the first). The extent to which such a slow temporal frequency could be related to our experimental manipulations would be very different in a design with 8 stimulus conditions and the same resting baseline. Because of the high number of conditions, it might take several minutes to have a repetition of a particular condition. Thus, in this second design we would prefer to be more conservative when deciding to filter away low temporal frequencies.

Another data operation that is often applied prior to the formal GLM involves a procedure to "whiten" the data. This procedure removes dependencies between data points that should not be there according to the statistical tests that will be applied to the data in a later step. The notion that statistical tests make assumptions should be familiar to most readers. For example, a simple t-test assumes that data points have a normal distribution and that each data point is independent from other data points (no dependencies). We know that fMRI data contain a lot of dependencies, one being a dependency or **temporal autocorrelation** among successive data points. This autocorrelation is reduced by removing such dependencies before applying the GLM.

7.1.5 The Efficiency of a Design and Correlation between Predictors

After fitting the GLM model to the fMRI signal in a particular voxel, we obtain an estimate for each column in the design matrix. These estimates are often referred to as beta values (cf. the notation of β in Section 7.1.2). The beta values tell us how much and in which direction the independent variable predicts changes in the fMRI signal. For example, a large positive beta for column 5 means that a small increase in independent variable 5 is related to a relatively large increase in the fMRI signal.

In a simple linear regression, there is a straightforward relationship between this beta and the correlation between the independent and the dependent variable. In a multiple linear regression, we also have to consider the correlations among the different regressors. Here we encounter the concept of a **partial correlation**, which is the correlation that remains between a particular regressor and the fMRI signal after taking into account the correlations with other regressors. Or, stated otherwise, the partial correlation captures the part of the fMRI signal that can only be explained by this particular regressor and not by other regressors. The beta value in a multiple linear regression is related to this partial correlation.

Problems emerge when regressors are highly correlated. In such a case, it becomes unclear which of the correlated regressors explains the fMRI signal. As a consequence, a particular regressor would explain very little variation in the fMRI signal that cannot be explained by other predictors. This is referred to as a low **efficiency**. In this context, high efficiency means that the variation predicted by a particular regressor cannot be explained by other regressors. Low efficiency results in other problems, too. In particular, the beta estimates and thus the model fitting becomes unstable, in the sense that small changes in the data can give rise to large changes in the estimated betas. For these reasons, it is preferred to have a design matrix with high efficiency, with small or no dependencies/correlations between the columns. Part of this is out of the control of the researcher, given that some of the columns in the design matrix might depend on unpredictable factors such as a subject's performance or head motion. However, the situation is different for the regressors of interests that are related to the timing of the different experimental conditions. The experimenter decides on this timing and thus can and should avoid correlations between the resulting regressors as much as possible. This can be achieved through a careful counterbalancing of condition order and timing. For example, if in an event-related design condition B would always follow condition A with a short and fixed time interval of less than 6 seconds, then the regressors for these two conditions would be highly correlated after convolution with the HRF (Poldrack et al., 2011).

Figure 7.2 illustrates a design matrix of a simple experiment in a commonly used graphical format. It represents a block design with three conditions presented in blocks of 15 seconds. The matrix at the left shows the actual design matrix. There

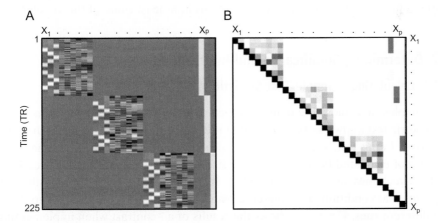

Figure 7.2 Visualization of the design of a block-design fMRI experiment. (A) The design matrix with the predictors as columns and time points as rows. The color scale from black to white indicates low to high values, respectively. (B) Matrix with correlations between the predictors in the design matrix. The color scale from white to black indicates low to high values, respectively. Images obtained through SPM12 software.

are three continuous time series, or "runs." In each run, each condition is presented 4 times/blocks, as visible from the design matrix in which the columns corresponding to the block onsets contain four white squares. Each run starts with a period of no stimulation (no white square in the first few time points in any of the runs). For each run, the first three columns represent the three stimulus conditions, which are the regressors of interest. The other six columns per run show the nuisance regressors, in this case the motion-correction parameters obtained through the alignment of the functional images during preprocessing. The last three columns in the design matrix model potential differences in fMRI signal between runs.

The right triangular matrix represents the absolute value of correlations between the columns from the design matrix (white = no correlation). As high efficiency can only be obtained with independent regressors, we would hope to see no or at most small correlations between columns. Of course, there are no correlations between regressors that refer to different runs. In addition, the experimenter did a good job avoiding correlations among the three regressors of interest. In individual runs there are some correlations with the nuisance regressors, but across runs there seems to be little systematicity in these correlations. If the same experimental condition would always be highly correlated with a particular motion-correction parameter, then this could have a detrimental effect on the researcher's ability to find and interpret any changes in the fMRI signal related to this experimental condition.

We mentioned before that the fitting of the GLM model per voxel provides us with a beta value per column in the design matrix per voxel. These beta values can be shown as a brain map, as is illustrated in Figure 7.3 for the first two columns in the design from Figure 7.2. Now the question comes up: Is the fMRI signal significantly different between these two conditions in at least some of the voxels?

7.2 Determining Significance and Interpreting It

7.2.1 Calculating a Simple Test Statistic: A *t*-Contrast

The simplest and most frequent approach to determine significance is to apply a parametric test known as the (student's) *t*-test. This test is applied for each individual voxel. In this test, a test statistic *t* is calculated that is proportional to the ratio of the size of estimated beta values to the size of the error term in that voxel. Often, multiple columns in the design matrix are combined if they refer to the same experimental condition, as is the case when a particular condition appeared in all the different runs. Figure 7.4 shows the results of a *t*-contrast when implementing a similar design as in Figure 7.2 comparing condition 3 (images of faces) with condition 1 (object images). The contrast terms for the different columns in the design matrix are shown on the right: +1 for each column with a regressor related to the occurrence of face images and -1 for each column related to object images. The brain maps on the left are shown in three formats, including a format that is a

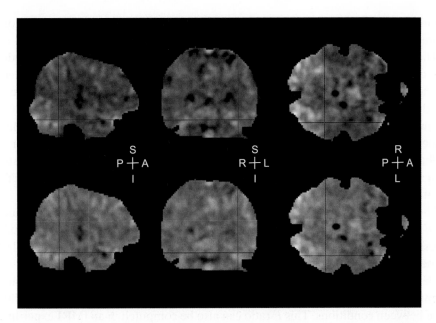

Figure 7.3 The beta values associated with the two first predictors of the design matrix in Figure 7.2 in one example participant. White indicates a high beta value. The outline of the gray area shows that in this case only part of the brain was imaged. A: anterior, P: posterior, R: right, L: left, S: superior, I: inferior.

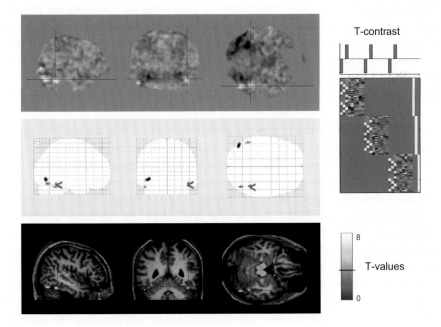

Figure 7.4 Visualization of the voxels with a high *t*-value in a simple *t*-contrast of visually presented faces minus object images. Brain maps represent the unthresholded *t*-maps (*top row*) and thresholded *t*-maps on glass brains (*middle row*) and on anatomical scans (*bottom row*). The threshold was put at a *t*-value of 3.79, corresponding to an uncorrected *p*-value of 0.0001, with cluster extent 20. Visualization performed with the SPM toolbox.

default in the SPM software and known as "glass brains." The gray level of voxels represents the calculated t-value in each voxel.

The distribution of t-values is well known and depends on the degrees of freedom. The degrees of freedom are related to the number of independent time points across all runs with the number of regressors subtracted. The higher the degrees of freedom, the narrower the distribution of t-values and the rarer it becomes to find t-values larger than a particular value if there is no effect. As such, each t-value is associated with a probability of occurrence. The higher the t-value, the lower this probability. When researchers say that a particular observed value of a test statistic is significant, they do this because the associated probability is very low, lower than a criterion value.

The t-maps shown in Figure 7.4 show only the t-values above a criterion value of 3.79, which is associated with a probability of a type-I error of $p = 0.0001$. Such a thresholding is standard practice in graphics in neuroimaging papers, although the chosen criterion probability might vary widely between studies.

Here we will introduce all concepts in the context of a simple parametric t-contrast. An alternative test includes an F-ratio to search for a significant difference between conditions. This F-ratio can also be computed in an fMRI experiment, and this is done in much the same way as computing a t-contrast. While a t-contrast signals not only the size of a difference between conditions but also the direction of this difference (only positive t-values are shown in the t-maps in Fig. 7.4), an F-ratio indicates only that there is an effect without providing any information about the direction of the effect. More complicated designs are also possible with more than two conditions, such as analysis of variance (ANOVA) with multiple levels of one factor (possibly with a parametric manipulation) and multifactorial designs (Friston et al., 1994).

Finally, while we restrict our discussion here to the use of parametric tests, these tests suffer from the same limitations as in other applications of statistics. Most researchers choose parametric hypothesis testing because it is the easiest approach to implement and they are most familiar with it, but parametric statistics make many assumptions that are often violated. The extent to which these violations will have a meaningful impact on the conclusions of a paper will vary case by case. For sure, if results are borderline significant, then they may very well fall at the other side (no longer being significant) with a test that is not subject to the same assumptions. Nonparametric permutation statistics are more computationally intensive, but would allow for more valid statistical inference (for a primer, see Nichols and Holmes, 2002). Furthermore, the dominant statistical approach of so-called null hypothesis significance testing (NHST) is also subject to criticism. Instead of trying to show that results are significant (meaning: very unlikely to appear under the null hypothesis), it is argued it is more fruitful to estimate and compare the amount of evidence in favor of both the null hypothesis and its alternative(s). This brings us into the territory of Bayesian statistics (Woolrich et al., 2009), which is a very valuable alternative for parametric tests.

7.2.2 Correction for Multiple Comparisons, or How to Avoid Brain Activity in Dead Salmon

Until this point, we have treated each voxel as a separate experiment: A GLM model was fitted per voxel, and the probability of differences between conditions was determined using a t-contrast calculated per voxel. However, it is problematic to stop at this point and claim to have found a significant result because some voxels are associated with a t-value beyond a criterion value, as used in Figure 7.4. Initially, the claim that the analysis is problematic might seem odd given that the criterion value used was associated with a probability of $p = 0.0001$. In many fields, researchers are happy with a p-value of 0.05 or 0.01, so why is 0.0001 not enough?

A thought experiment makes the issue clear. Let us first start with what these p-values mean. The p-value that we calculate reflects the probability with which we would make a statistical error known as a type-I error: making the claim that an effect is present while it is actually not there. For that we determine what the probability is to observe a certain t-value if the data would contain no effect. If this probability is very low, then we know that it is unlikely that there would be no effect. With a p-value of 0.0001, we know that we can expect to make an error of claiming a nonexistent effect in 1 out of 10 000 independent tests on data that have no effect in reality. Thus, if we run one GLM and use a criterion value associated with $p = 0.0001$, then the probability of making a type-I error is only 1 out of 10 000. However, we are not just running one GLM; instead, we are running a GLM for each voxel. If a dataset contains 200 000 voxels, then we would be fitting 200 000 GLMs. In each case, we have a probability of 0.0001 to make a type-I error (if there would be no effect in any of these voxels), so it would not be surprising to find 0.0001 x 200 000 = 20 voxels in which we would claim to have found an effect even though there would be none.

This issue is known in statistics as the **multiple comparisons problem**. If we run multiple tests, and we want to control the overall probability of making a type-I error, then we need to correct for the number of comparisons performed. Applying this reasoning to fMRI, we infer that the number of comparisons we need to correct for is the same as the number of voxels in the dataset.

Functional MRI researchers have been aware of this problem since the initial development of fMRI methodology. What would happen if we forgot about this, just for the sake of the argument? The consequences are shown most famously by Bennett and colleagues (Bennett, Miller and Wolford, 2009; Bennett, Wolford and Miller, 2009). They used a setup in which we can be quite sure that the experimental manipulation would not be associated with changes in the fMRI signal. They put a dead (!) salmon in an MRI scanner while showing it pictures with positive or negative emotional content. We do not expect any salmon to react to the emotional content of pictures, let alone a dead salmon. Thus, the signal measured in the salmon is sure to contain no systematic variations related to picture content. Still, the authors fitted a GLM to the data of each voxel in the salmon's brain and looked

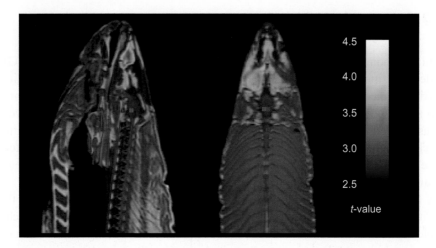

Figure 7.5 Spurious brain activity in a dead salmon related to the emotional content of pictures shown to it. This finding was awarded the IgNobel Prize in 2012. The tongue-in-cheek IgNobel Prize is not to be confused with the actual Nobel Prize.
Figure reproduced with permission from Bennett, Miller and Wolford, 2009

at how many voxels crossed a threshold associated with a low probability such as 0.001. Several voxels did (Fig. 7.5). Thus, using this approach, which includes no correction for multiple comparisons, we can seemingly "find" brain activity in a dead salmon.

Functional MRI researchers agree that a correction for multiple comparisons needs to be done and almost all papers in the literature perform such a correction. Multiple approaches exist, each with its own benefits and downsides, and each with its own believers and nonbelievers. Different software packages and subcommunities in the field have different defaults for performing this correction. We will describe three very important approaches below.

The first approach is based on a method known in statistics as a Bonferroni correction. In its simplest form, it involves dividing the desired probability for making a type-I error, such as 0.05, by the number of comparisons made—in our fMRI case, the number of voxels in a dataset. With 200 000 voxels, the new threshold would be 0.05/200 000, so 0.00000025.

However, this implementation of the Bonferroni is too conservative, because we do not necessarily need to correct for the total number of tests. Instead, we need to correct for the number of *independent* tests. In fMRI data, nearby voxels do not contain a fully independent signal. Instead, the signal in nearby voxels is correlated for several reasons: joined signal and noise during data acquisition and further correlations introduced during preprocessing (most explicitly in the step of spatial smoothing). When the data show such correlations among voxels, the true number of sources of variation is less than the number of voxels. This principle is central to many data-reduction techniques, such as factor analysis (FA) and principal component analysis (PCA). All these techniques capitalize on redundancies in data to find a small number of factors/components that can capture the shared variation in the data. The higher the redundancy and correlations among different variables in the data, the smaller the number of factors/components will be. The challenge for an appropriate level of Bonferroni correction in the context of fMRI is to estimate the number of sources of variation underlying the fMRI signal and correct for this number. With 200 000 voxels, this number is going to be much smaller than 200 000. The true number depends on the smoothness of the data, which is very much related to the amount of correlation between nearby voxels: the higher the smoothness, the higher the correlation and the smaller the number with which we need to correct. The researchers who developed the SPM software package proposed a theoretical framework known as random field theory as a principled approach to estimate the amount of correction needed, given the estimated smoothness of the fMRI dataset at hand (Friston et al., 1995). With this approach to Bonferroni correction, we control for the type-I error at the "family" level of all relevant voxels, and as such the resulting error is known as **family-wise error (FWE) correction**. If we have applied the FWE correction with a corrected $p = 0.05$, then the probability of finding one or more voxels with a lower p-value is 0.05 if the null hypothesis of no effect is true.

A second well-known approach to correct for multiple comparisons is the control of **false discovery rate (FDR)** (Genovese et al., 2002). In this approach, we control the proportion of incorrectly rejected null hypotheses based on the observed distribution of uncorrected p-values. If we apply the FDR correction with a corrected $p = 0.05$, then 1 out of 20 activated voxels/regions is a false positive. Mathematical analyses and simulations show that the FDR approach is less conservative than the FWE approach when effects are present (in that case, the null hypothesis is false). As such, it is more sensitive to existing differences. With random data in which no effects are present, the two approaches provide very similar levels of correction, although this might depend on the smoothness of the data.

Family-wise error and FDR are methods for voxel-wise correction for multiple comparisons. A third approach combines an uncorrected threshold at the voxel level with a further threshold incorporating cluster size: the number of adjacent voxels that cross the uncorrected threshold. The smoothness of fMRI data makes it more likely that nearby voxels might cross the threshold of significance together, but it might only be a few voxels if the apparently detected signal does not represent a real effect. For that reason, the choice to include a minimal cluster size should also prevent picking up spurious effects. Supporters of this cluster-wise correction approach point to the benefit that such methods are less conservative than voxel-wise FWE and FDR correction (Lieberman and Cunningham, 2009). However, the typical settings used for cluster-wise inference have also been criticized as leading to an inflation of false positives (Eklund et al., 2016). The suggestion was made to combine the cluster-wise correction approach with a sufficiently stringent initial voxel-wise threshold such as $p = 0.001$. The proper

Statistics: *p-values adjusted for search volume*

Set-level		cluster-level				peak-level					mm mm mm
p	c	$p_{FWE\text{-}corr}$	$q_{FDR\text{-}corr}$	k_E	p_{uncorr}	$p_{FWE\text{-}corr}$	$q_{FDR\text{-}corr}$	T	$(Z_\equiv)$	p_{uncorr}	
0.000	4	0.000	0.000	56	0.000	0.000	0.000	8.46	7.77	0.000	−42 −76 −10
		0.004	0.001	31	0.000	0.001	0.001	6.13	5.84	0.000	46 −50 −22
		0.004	0.001	32	0.000	0.001	0.001	5.95	5.68	0.000	46 −72 −20
		0.012	0.003	25	0.001	0.018	0.006	5.44	5.23	0.000	−50 −54 −28

Height threshold: T = 3.79, p = 0.000 (1.000) Degrees of freedom = [1.0, 186.0]
Extent threshold: k = 20 voxels, p = 0.003 (0.031) FWHM = 6.2 6.2 6.0 mm mm mm; 3.1 3.1 3.0 {voxels}
Expected voxels per cluster, <k> = 1.842 Volume: 1687960 = 210995 voxels = 6757.6 resels
Expected number of clusters, <c> = 0.03 Voxel size: 2.0 2.0 2.0 mm mm mm; (resel = 29.01 voxels)
FWEp: 5.221, FDRp: 4.997, FWEc: 18, FDRc: 18

Figure 7.6 Example table from SPM12 with *t*- and *p*-values associated with the contrast shown in Figure 7.4. The maps were thresholded with a voxel-wise threshold of 0.0001 and an extent threshold of 20 voxels. From left to right, the table shows the following values for the peak voxels in four clusters: for cluster-level statistics, the FWE-corrected and FDR-corrected probabilities, the number of voxels in the cluster, the uncorrected cluster *p*-value; for voxel-level statistics: the FWE-corrected and FDR-corrected probabilities, the *t*-value, the associated estimated standard-normal Z-value, the uncorrected *p*-value; and finally the X, Y, Z coordinates of the peak voxel. Below the table further information is given, including the threshold values for the voxel-wise and cluster-wise multiple comparison correction (*bottom left*), the estimated smoothness of the data (FWHM [full width at half maximum]) that determines the family-wise correction, and the number and average spatial extent of the sources of variance (resells [resolution elements]) estimated, given the smoothness of the data.

approach to cluster-wise inference is currently a highly debated topic (Cox et al., 2017; Slotnick, 2017). The problem of having to decide on the voxel-wise threshold can also be avoided altogether by resorting to so-called threshold-free cluster analysis (Oosterhof et al., 2016).

Figure 7.6 shows a table of *t*- and *p*-values for several voxels in the *t*-contrast from Figure 7.4. Several *p*-values are presented, after voxel-wise FWE and FDR correction, as well as cluster-wise correction. In this dataset, the example illustrates how the *p*-value becomes much less extreme after correction, an effect that is even more pronounced for FWE compared with FDR. The uncorrected *p*-value of 0.0001 that was used as the threshold value in Figure 7.4 is associated with an FWE- and FDR-corrected *p*-values of 1.0 and 0.7, respectively.

Below the table, several other parameters of this fMRI dataset are mentioned, including the estimated smoothness of the data expressed as the full width at half maximum (FWHM) of the data, which affects the required amount of FWE correction.

7.2.3 Combining Data across Participants: Second-Level Whole-Brain Analyses

Most neuroimaging studies test a sample of subjects and make inferences to the population level. To do this, we have to verify how effects vary across the subjects in the sample. The aforementioned *t*-tests do not do this, because they only test for variation across the time points obtained in a single subject. To make inferences at the population level, we need to test the effect size against the variability across subjects.

The standard approach is referred to as a **second-level (random-effects) group analysis**. The inputs to this analysis are the contrast maps that have been computed per participant, which is the first-level analysis. In a second-level analysis, we test for each voxel to see whether the contrast value is consistently different from zero across participants. The degrees of freedom of this new, second-level t-map are related to the number of subjects (N). In the simplest case this is $N-1$.

The simplest second-level analysis involves testing whether an effect in a group of subjects is significantly different from zero with a one-sample t-test. With a second-level analysis it is also possible to test whether a particular effect is different between groups of subjects, in which case we could use a two-sample t-test. More complex ANOVA designs might include factors with multiple conditions and multiple factors. Through a second-level analysis, we can also test whether the variation across subjects correlates with a factor or covariate that differs between subjects.

All these analyses are performed voxel by voxel. This is meaningful only if the data from a particular voxel relate to the same underlying brain region in the different subjects. To get a second-level analysis to work, we have to rely on the quality of the normalization and the inclusion of an appropriate level of smoothing during preprocessing. Given that we compute the test statistic for each voxel, we also have to correct for multiple comparisons after performing a second-level analysis. For this correction, we can resort to the same approaches that were described above in the context of a first-level analysis.

7.2.4 Region-of-Interest Analyses

Researchers typically make predictions about how an experimental condition might recruit particular brain regions. In some cases, their manipulations might even target questions about very specific representations of which the researchers already know the anatomical location. Making such a priori decisions is inherent to many neuroscientific approaches because many of them do not provide whole-brain coverage. For example, researchers wishing to obtain data with single-neuron resolution through a technique such as extracellular recordings or two-photon imaging will have to decide where to place electrodes or where to perform a craniotomy to study the underlying tissue. For such methods, the decision to target a specific brain region has to be made prior to performing the experiment and is irreversible. After making the decision to put electrodes in the primary visual cortex, the study can only investigate the primary visual cortex.

The situation is different in human noninvasive imaging techniques that provide a relatively large coverage of the brain. Still, even in a study with whole-brain coverage, the researchers might have predictions about specific brain regions. In such a case, many studies employ a **region-of-interest (ROI)** approach (Poldrack, 2007; Saxe et al., 2006). For this approach, one or more ROIs are first defined using established criteria. These criteria could relate to anatomy. For example, if the studied hypothesis were to relate specifically to a primary sensory area, then this area might be defined using a probabilistic brain atlas. The ROI might come from another study that published its MNI coordinates, which could then be used to define the ROI in the current study. Alternatively, the ROI could be based on functional criteria, often combined with anatomical criteria. For example, a region such as the fusiform face area (FFA) is defined by a functional contrast (higher response to faces compared with objects) combined with an anatomical criterion (located within the fusiform gyrus).

A valid ROI approach requires that the ROI is defined using criteria that are independent of the effects of interest. This is relatively straightforward for an anatomical ROI, in which case the ROI is defined anatomically and the effects of interest are of a functional nature. For a functional ROI, many studies include separate **functional localizer** runs of which the data are used to define the ROI and experimental runs that contain the conditions that are the primary interest of the current study (Saxe et al., 2006). The design and conditions of the localizer runs might be shared among many different studies that are interested in the same ROIs. For example, there are numerous fMRI studies that have focused on the FFA defined through a contrast of faces with object images, or the human MT/V5+ area that is defined through a contrast of moving versus stationary images.

Some studies define a functional ROI using the same data used for testing effects, but with a different contrast. In such a case, it is important that the contrast used to define the ROI is statistically independent from the tested effects. For example, the design could contain two factors, the ROI could be defined based on the existence of a main effect of one of those factors, and the critical test could be whether there is also a main effect of the other factor or an interaction between the two factors. In this approach, it is important that the experimental design be well balanced (e.g., equal number of blocks of each condition), because otherwise the use of orthogonal contrasts (e.g., main effect versus interaction effect) does not guarantee statistical independence (Kriegeskorte et al., 2009).

Figure 7.7 illustrates the ROI approach with data from Yovel and Kanwisher (2005). The authors defined several face-selective regions, including the FFA. They localized these regions using data from a set of localizer runs that consisted of blocks of different stimulus conditions, including the two conditions involved in the contrast to find face selectivity: faces minus objects. In the resulting ROIs, the authors tested for the effect of interest: how the signal would be affected by inverting face images. The data included to test this effect did not come from the runs used to define the ROIs. The results showed that the size of the face inversion effect in the FFA is correlated across subjects with the effect of face inversion on the behavioral performance of subjects in a face recognition task.

The literature contains arguments in favor of and against ROI approaches (Friston et al., 2006; Saxe et al., 2006). A first benefit of the ROI approach is that it allows for a definition of ROIs at the level of a single subject, and so avoids the problem of

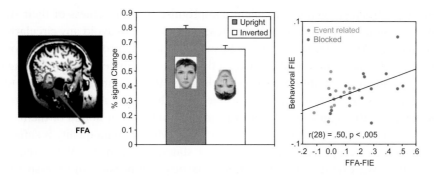

Figure 7.7 Illustration of the region-of-interest approach. The percent signal change is shown in the FFA for two experimental conditions: upright and inverted faces. The scatterplot shows the relationship across subjects between the difference in fMRI signal for these two conditions in FFA (upright – inverted, FFA-RE) and the behavioral difference in accuracy.
Adapted with permission from Yovel and Kanwisher, 2005

inter-individual variability in anatomy and provides more anatomical specificity. A second benefit is that it circumvents the problem of multiple comparisons. If researchers are interested only in the overall effect in one or a few ROIs, then they perform fewer statistical tests and do not need to correct for a high number of multiple comparisons. Note that this reasoning applies only if the ROIs were chosen in advance.

One major disadvantage of the ROI approach is that the analyses only provide a very local view of the data. Researchers depend on the validity of the functional and anatomical specificity of their prior hypothesis. Some functional contrasts might only make sense if they were tested in a particular functional region. For example, if there is a theoretically relevant hypothesis about how visual stimuli might be processed in the region in which visual information enters the cortex, then it is clear that the primary visual cortex is *the* region to study. However, in some cases the specificity of the hypothesis might be less clear, and one might wonder whether there might be any effects in other brain regions. Suppose that many other brain regions were to show similar effects or even larger effects than the primary visual cortex; that knowledge, then, might qualify our interpretation of the effect in primary visual cortex.

There have been combined approaches trying to retain the benefits of an ROI approach but avoiding its disadvantages. One approach involves performing a standard ROI approach and complementing it with an exploratory whole-brain analysis to test whether any effects in other brain regions might be missed.

7.2.5 Another Statistical Caveat: Double Dipping and Circular Analyses

The statistical analysis of fMRI data is complex. Many steps are involved, and researchers have to be aware of possible errors that they could make in each of those steps, because such errors might compromise the correctness of their statistical conclusions. A major caveat is that researchers have to avoid any circularity in their analyses. Many decisions have to be made during the process. Ideally, most or all of these decisions are based on criteria that were already set prior to starting the study. This ideal is not always easy to reach, given that research studies tend to be innovative, and as such unexpected problems might occur. A standard operating procedure (SOP) might exist to deal with some problems but not all of them.

As an example, we can refer to decisions about whether data quality is sufficient. In many published studies, one can read a statement such as "We scanned 20 participants. We excluded the data from 2 participants because of excessive head motion." How and when did the authors make this decision? The decision should be based on transparent criteria, which are often developed from experience in other studies in the same lab and other labs. A common criterion is that data are problematic if the participant moved more than the size of a voxel. This decision should be made prior to looking at the effects of interest. It would be unacceptable if the decision depended on information about the effects of interest. Suppose, for example, that of the 20 participants there were three participants with excessive head motion but only the two that did not show the effect of interest would be excluded. Decisions about how to analyze data should not be influenced by information about the effects of interest in the current dataset.

Kriegeskorte and colleagues (2009) provided an overview of bad practices that should be avoided and that can be grouped under umbrella terms such as **circular analyses** and **double dipping**. Note that these caveats are not specific to the field of brain imaging and are common to all empirical research. Related to the previous example with excessive motion, a researcher working with behavioral data might also be confronted with "outlier" participants with low data quality.

Figure 7.8 illustrates the problem of double dipping or circularity as it might occur in an ROI analysis when researchers are not careful. The middle matrix shows a set of voxels containing simulated fMRI data. The simulated data contain a particular effect and added noise. The "true" effect embedded in the data is shown at the left: Some voxels are more active for conditions A and B than for conditions C and D. This effect was embedded in the voxels enclosed by the blue contour in the matrix. It is not straightforward to detect these voxels due to noise in the data. The authors resort to a functional contrast to define the ROI, and this includes the contrast of conditions A and D (A > D).

The correct, noncircular approach involves taking a separate set of data to define the ROI. This is how the voxels in the green contour are selected. Then the researchers test in this independent-data ROI what the difference in response is between the four conditions. The data show an (equally) high response in conditions A and B and an (equally) low response in conditions C and D. This is exactly the "true" effect that was embedded in the simulated data on the left.

An incorrect, circular approach involves using the same data to define the ROI and to test for effects. Using these data to define the ROI, the simulated data

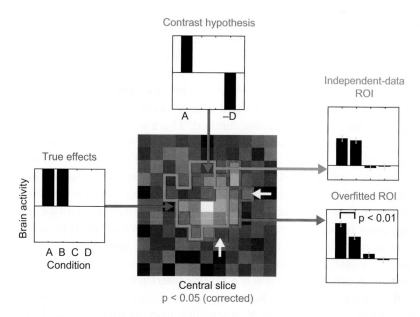

Figure 7.8 The effect of circular analyses in a region-of-interest analysis. See text for more explanation. Adapted with permission from Kriegeskorte et al., 2009

indicate that the voxels in the purple contour show a difference in the contrast of A–D. Then the researchers test in this ROI what the difference in response is between the four conditions. The data show a linear decline in simulated brain activity across the four conditions: $A > B > C > D$. This is not the same as the "true" effect that was embedded in the simulated data, as the true effect does not show a difference between conditions A and B. The detected effect is a mixture of the true effect ($A = B > C = D$) and the contrast hypothesis used to define the ROI ($A > D$). In general, the more noisy the data are and the smaller the effect size of the true effects is, the more such circularity in the analyses can affect the outcome of the analyses.

7.2.6 Statistical Inference

Once a statistical test has resulted in a truly (corrected) significant effect in a set of voxels, the question becomes, What does the result mean? The extent to which this statistical inference is straightforward depends on the design that was used, a point that was emphasized already in the context of Figure 6.1. In the simplest case, the statistical test involved the comparison of two experimental conditions A and B. What does it mean that condition A is associated with a significantly higher fMRI signal in a particular brain region R?

If the experimental design obeyed all the requirements in the context of the Donders subtraction method (see Chapter 5), then the two conditions are different in just one identifiable cognitive/neural process. Suppose that condition A involves cognitive process X and condition B does not, and the two conditions are equivalent in all other aspects. The statistical inference would then be: If process X is manipulated, then region R is activated; thus, activation of region R is related to process X. This type of reasoning is often referred to as a **forward inference**.

However, in many paradigms it might turn out to be difficult to strictly adhere to the requirements of the subtraction method. There are countless examples in the literature where conditions are compared that differ in more than one cognitive process. In this case, we can no longer make a forward inference. If we were to do so, it would sound like this: If processes X, Y, Z, ... are manipulated, then region R is activated. With this inference, we do not know which process is related to the activation of region R. In fact, in such a case we are likely to see more than one activated brain region, resulting in a forward inference such as: If processes X, Y, Z, ... are manipulated, then regions R, S, T, U, ... are activated.

In the latter case, researchers often resort to another type of inference to draw more specific conclusions, known as a **reverse inference**. It goes as follows. Results show an activation of region R, among other activations. Other studies in the literature have activated region R when they manipulated process X. Thus, the activation of region R in the current study is related to process X.

Russell Poldrack was the first researcher who explicitly dissociated these two types of inferences and highlighted the potential drawbacks of a reverse inference (Poldrack, 2006). In particular, Poldrack points out that a reverse inference is problematic when region R is involved in more than one cognitive process. This is a realistic problem because it is clear from the literature that the fMRI signal in most brain regions is modulated by more than one experimental manipulation and more than one cognitive process. The more this happens, the less certain we are about the conclusion from a reverse inference that the activation of a region such as R is due to the involvement of one of these cognitive processes. For this reason, conclusions from reverse inferences should be more cautious compared with conclusions from forward inferences.

The importance of the caveats with reverse inference cannot be emphasized enough, given that these improper conclusions constitute a frequent cause of inappropriate media coverage of brain imaging studies. One example is the proposal that fMRI can be used for lie detection. The areas of the brain that are more activated when participants are not truthful in an experimental paradigm, chiefly in the parietal and frontal cortex, are all general-purpose areas that are known to be involved in multiple processes. In fact, the increased activation when telling a lie does not occur because of the lie itself, but because lying is associated with other, more general monitoring and conflict processes. For these reasons, an increased activity in this frontoparietal network is a very unreliable reverse inference indicator of telling a lie.

Nevertheless, even high-quality neuroimaging studies often include a reverse inference at some point. Even if the design is perfected to isolate one or a few cognitive processes in a very specific way, there are often other, less specific

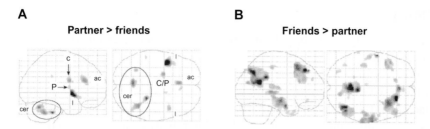

Figure 7.9 The investigation of the neural basis of romantic love through reverse inference. (A) Significantly activated voxels in the contrast partner minus friends. Activated regions include medial insula (I), anterior cingulate cortex (ac), caudate nucleus (C), putamen (P), and cerebellum (cer), all bilaterally. (B) Contrast friends minus partner. Activated areas include posterior cingulate gyrus and amygdala, and on the right prefrontal, parietal, and middle temporal regions.
Figure reproduced with permission from Bartels and Zeki, 2000

contrasts computed, of which the findings are interesting to mention but are not specific enough to isolate a particular cognitive process. In such a case, even the very best researchers might cautiously hint at the possible ways in which the related brain activations might be associated with particular cognitive processes. Such observations might often motivate subsequent experiments in which the design allows the testing of the hypotheses inspired by reverse inference through a forward inference.

Figure 7.9 gives an example of a study for which it can be claimed that even the comparison that is most central to the study can be interpreted only by resorting to reverse inferences. This study by Bartels and Zeki (2000) investigated the neural basis of romantic love. Participants looked at pictures of two conditions: (i) pictures showing their partner with whom they were in love and (ii) pictures showing good friends. They contrasted these two conditions and found several brain regions that were more active when participants were presented with pictures of the partner, and a range of other brain regions that were more active when participants viewed pictures of good friends.

It is obvious that there are several cognitive and emotional processes and reactions that might be very differently activated in these two conditions. The emotional responses can be very different in various ways (valence, intensity, etc.), as might several other cognitive and neurobiological reactions. A reverse inference can provide us with some hints about which process(es) is/are responsible for the higher activation of, for example, the cerebellum and the anterior cingulate when presented with a picture of a beloved partner. This might be fine as a first exploratory approach to develop finer hypotheses and test them in further studies. From this perspective, there is nothing wrong with studies such as this example used as a first step in a research program. However, we should be cautious when drawing conclusions in such a case. In and of itself, a reverse inference does not yet provide very strong experimental evidence about relationships between target cognitive processes and specific brain regions.

Summary

- Statistics are typically based on a regression model referred to as the general linear model.
- Correction for multiple comparisons is needed when determining the significance of the results.
- One should avoid performing circular analyses in which knowledge about the results of initial analyses influences how later analyses are performed.
- Statistical inference is preferably based on forward inference, and proper caution should be used in the case of reverse inference.

Review Questions

1. Explain the regressors that are typically included in the general linear model used to analyze functional magnetic resonance imaging (fMRI) data.
2. Explain the rationale behind and the differences between the methods to correct for multiple comparisons when analyzing an fMRI dataset.
3. Explain the distinction between forward and reverse inference.
4. A researcher computes a whole-brain second-level contrast of condition X minus condition Y. He finds two clusters of voxels with a threshold p-value that is not corrected for multiple comparisons, but none of these clusters survives an FWE-corrected threshold. One cluster is in the medial prefrontal cortex (MPC), the other in the intraparietal sulcus (IPS). This observation motivates the researcher to define two anatomical regions of interest (ROIs), MPC and IPS. He averages the signal across all voxels in these two ROIs and performs a t-test (X - Y) in each ROI. He corrects the observed p-value for the fact that he has performed the t-test in two ROIs (corrected p = uncorrected $p/2$). Based on this corrected p-value, he concludes that there is a significant effect of X > Y in IPS (corrected p-value 0.007). Do you agree with this statistical inference? Why (not)?

Further Reading

Ashby, F. G. (2011). *Statistical Analysis of fMRI Data*. Cambridge, MA: MIT Press. (This is an in-depth book and very useful for students with sufficient statistical background.)

Poldrack, R. A., Mumford, J. A. & Nichols, T. E. (2011). *Handbook of Functional MRI Data Analysis*. Cambridge: Cambridge University Press. (This is an in-depth and very concrete explanation of the important concepts and steps involved when analyzing fMRI data.)

CHAPTER EIGHT

Advanced Statistical Analyses

Learning Objectives

- Being aware that experimental design and statistical analyses are closely intertwined
- Understanding the concept of functional connectivity and how to analyze it
- Knowing the basics of multi-voxel pattern analyses and how they differ from voxel-wise analyses
- Understanding adaptation paradigms and their assumptions

The spectrum of data analyses that can be performed on a large dataset such as a functional magnetic resonance imaging (fMRI) experiment is daunting. The data analyses that were introduced in Chapter 7 were described as "basic," but that is not doing justice to their complexity or the importance of their underlying assumptions. Now we move to analyses that are "advanced," meaning that the analyses are even more complicated and often have been introduced more recently.

The "basic" analyses were very well suited for the experimental designs that were introduced in Chapter 5. The "advanced" analyses in this chapter require specific design choices, and therefore we will also discuss the implications at the level of experimental design. We focus on three types of analyses: functional connectivity, multivariate pattern analyses, and adaptation. The current chapter primarily serves as an introduction to these methods to explain the most basic variations of them and to help the reader to understand a nontechnical article describing such results. It would bring us into too much depth, and require much more space, to discuss all advanced methods at the same level of detail as we did for more basic concepts (e.g., the general linear model).

8.1 Functional Connectivity: Designs and Analyses

Previous chapters chiefly focused on functional localization: What is the function of specific brain regions? Which brain regions are involved in which cognitive function? However, no brain region works in isolation from other brain regions. Take, for example, the previously mentioned fusiform face area (FFA), which is defined functionally by a stronger response to face images than to images of other objects. This brain region needs other regions to receive input. Without the retina, thalamus, and primary visual cortex, the FFA would receive no input and its neurons would not be able to respond differently to faces and nonface stimuli. Furthermore, if there were no other brain regions receiving the output of the FFA, then the processing happening within the FFA would be of no further consequence and irrelevant to behavior and cognition. Finally, given that the FFA is only one of several face-selective regions, those regions must be communicating with each other to result in an overall representation of a presented face and its properties.

Thus, to understand how the brain works, not only do we need to know about what happens in each brain region, we also need to understand which brain regions communicate and how these brain regions form systems or networks.

Functional connectivity is not the same as anatomical connectivity. Two regions are anatomically connected when there are axons leaving from one of the two regions and ending in the other region. Large anatomical connections can be investigated through methods such as diffusion tension imaging (DTI; see Chapter 3). Functional connectivity refers to a relationship between the functional activity of different brain regions.

8.1.1 Correlations in Brain Activity

The simplest index for functional connectivity is the correlation between the activity of two brain regions across time. A straightforward approach (Fig. 8.1) is to take one particular region of interest, in this context referred to as a **seed region**, take the time-varying signal averaged across all voxels in this seed region, and correlate it with the signal in all voxels of the brain. Figure 8.1A shows the seed region, and Figure 8.1B shows the signal in this region over time. In contrast to earlier chapters, we are less interested in the relationship between this signal and a prespecified manipulation or predictor. Instead, we relate this time-varying signal in the seed region to the signal in other voxels. Figure 8.1C shows the voxels that are correlated with the seed region in this particular study of Buckner and colleagues (2013). One could say that all these colored voxels form a network of functionally connected voxels. The resulting brain map can be analyzed statistically in the same way as described in Chapter 6 through a GLM, now with the regressor being an fMRI signal (from the seed region) rather than an experimental condition. Further statistical considerations (e.g., procedures for correcting for multiple comparisons) apply here as well.

We have to consider the time scale at which such correlations unfold. Neuronal communication often happens in the milliseconds range. When neurons in one cortical area fire action potentials that are transported by the axons to a second cortical area, these action potentials will influence the second area after a few milliseconds and might result in action potentials in the second area roughly 10 milliseconds later. Cortical layers and areas might also be involved in back-and-forth communication at temporal frequencies far above 1 Hz. To capture neuronal communication at these speeds, we need to perform electrophysiological imaging (see Chapters 9–12). With hemodynamic imaging, we are restricted to the study of

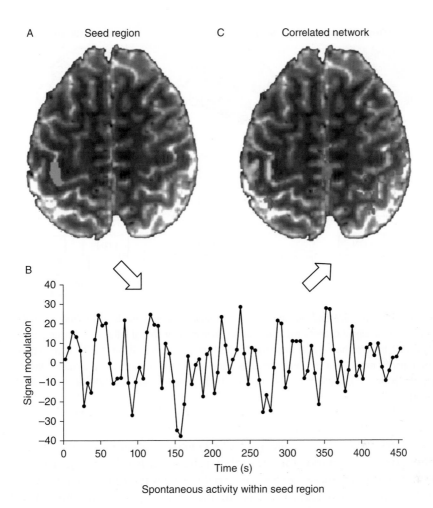

Figure 8.1 Seed-based functional connectivity: (A) the anatomical location of the seed region; (B) the temporal fluctuation in the fMRI signal in this seed region; (C) voxels with above-threshold correlation with the seed region in the fMRI signal across time.

Figure reproduced with permission from Buckner et al., 2013

much slower changes in the signal. A typical analysis stream for functional connectivity will include a low-pass filtering with a high cutoff around 0.1 Hz. The signal of interest is primarily at these slower frequencies, as higher frequencies are dominated by noise (Cordes et al., 2001).

8.1.2 The Interpretation of Correlations in Brain Activity

There could be many causes for a correlation in fMRI signals between two voxels or regions. As with the aforementioned GLM-related approach, we can distinguish between causes that are of interest to us versus those that are annoying confounds.

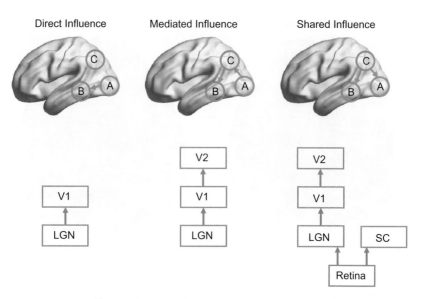

Figure 8.2 Three possible explanations for why two brain regions A and B might show a correlation in how their fMRI signal changes over time: direct, mediated, or shared influence. The top panel illustrates the three scenarios with three hypothetical cortical areas A, B, and C. The bottom panel shows a specific example of the three scenarios using part of the visual circuitry, including the retina, superior colliculus (SC), lateral geniculate nucleus (LGN), primary visual area (V1), and secondary visual area (V2).

We follow Poldrack and colleagues (2011) and others in differentiating between three interesting scenarios for a correlation between two brain regions A and B. Figure 8.2 illustrates these scenarios in two different ways. In the top panels we refer to three hypothetical cortical areas. In the bottom panels we show flowcharts referring to specific examples of areas of which the connectivity is well known from a range of methods, including the use of anatomical tracers in animals.

First, there might be a **direct influence** from region A to region B. At the neuronal level, this would imply that neurons in region B receive direct input from neurons in region A. This is the situation for region A = lateral geniculate nucleus (LGN in the thalamus) and region B = primary visual cortex (visual area 1). The LGN is the primary source for input to V1, and V1 neurons inherit most of their tuning properties from this LGN input.

A second scenario involves no direct influence from A to B, but a **mediated influence** through a third area C. This situation implies a direct influence from A to C and then from C to B. An example of this is the influence of the aforementioned LGN on the second visual area V2. Visual area V2 receives most of its input from area V1, and V1 receives most of its input from LGN. Therefore, if we find a correlation between LGN and V2, then this is in large part an influence of LGN on V2, which is mediated by area V1.

A third scenario is referred to as a **shared influence**, in which areas A and B receive input from a common area C. Remaining with our earlier example, visual signals from the retina are sent not only to the LGN-V1 pathway, but also to other structures such as the superior colliculus. In a paradigm where light is going on and off, LGN/V1 and the superior colliculus would show a strong correlation in activity based on the shared input from the retina.

It is not easy to differentiate among those interesting causal relations. However, before we can even start to try, we should consider the possibility that correlations might be induced by less interesting, confounding factors that have nothing to do with brain functioning. There are many other factors that might induce changes in functional activity. We could refer to such factors as another type of shared influence, but one not from a neural source.

One very important possible confound is **subject motion**. Subject motion can induce very strong correlations in fMRI signal. Take the example of two voxels at the left side of the brain that are both centered on gray matter. On the left of each of these voxels, we have no brain tissue and a much lower fMRI signal. On the right, we have white matter and a much higher fMRI signal than in the center of the voxel. If the subject would sometimes move to the left, then these two fMRI voxels would start picking up fMRI signal from white matter. If the subject would move to the right, then the voxels would pick up the lower signal from outside the brain. So, for these two voxels, left/right subject motion would induce very strong correlations. These correlations would dominate correlations based on neural activity because the magnitude of the motion-related signal changes could be much larger than the 1–3% signal changes that we typically see with the blood-oxygenation-level dependent (BOLD) contrast.

The example illustrates that one does not have to be a rocket scientist to understand that subject motion is an important factor to control for. As for other types of fMRI analyses, the standard approach for dealing with subject motion used to be to calculate misalignments during preprocessing, realign the functional images, and include the motion parameters as regressors in further analyses. However, this approach turned out to be insufficient for avoiding motion-related artifacts.

Figure 8.3, from Power and colleagues (2012), illustrates this problem. Figure 8.3A shows the fMRI signal as a percent difference from the mean signal in three regions of interest. These data were obtained from motion-corrected data, and the motion-correction parameters have already been taken into account in the analyses. These motion-correction parameters are shown in Figure 8.3B. There is some motion, but according to common practice at that time the data might be used. Figure 8.3C and D are derived from the data from Figure 8.3A and B, respectively, but now the plot shows the change from one time point to the next (the differential) in terms of absolute values (negative values are made positive). There is an obvious correspondence between the changes in the BOLD signal (Fig. 8.3C) and the changes in head position, or so-called frame-wise displacement (FD) (Fig. 8.3D). The standard analyses steps turned out not to be enough to avoid motion-induced

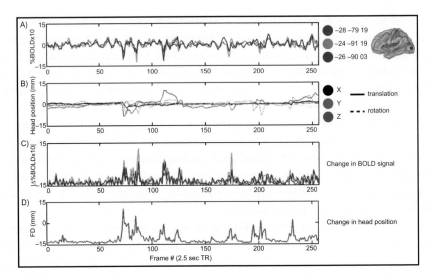

Figure 8.3 Correlations in fMRI signal between regions can be caused by subject motion. See text for more information.

Figure reproduced with permission from Power et al., 2012

changes in BOLD signal. The three regions show a very high correlation in activity, but this correlation is induced by subject motion, not by neural activity. Since 2012, studies on functional connectivity have been more careful to avoid motion artifacts by including extra steps in the analyses. One rather successful approach is to include only those time intervals in the data in which there is no or almost no motion, a method referred to as "**scrubbing**."

The analyses of Power and colleagues (2012) also showed what the typical overall effect is of subject motion on functional connectivity. Subject motion will typically increase the correlation between nearby regions/voxels. Long-range correlations between faraway regions will decrease due to subject motion. Suppose that a researcher compared two groups of subjects, with one group moving slightly more than the other. The results might reveal stronger short-range and weaker long-range functional connectivity in the group with more motion, without there being any existing differences in real brain connectivity.

8.1.3 Modeling Directional Functional Connectivity

To the extent that we have been able to avoid the confounds mentioned in the previous section, we can start with trying to differentiate among the more interesting causes, such as a direct influence, indirect influence, or shared influence. Here we have to deal with several challenges.

A first challenge is directionality. Even if we have arguments in favor of a direct influence, a simple correlation between A and B does not by itself provide information about whether it is A that drives B or B that drives A (in the case of a direct influence). Here we jump from functional connectivity, represented by the correlation, to **effective connectivity**, implying a causal direction.

In order to infer effective connectivity, we need information over and above the available correlation between A and B to make inferences about directionality. It was not a coincidence that we illustrated the (in)direct influences with a well-known basic sensory circuit involving LGN and cortical area V1. We know from animal physiology that LGN drives V1 and not the other way around. Thus, in this example we have ample evidence to assume a directionality when we observe a correlation between these regions. Apart from empirical evidence from animal models, the evidence might be of a more theoretical and conceptual nature. The researchers might have a few hypotheses about how multiple brain regions might be connected, and these models might imply directionality. If a model were then supported by the data, then this is taken as evidence of directionality. However, we should keep in mind that the evidence for directionality depends on the correctness of the theoretical assumptions.

Several methods have been applied to investigate effective connectivity, for example, structural equation modeling (SEM), dynamic causal modeling, and Granger causality. The first type, SEM, might be familiar to scientists from various fields, including behavioral sciences, because it is widely applied to correlational data that can be modeled as a complex graph model no matter where those data come from (psychometric tests, models of climate change, imaging data, ...).

An example of SEM from the field of human imaging is shown in Figure 8.4, taken from a study by Santens and colleagues (2010). The authors studied numerical representations, which are involved when we process numbers that are presented in various formats, such as Arabic symbols or patterns of dots (as on a dice). Through a series of experiments the authors identified three regions of interest: (1) Visual representations of the visual characteristics of a presented number symbol or dot pattern; (2) number-sensitive representations characterized by a response that increased monotonically with larger numbers; and (3) number-selective representations in which neurons are tuned for specific numerosities. The authors assumed two pathways by which the visual representations could provide input to the number-selective representations: a direct pathway and an indirect pathway going through the number-sensitive representations. The authors compared these two models and found that the relative importance of the two pathways was modulated by the format in which the numbers were presented. For symbols, there was a direct influence from vision to the number-selective representations in addition to an indirect influence. For nonsymbolic formats, namely dot patterns, the pattern of correlations could be fully explained by only the indirect influence through number-sensitive representations. Figure 8.4E shows the actual correlations to which the models were applied.

Note that the available data allow one to test for the relative importance of the two involved pathways, but do not by themselves prove the directionality of the

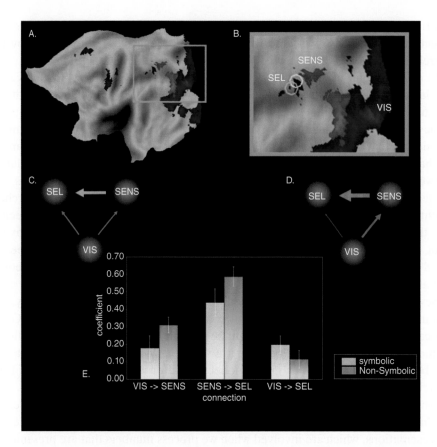

Figure 8.4 Structural equation modeling in the domain of numerical cognition. (A–B) Flatmaps with functional regions of interest. Regions in blue are activated by digits (symbolic) as well as dot patterns (nonsymbolic). Regions in red show an increase in activation as a function of the number of dots in nonsymbolic numbers. This effect was used to delineate number-sensitive regions (SENS) in the superior parietal lobe. The cyan and yellow circles in (B) reveal the likely location of number-selective regions (SEL) based on other studies. The third region of interest was primary visual cortex (VIS). (C) and (D) show a graphical illustration of the modeling results in, respectively, the symbolic and the nonsymbolic condition. (E) The coefficient representing the modeled strength of connectivity between pairs of regions of interest (ROIs) in the two stimulus conditions.
Figure reproduced from Santens et al., 2010

connectivity. The same model with all the arrows reversed would fit the data equally well. However, such a model would not make sense theoretically from an information processing perspective, given that visually presented numbers first have to be processed visually before they can inform about numerosity.

If the temporal resolution of fMRI had been better, then there would have been a very important additional piece of information to infer directionality: the leading signal. If the signal in B goes up or down after the signal in A, then we know that A is the leading signal and the cause of the signal changes in B. To get this to work, we need a very high temporal resolution that is beyond the reach of hemodynamic imaging. Methods that depend on such time-relative analyses, such as Granger causality, have only limited applicability with fMRI and are much more useful in the context of other methods such as electroencephalography (EEG) and magnetoencephalography (MEG), as we will show in Chapter 12.

The second challenge that we face when we want to discriminate between options such as a direct, indirect, and shared influence is that the number of alternative situations increases dramatically when we consider a greater number of regions. With just two brain regions, we only have to consider a direct influence. With three brain regions, the influences can already run in several different directions. With tens or hundreds of regions, which is what we deal with in the real brain, the number of alternative models is massive. Researchers typically simplify reality by focusing on a small number of prior predictions and hypotheses which include a small number of previously decided regions of interest (ROIs). This approach is again illustrated by the example from Santens and colleagues (2010).

8.1.4 Task-Related Modulations of Connectivity

The example of Santens and colleagues (2010) already illustrates that the functional connectivity between brain regions might depend on the experimental condition, otherwise known as a task-related modulation of connectivity.

In some cases, researchers have specific predictions that the functional connectivity between regions would depend on the degree to which brain regions are modulated by an experimental manipulation. Often this is referred to as a **psychophysiological interaction (PPI)** (Friston et al., 1997). Such interactions between experimental manipulations and connectivity can be tested directly.

If the experimental manipulation is induced across time series or runs or even across experiments, then the initial analysis can be done separately for the two conditions. Afterward, the results are statistically compared. For example, with per participant separate runs for each task condition, a paired *t*-test across participants could be used to compare the connectivity index (e.g., a correlation) between tasks.

However, in most experiments tasks are interleaved within runs. In the most extreme case of an event-related design, trials of the different task conditions are succeeding rapidly. In such cases, it becomes difficult to investigate the functional connectivity in one task independently from the other task. This is due to the delayed and temporally smoothed hemodynamic signal. A correlation in fMRI signal between two voxels could be caused not by the current condition but by the one presented 6 seconds ago. This problem is solved by first modeling the activity of individual events with a general linear model (Gitelman et al., 2003; Rissman et al., 2004). As a consequence, we have a beta estimate of the task effect for each event. Next, we can correlate the variation of these beta estimates across events, separately for each task condition. This procedure is referred to as **beta-series correlations**.

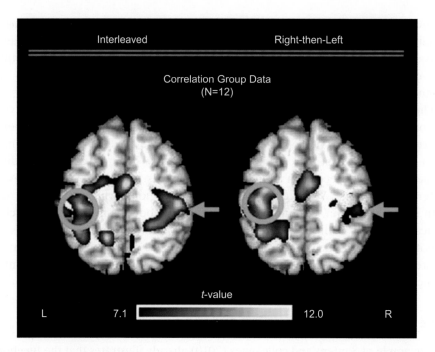

Figure 8.5 Task-based modulation of functional connectivity. Connectivity is calculated in two tasks, referred to as "interleaved" and "right-then-left." The seed region in the left primary motor cortex (M1) is identified by the blue circle, and right M1 is indicated by the blue arrow. The color map shows the *t*-values from a second-level random-effects analysis thresholded at a Bonferroni-corrected $p = 0.01$.
Figure reproduced with permission from Rissman et al., 2004

An early application of beta-series correlations is shown in Figure 8.5 (Rissman et al., 2004). The researchers compared two simple motor tasks that differed in the degree of coordination needed between the right and left hand. In one condition, the "interleaved" condition, participants had to alternate between tapping with left-hand fingers and with right-hand fingers. In the second condition, the "right-then-left" condition, participants first tapped with several left-hand fingers and then with several right-hand fingers. Univariate statistics comparing the overall fMRI signal between these two conditions revealed no significant differences. The researchers expected a greater need for intercallosal communication in the interleaved condition and thus more functional connectivity between left and right hemispheres. To test this, they used beta-series correlations to investigate functional connectivity between left and right primary motor cortex (M1). Connectivity was indeed significantly higher in the interleaved condition compared with the right-then-left condition.

The possibility that task influences functional connectivity reminds us of an important difference between functional and anatomical connectivity (Gillebert and Mantini, 2013). In the case of a PPI, we see a change in functional connectivity, while the anatomical connectivity between the two areas must be static at this time scale. Also, two regions might appear not to be functionally connected while there is a direct anatomical connection. Of course, there must also be some relationship between functional and anatomical connectivity. In particular, the inference of a direct influence from region A to region B implies a direct anatomical connection from A to B. Damoiseaux and Greicius (2009) reviewed the literature and concluded that overall functional connectivity is positively correlated with structural connectivity strength. Nevertheless, there are discrepancies, such as the existence of pairs of regions with strong functional connectivity, that have little or no structural connectivity. In such cases the most likely explanation is that the functional connectivity reflects a (perhaps unknown) mediating influence.

8.1.5 Resting-State fMRI (RS fMRI)

The Implementation and Analysis of RS fMRI

Most studies of functional connectivity are not interested in task-based effects or want to avoid such effects. These studies primarily utilize **resting-state fMRI (RS fMRI)**. During an RS fMRI scan, a subject is asked to rest and try to think of nothing in particular. A scan session might include only 1 or 2 scans of 8 minutes. This is a very efficient type of scan, and it is particularly useful in patient populations in which it would be difficult to explain an explicit task and ensure full compliance with the task requirements. Similar analyses are often also performed on a task fMRI experiment, in which case the task-related activity is subtracted from the BOLD signal through a regression analysis. The extent to which this approach gives results similar to an RS fMRI will depend on the presence of task-related modulations of connectivity.

Resting-state fMRI analyses share the initial preprocessing stages with task-based fMRI, with a few additional steps such as data scrubbing (see Section 8.1.2) and temporal low-pass filtering (see Section 8.1.1). The full dataset for the analyses could be considered as a two-dimensional matrix of size $V \times T$, with all relevant voxels (e.g., all gray matter voxels) as rows and the time points as columns. The number of voxels V in this matrix is daunting.

One solution for the size of this matrix is to restrict the analysis to a lower number of previously selected regions of interest. In some studies, only a few ROIs might be chosen, but in principle they could also number in the hundreds, or even thousands, and include fine-grained local regions or vertices spanning the whole cortex. With a reasonably small number of ROIs, study authors might restrict the further analysis to the calculation of the correlation in RS fMRI signal between all of them, which would result in a correlation matrix of size $N \times N$, with N being the number of ROIs. There are various methods to analyze the structure in such a matrix, including **principal component analysis (PCA)**, which is based on the same principles as the method of factor analysis that might be more familiar to behavioral scientists. These methods are used to identify a small number of components (or factors) that explain most of the variance in the data. For example, if a subset of regions shows very high correlations in activity, then their activity fluctuations can be summarized to a large extent by one component. Statistical analyses can also focus on individual values in this correlation matrix, for example, to infer whether there are pairs of ROIs for which the connectivity is different between two groups of subjects. Here we again have a need to correct for multiple comparisons, which is now related to the number of cells in the N x N matrix.

As an alternative approach for the selection and delineation of regions of interest, the voxels could be clustered into regions in a data driven manner, based on the correlations between the signals. For this we need methods that can handle the large number of voxels V in such a dataset. One such method is **independent component analysis (ICA)** (Beckmann et al., 2005), which identifies components that are statistically independent. These components can be used for clustering nearby voxels into regions and to identify the networks formed by these regions.

It is not easy to summarize the findings from connectivity analyses based on large datasets involving many voxels or ROIs. An important insight has been that a small set of parameters from a theoretical framework known as **graph theory** is extremely useful for describing the behavior of many complex systems and datasets, including function connectivity data as well as those from other imaging modalities (structural MRI, DTI, MEG, EEG, etc.). Graph theory provides a framework for the study of graphs that are composed of nodes with pair-wise connections. A graph theoretical analysis leads to the computation of network parameters, which summarize important properties of the network (for an introduction and review, see Bullmore and Sporns, 2009). Examples include node degree, the number of nodes a node is connected to; the distribution of node degree across voxels; and path length (with efficiency, which is inversely related to it), the number of nodes that have to be passed to move from one node to another.

Findings Obtained with RS fMRI

The first network that often emerges in resting-state analyses is referred to as the **default mode network** (DMN), as shown in Figure 8.6. Interestingly, this network also emerges in almost the same form in task-based fMRI when looking for regions that are more active during a rest condition compared with an active task condition (as described in Chapter 5; compare the regions activated in Fig. 8.6 with the blue regions in Fig. 5.9). The DMN network is also consistently found through the different approaches for analyzing functional connectivity, such as independent component analysis (Fig. 8.6A) and correlation-based analyses (Fig. 8.6B). Given the consistency with which this network emerges in relatively short and easy-to-administer RS fMRI datasets, changes in DMN connectivity have been investigated in a wide range of clinical populations such as major depression (Greicius et al., 2007), schizophrenia (Garrity et al., 2007), and autism (Di Martino et al., 2014).

In addition to the DMN, several other networks have been identified in resting-state data, such as parietal-frontal attention networks, a motor network, and visual

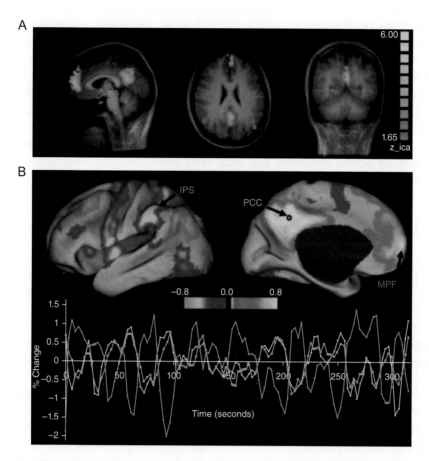

Figure 8.6 The default mode network (DMN) identified through the analysis of functional connectivity in resting-state fMRI. (A) The DMN as identified through independent component analysis. Reproduced with permission from Meindl et al., 2010. (B) The DMN as identified by taking one of the DMN regions, the posterior cingulate cortex (PCC), as seed region and performing a whole-brain correlational analysis in a single subject. The time series represent the fMRI signal fluctuations in one run for the PCC (yellow), for another DMN region (medial prefrontal cortex or MPC; orange), and a region that does not belong to the DMN, the intraparietal sulcus or IPS (blue).
Reproduced with permission from Fox et al., 2005, Copyright (2005) National Academy of Sciences, U.S.A.

networks. The distinctions between these networks are less prominent, which is reflected in the fact that they typically all show higher activity in task conditions, in contrast to the DMN. With correlation-based approaches, it is even common to observe negative correlations or so-called anticorrelations between the DMN and the other networks (see Fig. 8.6B)(Fox et al., 2005). However, whether this implies negative connectivity at the neural level is less clear given that some analysis steps (e.g., normalization for whole-brain correlations) could turn lower-than-average positive correlations into negative correlations (Hampson et al., 2010).

There has been discussion about whether these resting-state networks and the underlying correlations in temporal signal variation do in fact reflect a neural signal such as synaptic processing or action potentials, or instead a number of potential confounds (motion, and respiratory and cardiac modulations) (for review, see van den Heuvel and Hulshoff Pol, 2010). The observation that the networks make sense given our knowledge gained from other neuroscientific methods is one argument in favor of an interpretation in terms of neural signals. Importantly, monkey studies have directly compared resting-state BOLD fluctuations with simultaneous measurements of action potentials and local field potentials, and observed a robust relationship (Shmuel and Leopold, 2008, Shmuel et al., 2002).

8.2 Multi-voxel Pattern Analyses

Multi-voxel pattern analyses (MVPA) are most easily defined by contrasting them with the standard analyses that we refer to as voxel-wise analyses. As explained, fMRI analyses are typically done voxel by voxel, often by applying a GLM model on the data of each voxel. As far as these analyses combine information across voxels, they assume that *nearby voxels show a similar signal*. This was apparent in several analysis steps explained earlier. During preprocessing, researchers often apply spatial smoothing based on the assumption that this will increase the signal-to-noise ratio in the data. When inferring significance, researchers might use the smoothness of the data to properly control for multiple comparisons. In ROI-based analysis, a researcher would average the signal across all voxels in an ROI and use this average in further analyses. All these smoothing and averaging operations show that even voxel-wise analyses are often based on signals originating from multiple voxels, but always under the assumption that nearby voxels are similar in their response. In contrast, with MVPA researchers instead *search for differences between voxels* and whether such differences replicate across independent data points.

Apart from the nomenclature of multi-voxel pattern analyses, the same analyses are often referred to as multivariate pattern analyses to denote the fact that they involve the analysis of multiple dependent variables. The alternative approach, such as in all the examples in Chapter 7, involves univariate analyses.

8.2.1 A Schematic Tutorial of MVPA

The general approach taken with MVPA is illustrated in Figure 8.7. Consider a small schematic region of interest with nine voxels. We want to investigate whether this ROI responds differently to the presentation of two different exemplars of Tamagotchis: Kuchipatchi and Kuchitamatchi. With univariate analyses, we average the signal across all nine voxels and test whether there would be any significant difference in mean activation between these two conditions. In this schematic example, there is no difference and the ROI shows the same overall activation for

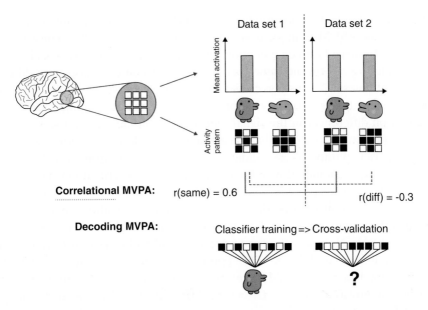

Figure 8.7 Schematic illustration of multi-voxel pattern analyses. See text for further information.
Figure inspired by Mur et al., 2009

the two Tamagotchis, both in the full dataset and when we divide the dataset in two subsets 1 and 2.

With MVPA, we investigate whether the pattern of activation across voxels is systematically different between the two conditions. The simplest approach is to take the nine values and correlate them between conditions and between datasets. We refer to this approach as **correlational MVPA**. In the schematic example, most voxels show a similar activation when Kuchipatchis are presented in dataset 1 and in dataset 2, resulting in an across-voxel correlation of 0.6. When we correlate the activation for Kuchipatchi in dataset 1 with the activation for Kuchitamatchi in dataset 2, this correlation between different conditions is much lower, -0.3. If statistical testing showed that the within-condition correlation was systematically higher than the between-condition correlation, then we could infer that the pattern of response across voxels is systematically different between the two Tamagotchis. Thus, despite the same overall activation, there is clear evidence that this region of nine voxels differentiates between Kuchipatchi and Kuchitamatchi.

Many studies use more complicated MVPA methods, which can be grouped under the label of **decoding MVPA**. In this approach, the measured across-voxel activity patterns in dataset 1 are used to train a pattern classifier on the difference between two conditions (Cox and Savoy, 2003). A pattern classifier takes multiple input dimensions, such as data coming from different voxels, and tries to find a function or decision boundary in this multidimensional input space that separates these conditions as well as possible. We have already seen a graphical example in Figure 3.5B. Many types of classifiers are used that differ in the mathematical approach used to find this decision boundary, including linear discriminants, support vector machines (SVMs), and neural networks. If there were to be a consistent and replicable difference between conditions, we would expect that this classifier would then be able to perform the same classification between conditions in a different, independent dataset 2. This is a cross-validation procedure. Cross-validation is an important step that is necessary before one can conclude that the classifier has picked up on differences in the signal that replicate in independent subsets of the data. The alternative would be that the classifier would have over-fitted noise in the training dataset. Without cross-validation, we would be confronted with problems similar to those encountered with the circular analyses described in Chapter 7.

In a simple two-class problem, chance performance would be 50%. If the classifier performance was consistently above 50% after cross-validation, then this would imply that the activity pattern in this region of nine voxels differentiates between the two Tamagotchis. Note that the use of decoding and multivariate pattern classification is not limited to MVPA. This approach is widespread in the analysis of neuroimaging data, and it could be referred to in the context of every method that involves a multivariate dataset (structural MRI, functional connectivity analyses, MEG, EEG, . . .).

Thus far, we have focused on ROI-based MVPA. This is a very powerful approach if there are valid hypotheses about the location and the size of the region where particular representations might reside. If this location is unknown a priori, then it is possible to perform MVPA at each location in the brain, each time defining a small spherical ROI at that location. This approach is known as a whole-brain searchlight analysis (Kriegeskorte, Goebel & Bandettini, 2006). The values that are obtained through this approach can be analyzed statistically in a way similar to a second-level univariate analysis (including correction for multiple comparisons). If the size of the region that would contain the representations is unknown, then the size of the searchlight spheres can be adapted. This approach still assumes that the representations are relatively local. This is not necessarily the case, as it may be that a representation would be distributed across a wide cortical region, potentially covering a whole lobe or even multiple lobes. It has been shown that in such cases both the ROI-based and the searchlight analyses are suboptimal (Bulthe, Van den Hurk, Daniels, et al., 2014). Here the best method is a multi-scale approach that combines MVPA in a large, whole-brain ROI, MVPA in smaller ROIs, and a whole-brain searchlight approach.

8.2.2 A Specific Example of MVPA

Figures 8.8–8.10 illustrate MVPA with a specific example from a relatively simple study by Op de Beeck and colleagues (2008). The study aimed to test the hypothesis that higher regions in the visual processing hierarchy would represent the shape features that human subjects rely on when they judge the shape similarity between objects. Thus, the researchers predicted a correspondence between the difference in neural response between two objects and the difference in shape as judged by human observers. This hypothesis could not be tested with univariate analyses, given that all objects tend to activate the same high-level visual region known as the lateral occipital complex (see Chapter 5). This region is defined by taking voxels that are more activated in a functional localizer by intact object images than by scrambled object images or textures (Figure 8.8B).

The study included nine conditions, each referring to a specific class of objects (Figure 8.8A). The nine conditions differed in the overall shape envelope, which is less relevant for human shape judgments, and in shape features that are very relevant for human shape judgments. The study included a block design, and data were collected from 12 subjects. In terms of univariate analyses, these nine conditions do not show differences in overall activation in the lateral occipital cortex.

Figure 8.8C illustrates the MVPA methodology. The data were divided in two datasets, one containing the odd scan runs and the other the even scan runs. The

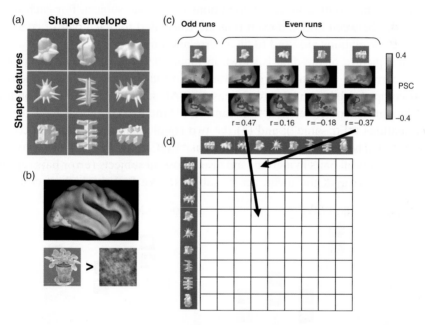

Figure 8.8 Illustration of the design and analysis approach in an MVPA fMRI study. (A) The experimental design included 9 shape conditions, which varied by 2 factors with 3 levels each: features x envelope. (B) The region of interest as defined in a single subject from the contrast of intact minus scrambled images, using a threshold of $p < 0.0001$, uncorrected for multiple comparisons. (C) Patterns of selectivity in the same subject, with selectivity expressed as the response to a particular condition minus the mean response to all conditions (all responses expressed as percent signal change). Note that these selectivity maps are not thresholded for significance and only show very weak selectivity in individual voxels. Maps are shown for one condition in odd runs and for four conditions in even runs. Below is the correlation of the odd-run selectivity map for each of the four even-run selectivity maps. (D) The correlations in (C) are used to construct a 9x9 correlation matrix that serves as the input for further analyses.
Adapted with permission from Op de Beeck et al., 2008

activity patterns per dataset were first converted into selectivity patterns by sub-tracting the mean response in a voxel across all nine conditions. The color maps represent the response relative to this mean response, with green/blue meaning less and red/yellow meaning more activation compared with the mean. The selectivity pattern is shown for one condition in the odd runs and for four conditions in the even runs. It is important to emphasize that the selectivity maps and the color scale are not thresholded for significance. In fact, none of the individual voxels shows a significant difference in response between the conditions. The power and sensitivity in MVPA reside in its ability to combine information across voxels, and the pattern of response across many voxels can be meaningful and significant even if no single voxel yields significant differences. Below the color maps we find the correlation between a particular selectivity pattern in the even runs and the shown selectivity pattern in the odd runs. The correlations range from positive when we compare the same condition between datasets, to less positive and negative. These maps and correlations show only a subset of conditions in just one subject. For each subject, correlations between odd and even runs are calculated for each pair of conditions, and these correlations are used to fill a correlation matrix (Fig 8.8D).

A fuller picture of the data is shown in Figure 8.9 (left plot). For this plot, the pairs of correlated conditions are separated into four groups: (1) The same condi-tion is compared between the two datasets ("All same"); (2) the two conditions have the same shape envelope ("Env same"); (3) the two conditions have the same shape features ("Ftr same"); and (4) the two conditions have nothing in common ("All diff."). The correlations (referred to as "LOC similarity" on the Y-axis) are averaged across all pairs in a group and also across all subjects (error bars represent the standard error of the mean across subjects). We find the highest correlation

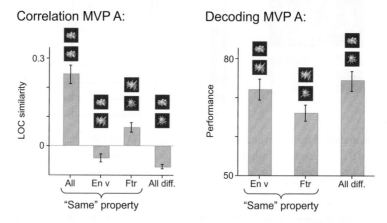

Figure 8.9 MVPA results obtained through correlational MVPA (*left*) and decoding MVPA (*right*). The MVPA measure of (dis)similarity is shown as a function of the difference between stimulus conditions: all shape factors the same (All same), same shape envelope (Env same), same shape features (Ftr same), and all shape factors different (All diff.).

Adapted with permission from Op de Beeck et al., 2008

when we compare the same condition in the two datasets, which is the primary evidence that there is a reproducible selectivity pattern associated with each condition. The other conditions also show consistent differences among them, and these differences provide evidence that some conditions are more similar to each other than others. The highest correlation is found when two conditions share shape features, implying that such conditions are most similar in their selectivity pattern. Note that this result confirms the prediction of the researchers, given that those shape features are also very important for human observers who judge objects that share the same feature to be very similar.

The right plot in Figure 8.9 shows that a very similar result is obtained with decoding MVPA using a classifier known as a support vector machine. We expect that a classifier will show a lower cross-validation performance when two conditions are very similar in terms of fMRI selectivity pattern. Therefore, we expect the reverse pattern as with correlational MVPA: Higher similarity means a higher correlation in correlational MVPA, which corresponds to a lower performance of a classifier. This is indeed what we see when we compare the left and the right plot in Figure 8.9. For many questions, correlational MVPA and decoding MVPA provide complementary results.

8.2.3 The Potential of MVPA to Move beyond Neophrenology

The example in the previous section illustrates two marked benefits of MVPA. First, MVPA often provides sensitivity to detect differences between conditions that cannot be differentiated with univariate analyses. Second, MVPA provides a graded measure of the size of the differences in across-voxel activity patterns.

Because of these two advantages, MVPA studies illustrate the power of fMRI to be more than a new sort of phrenology. Take, for example, a cognitive scientist who is interested in how humans represent objects. She would not be very interested by the finding of Malach and colleagues (1995) that there is a region in the brain that shows a preference for object images over texture patterns. The scientist would want to know how this region represents objects and whether this object representation at the neural level would show characteristics that are predicted by cognitive models of object representations. The univariate analyses give an indication about *where* these representations might be located in the brain, but MVPA is very helpful in investigating *what* the properties are of these representations.

The example of Op de Beeck and colleagues (2008) is just one of the many studies in the literature that have gone beyond localization by using the ability of MVPA to discriminate between stimuli of the same kind – in our example, among different objects. Cognitive models of object recognition make specific predictions about which objects should be represented similarly, and which not. These predictions can be tested once we can differentiate among different objects.

Figure 8.10 illustrates this mapping between the sort of data a behavioral scientist would be interested in and the results from MVPA. The behavioral scientist might

Perceived shape   **Neural shape (LOC)**   **Deep shape (GoogLeNet)**

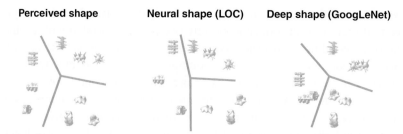

Figure 8.10 Shape representations derived from human similarity judgments (perceived shape), MVPA (neural shape), and artificial "deep" neural networks (deep shape). The plots are constructed by applying multidimensional scaling to a (dis)similarity matrix.
The left and right panels are adapted from Kubilius et al., 2016, and the middle panel is based on the data of Op de Beeck et al., 2008

ask human observers to rate the similarity among objects and apply a similarity analysis technique such as multidimensional scaling (MDS) to the resulting similarity matrix to get an insight about the dimensions that underlie these human judgments. The results from MDS are shown on the left of Figure 8.10 in a two-dimensional space. Stimuli that are judged to be similar are presented near each other. When we inspect this diagram visually, we notice that objects that have the same shape features (the rows from Fig. 8.8) are close to each other in this behavior-based MDS space. From this result, the behavioral scientist would conclude that these shape features play an important role in the shape representations of human observers.

The (cognitive/behavioral) neuroscientist can test this prediction by starting from the results of MVPA. Correlational MVPA gives us a matrix of correlations in multi-voxel patterns among all pairs of stimuli. These correlations are an index of similarity at the neural level, just as the human judgments were a measure of similarity at the behavioral level. Thus, this correlation matrix can also be analyzed through the technique of MDS, resulting in the plot shown in the middle of Figure 8.10. Interestingly, objects with the same shape feature also tend to be near each other in this neural MDS space. The comparison of the behavior-based and the neural MDS space provides an important test for the models and predictions of the behavioral scientist, going far beyond simple localization.

Apart from allowing a direct comparison of neural data with behavioral data, the same principles can be applied to data from many different sources. For example, a similarity matrix and an MDS space can also be constructed from the responses of mathematical units in an artificial neural network, such as the deep neural network of Google (Figure 8.10, right panel; see Kubilius et al., 2016). As emphasized by Kriegeskorte, Mur and Bandettini (2008), this is made possible because the comparisons are made at the level of similarity matrices, which have the same format no matter the format of the input data (behavioral judgments, voxel responses, computer models, ...). These authors called this approach **representational similarity analysis (RSA)**.

The advent of MVPA and RSA have affected the design of experiments. Given the high sensitivity of these methods and the benefits of similarity-based methods when a sufficient number of conditions are compared, MVPA/RSA studies typically include many more conditions than one would expect based on our introduction of experimental designs in Chapter 5. Figure 8.11 illustrates the first and most famous application of such a **condition-rich design**, in which 92 conditions were included (Kriegeskorte, Mur, Ruff, et al., 2008). Given that more conditions lead to less repetitions per condition (when holding scan time constant), one would expect that the signal in each condition would be measured with much less reliability. Still, MVPA and RSA are often able to provide meaningful results with such designs, in particular in cases in which some of the conditions would already be differentiable through univariate analyses. This is the case in this particular example, given that the stimulus set includes exemplars from conditions such as faces, body parts, and other objects.

The correlation matrix (left) and the MDS space (right) illustrate that for this stimulus set there is a dominant dimension related to whether a stimulus is an animate object (faces, bodies, animals) or not. This finding confirms predictions from long-standing cognitive, neuropsychological, and connectionist models of object recognition.

8.2.4 What Do We Measure with MVPA?

Multi-voxel pattern analysis has repeatedly been shown to pick up differences between conditions that cannot be differentiated by univariate analyses. With univariate analyses, it is conventional wisdom that the sensitivity of fMRI is limited by the spatial resolution of the underlying signal. Given that the hemodynamic response at 3T field strength is typically spread out over millimeters of cortex, we do not have access to signals that have a higher spatial resolution. With multi-voxel analyses, there is more controversy about the spatial specificity of the signals. The most conservative hypothesis would be that MVPA is limited by the same spatial resolution (Op de Beeck, 2010). After all, it is based on the same BOLD signal as univariate analyses. Whether or not we make this assumption might have effects on how we analyze the data. In particular, under this hypothesis, and referring back to the Matched Filter theorem, it would make sense to include a spatial smoothing step during preprocessing.

However, there is another hypothesis, sometimes referred to as **hyperacuity** (Op de Beeck, 2010), which suggests that MVPA might give the researcher access to a finer scale of spatial organization (Haynes and Rees, 2005; Kamitani and Tong, 2005). If true, then spatial smoothing would hurt the ability to pick up these signals. The rationale behind this hypothesis is illustrated in Figure 8.12. A well-known organization in the primary visual cortex is shown in Figure 8.12A, where neurons with a preference for lines with a similar orientation are clustered in so-called orientation columns. This organization happens at such a fine scale that a typical

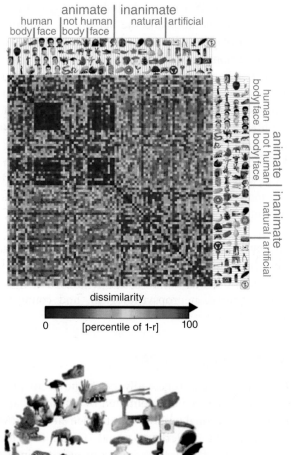

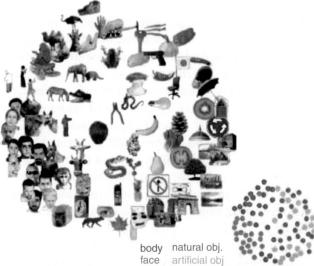

Figure 8.11 Results from a condition-rich fMRI experiment with 92 stimulus conditions. The spatial configuration at the bottom is obtained by applying MDS to the (dis)similarity matrix in the top panel.

Figures reproduced with permission from Kriegeskorte, Mur, Ruff, et al., 2008

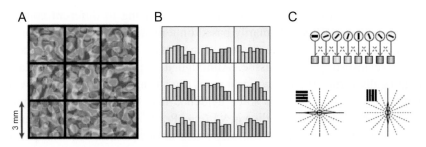

Figure 8.12 The principle of hyperacuity. (A) Orientation columns visualized through invasive optical imaging. The color scale represents the preferred orientation at each location in the map. The 3x3 grid shows a typical sampling resolution of fMRI, with a voxel size of 3x3x3 mm. (B) Response to the different orientations per voxel or grid cell, with responses derived from the map in (A). (C) Classification performance of a classifier trained on the pattern of response across multiple voxels with weak orientation selectivity. The polar plots illustrate the decisions made by the classifier for trials with a horizontal orientation (*left*) or vertical orientation (*right*). The radial dimension in the plots reflects the combination of orientation and direction of motion, so that the same orientation moving in an opposite direction is represented 180° apart. The distance from the center of the plot reflects how often a particular classification decision was made. Almost all trials are classified correctly, namely, as horizontal and as vertical trials in the left and right polar plots, respectively.
Figure adapted from Haynes and Rees, 2006

fMRI voxel of 3x3x3 mm would contain many such orientation columns, and as such the clear selectivity of individual columns would be averaged away at the level of a voxel. This is shown in Figure 8.12B, where very little selectivity can be seen for differences in orientation. Individual voxels would not show enough selectivity to indicate which orientation would be shown in which trial. However, in combination, many such voxels provide much more information. Figure 8.12C shows what happens when the fMRI signal in all these voxels is given as input to a pattern classifier (i.e., a neural network), and this classifier is trained and cross-validated in the task of differentiating between different orientations. When the classifier is trained to discriminate a vertical from other orientations, it only classifies a vertical orientation as "vertical" and makes almost no mistakes for other orientations. The classifier output is very selective. Based on this rationale, it seems theoretically possible to detect signals from a functional organization that is at such a small scale that very little selectivity is left at the voxel level.

Given these theoretical considerations, we need to ask, What does the fMRI signal and the outcome of MVPA reflect in practice: large-scale or small-scale patterns of selectivity? One approach to investigate this question is to spatially smooth the fMRI data and see whether such smoothing deteriorates the outcome of MVPA. If so, then MVPA is most likely based on relatively fine-scale signals that are weakened by smoothing. In the first test of this prediction, the opposite pattern of results was observed (Op de Beeck, 2010). Smoothing tends to increase the correlation among multi-voxel patterns belonging to the same orientation condition (and decrease the correlation among patterns belonging to different conditions). This suggests that MVPA is primarily based on a relatively large scale of organization that survives some degree of smoothing. After this first test, several other studies have investigated this issue. Although it is theoretically understandable and empirically verified that large-scale maps can strongly determine MVPA results (Freeman et al., 2011), there is some evidence that hyperacuity can be partially responsible for orientation decoding in V1 (e.g., Pratte et al., 2016). Representations in other brain regions might be coarser, which illustrates how the best parameter settings (in this case, voxel size and spatial smoothing) might depend on the question and region of interest (Coutanche et al., 2016).

Independently from the issue of hyperacuity, MVPA as an fMRI-based method will always depend on the presence of a clear mapping/organization/clustering. If a region contains neurons that are very selective for a certain stimulus property, but neurons with a similar preference are not clustered together, then this lack of a spatial organization would result in no sensitivity in MVPA. Thus, lack of MVPA sensitivity does not imply lack of neural selectivity. A recent example of a dissociation between single-neuron selectivity and MVPA sensitivity can be found in a paper by Dubois and colleagues (2015), who showed a lack of MVPA sensitivity in a face-selective region in which the single neurons were very selective.

When MVPA shows a positive finding, there are other interpretational problems. A positive finding indicates that there is information in the multi-voxel patterns about the stimulus/task conditions in the experiment. However, by itself this finding does not tell us what this information is about, and further tests or even experiments might be needed to shed light on this issue. The problem is related to the distinction between forward and reverse inference (Chapter 7) and the need to have conditions that differ in only one cognitive process (Chapter 5). Suppose we have results from a condition-rich experiment such as is shown in Figure 8.11. The stimuli in this experiment vary on many dimensions, including shape, color, and semantic associations. Several dimensions are correlated with each other, for example, stimuli from different semantic categories are also different in their shape. How can we find out which dimensions explain the findings? To this end, researchers perform specific comparisons to find out to what extent the results can be explained by each of these dimensions. For example, they can compute a similarity matrix based on some sort of shape metric and see to what extent this metric can explain the findings. In addition, authors can design further experiments in which multiple dimensions are more clearly controlled and/or dissociated (for further discussion, see Bracci et al., 2017).

In addition, the fact that a classifier "finds" information does not by itself prove that the brain uses this information (de-Wit et al., 2016). We will illustrate this with a specific example. Williams and colleagues (2007) showed their participants object images for only a few tens of milliseconds, followed by a masking pattern. They found that multi-voxel patterns in both V1 and object-selective area LOC differentiated objects. However, only in the LOC was the pattern stronger for correct than

Box 8.1 From Group Studies to Individual Diagnostics Using Advanced Methods

Functional imaging studies often compare different groups of subjects. In Chapter 3, we mentioned some caveats about the typical effect size in anatomical imaging and the consequence for making inferences at the level of individual subjects. We used the measure for effect size known as Cohen's *d*, and related the typical effect size in research studies to how much information the anatomy would provide about to which group a particular individual would belong. It turned out that typical effect sizes do not provide much confidence about what is going on at the individual level. Sometimes we can say with 70% accuracy to which group a participant belongs; often, however, the accuracy is even lower.

This reasoning also applies to functional imaging, whether hemodynamic or electrophysiological, and independently of the degree of sophistication of the analysis. To take one example, Kassraian-Fard and colleagues (2016) applied various classifiers of the type frequently used in MVPA, but in this case the classifiers were trained on a large resting-state dataset. The task was to distinguish between individuals with and without the diagnosis of autism. The achieved accuracy of the classifiers was about 60–70%. From the perspective of fundamental neuroscience, this accuracy is more than sufficient to learn something about the neural basis of autism by studying which features the classifier uses to achieve this performance.

However, an accuracy of 60–70% is not sufficient to use the classifiers for individual diagnostics. There are numerous functional imaging studies on a wide range of mental disorders, such as depression, schizophrenia, autism, ADHD, and many of these studies have been very successful in identifying various neural changes associated with these disorders at the group level. Despite these successes, functional imaging is not used to diagnose these disorders at the individual level. Type "autism fMRI" in the freely accessible search engine of the scientific literature at http://scholar.google.be/, and you get hundreds of studies, most of which document significant differences, and many of which are cited hundreds of time. Nevertheless, we cannot put a child in an MRI scanner and use the functional or anatomical images to help diagnose the child with autism. Psychiatrists know not to jump to conclusions based on imaging results. However, the careless extrapolation toward the individual level is one of the primary mistakes made when human imaging results are broadcasted widely in the popular media, as was the case in several of the examples in Chapter 1. It remains to be seen whether this limitation can be remediated by further progress.

Progress can result from even better and more sensitive measurements, as well as from advanced analysis methods that can capture the full information contained in the multivariate signals such as MVPA. An example of the latter is provided in Chapter 3 in the context of structural imaging of the neural correlates of sex. However, for now, we have to live with the fact that noninvasive, and thus coarse, imaging of a complex system such as the brain does not provide the level of detail needed for sufficiently sensitive and specific prediction at the level of individual participants.

for incorrectly recognized objects. Thus, not all multi-voxel patterns seem to be related to and read out during task performance.

In sum, despite the widespread use of MVPA in the recent fMRI literature, questions remain about the spatial scale of the underlying signals, their relationship to neuronal selectivity (e.g., in the case of null findings), the interpretation of the results in the sense of implicated cognitive processes and relevance for neural information processing and the potential for diagnostics (see Box 8.1).

8.3 Functional MRI Adaptation

In addition to MVPA, there is another approach used to measure neural selectivity and overcome the limitations imposed by the spatial resolution of fMRI. This alternative approach does *not* depend on clustering of response properties and thus provides a way to pick up neural selectivity even in cases where neuronal populations with different preferences are spatially intermingled. This alternative approach is known as fMRI adaptation (Grill-Spector and Malach, 2001).

Functional MRI adaptation infers neural selectivity from the extent to which neural responses depend on whether successive stimuli are the same or not. Typically, the neural responses for each individual stimulus event decreases when one and the same stimulus is repeated over and over again. This response "suppression" is not seen or is not as clear when a different stimulus is presented. The difference between a repeat stimulus and a different stimulus is the basic measure of fMRI adaptation. It is taken as a measure of selectivity of neurons in a voxel based on the assumption that the difference in response only appears in neurons that are selective to the difference between the two stimuli. The amount of fMRI adaptation in a particular voxel will depend on (1) the proportion of neurons in that voxel that are selective to the stimulus difference, and (2) how selective the individual neurons are to the difference.

Figure 8.13 illustrates the rationale of fMRI adaptation with an experiment including our two Tamagotchis, Kuchipatchi (green) and Kuchitamatchi (orange). In each panel, the first stimulus is green, as such activating neurons prefer the green stimulus. Neurons that prefer the orange are not activated. In Figure 8.13A, the second stimulus is the orange Kuchitamatchi, thus a different stimulus compared with the first. Now the orange neurons are responding heavily to this preferred stimulus, which results in a strong BOLD response that matches the response to the first stimulus. At the voxel level, the two stimuli would evoke the same overall response. In Figure 8.13B, the second stimulus is the same as the first, the green Kuchipatchi. This stimulus again activates the green neurons, but less so compared with the first stimulus because of adaptation. As a result, the overall fMRI activation is reduced. By comparing the responses in the two situations, fMRI adaptation allows us to measure stimulus selectivity even though the voxel as a whole shows the same overall response to the two stimuli when presented in isolation.

Functional MRI adaptation is a direct measure of a voxel's sensitivity to temporal changes in the stimuli. Typically, researchers who use fMRI adaptation want to

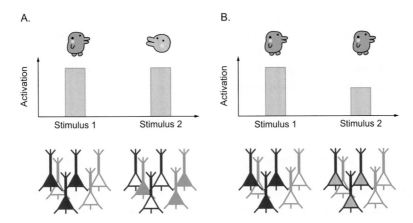

Figure 8.13 Functional MRI adaptation as a method used to detect neuronal selectivity. The illustrated case is a design with two stimuli per trial: (A) shows a trial with two different stimuli, while (B) represents a trial with a repetition of a stimulus. The top graphs illustrate the overall activation at the voxel level. The bottom images show two subpopulations of neurons within the voxel, one set of neurons that responds most strongly to the green Kuchipatchi (neurons colored in green), and another set of neurons that prefers the orange Kuchitamatchi (neurons in orange). Neurons that are not responding to a stimulus are shown with a white cell body; responsive neurons are colored to a degree that reflects the strength of their response.
The figure is adapted with permission from Krekelberg et al., 2006

make a further inference, based on the reasoning above, and use this sensitivity for temporal statistics to infer the overall single-unit selectivity in a region. It is import-ant to keep in mind that fMRI adaptation is at best an indirect measure of such single-unit selectivity. There are several factors that might influence the sensitivity to temporal changes in a different way compared with single-unit selectivity. Each possible dissociation between temporal sensitivity and single-unit selectivity limits the possible use of fMRI adaptation as a measure of single-unit selectivity.

Studies using monkey electrophysiology have illustrated such dissociations. For example, Sawamura and colleagues (2006) have shown that some neurons can have the same response to two different stimuli, A and B, thus not revealing any single-neuron selectivity, but still showing release from adaptation when a repetition of A (or B) is interrupted by the other stimulus.

Summerfield and colleagues (2008) provide another example. The authors pre-sented trials with two face stimuli that typically elicit adaptation when the same face is repeated in the trial (repeat trials) and release from adaptation when a different face is shown (non-repeat trials). They found this expected adaptation and release from adaptation when repeat trials were relatively frequent (the so-called repeat blocks that contained a high proportion of repeat trials). However, their study also included non-repeat blocks in which repeat trials were rare and thus unexpected or "surprising." In the non-repeat blocks, there was a much smaller difference in fMRI signal between repeat trials and non-repeat trials. Thus, the size of the adaptation effect depended on the proportion of repeat trials. Given that the underlying single-neuron selectivity for the differences between faces would probably not be different between the two block types, this study shows another dissociation between the sensitivity for temporal statistics and single-neuron selectivity.

Summary

- This chapter introduced several more advanced analysis methods that allow the use of fMRI to investigate not only where different psychological processes are localized, but also how the identified regions interact, as well as, to a certain extent, the properties of the representations within these regions.
- The study of functional connectivity provides the opportunity to study how brain regions interact and form networks.
- We have introduced two approaches to measure neural selectivity, MVPA and fMRI adaptation. Each approach depends on particular assumptions and each has its own weaknesses, but together they give fMRI the potential to be highly relevant for testing models of cognition and mental functioning.

Review Questions

1. Give an overview of analysis approaches that can be applied to data from an RS fMRI scan.
2. A researcher has found a positive correlation across time between the fMRI signal in the lateral occipital cortex and in the intraparietal sulcus. To what extent does this finding prove that there is a direct connection between these two brain regions? Why?
3. How is it possible to obtain reliable results with condition-rich designs even though the number of time points measured for each condition is too low for detecting any significant differences in a voxel-wise analysis?

Further Reading

Haxby, J. V., Connolly, A. C. & Guntupalli, J. S. (2014). Decoding neural representational spaces using multivariate pattern analysis. *Annual Review of Neuroscience*, **37**, 435–456.

Pereira, F., Mitchell, T. & Botvinick, M. (2009). Machine learning classifiers and fMRI: a tutorial overview. *Neuroimage*, **45**(1), S199–S209. (This paper provides a short tutorial in how to apply pattern classifiers and decoding to fMRI data.)

Van Den Heuvel, M. P. & Pol, H. E. H. (2010). Exploring the brain network: a review on resting-state fMRI functional connectivity. *European Neuropsychopharmacology*, **20**(8), 519–534. (This paper provides an overview of the analysis of functional connectivity in resting-state fMRI.)

PART III
Electrophysiological Neuroimaging

[For an electric stimulation experiment] I dissected and prepared a frog. I placed it on a table where the electric machine [a hand-cranked generator] was placed. . . . The conducting wires of the machine were not in contact with, but distanced from the frog. By accident, one of my assistants touched the internal crural nerves of the frog lightly with the tip of a surgical knife. Suddenly, all the muscles of the limbs contracted convulsively as if they were touched by the worst toxin. . . . Another assistant of mine reported that the phenomenon seemed to happen when the conducting wires sparked. . . . I was completely engrossed by this new phenomenon. Incredible desire was burning me; I just wanted to repeat the experience, and to bring what is hidden into light.

Luigi Galvani, 1791

A translated excerpt from *De viribus electricitatis in motu musculari commentarius.* (The original Latin text is available at https://archive.org/stream/ AloysiiGalvaniD00Galv#page/4/mode/2up.)

Volt, ampere, ohm . . . Units of electricity feature the names of pioneers of the late eighteenth and nineteenth centuries when an understanding of the physics of electricity was developing. On the cusp of this, Italian physician/physicist/anatomist Luigi Aloisio Galvani was studying the relationship between electricity and a physiological phenomenon, the contraction of the leg muscles of frogs. Through a series of experiments, he concluded that "animal electricity," which was considered a specific type of electricity generated and stored in the muscle, caused the contraction. His study inspired many others, including Alessandro Giuseppe Antonio Anastasio Volta, an Italian physicist. Volta challenged Galvani's claim of animal electricity. He invented a battery that generates electricity via a chemical reaction and showed that non-animal electricity also contracted the muscles. His work showed that electricity, regardless of how it is generated, caused the contraction. With this and other work, Volta established research methods for electrostatic capacity. For this, the unit of electric potential was named for him.

Parallel to the emergence of electrophysiology, in the Romantic era, a somewhat mystical view of electricity – energetic presence without a concrete shape – was often related to *psyche*, a philosophical notion of what makes us animated and willful. Over the centuries, however, no scientific relationship was confirmed between electricity and psyche. Instead, we've learned that what makes us the way we are is related to brain activity, which is, in large part, electric. This is the basis of electrophysiological brain imaging, the topic of Part III of this book.

PART III
Electrophysiological Neuroimaging

CHAPTER NINE

Electromagnetic Field of the Brain

Learning Objectives

- Explaining the relationship between neural activity in the brain and electromagnetic field signals from the brain
- Explaining the advantages and disadvantages of the different noninvasive methods for measuring electrophysiological signals
- Explaining the dynamic approach to the mind-brain problem

As a result of physiological activity, electrical activity can be observed in cells, tissues, and organs. This activity, known as electrophysiological activity, particularly characterizes the brain. It reflects the brain's condition, for instance, its health, but it does more than that; it also correlates with various psychological processes, such as perception, memory, and emotion, and with states of consciousness. This is why the electrophysiological activity of the brain is of interest not only to medical, biological, and behavioral scientists and professionals, but is also a source of fascination to philosophers, artists, educators, students, and the general public.

The first electrophysiological brain signal was reported in 1875 by Richard Caton, a British physiologist, from electrodes placed on the cortical surface in a rabbit and monkey (Caton, 1875). Vladimir Pravdich-Neminsky, a Ukrainian and then Soviet physiologist, reported in 1913 how he recorded brain activity from electrodes placed on the skull of a dog (Pravdich-Neminsky, 1913). The first electrophysiological brain signals recorded from electrodes on the scalp of human participants were reported by Hans Berger in 1929 (Berger, 1929). Berger, a German psychiatrist and psychophysicist, was driven by a passion to understand the relationship between mind and brain throughout his career. His biography reports a bizarre but critical incident in 1892, when he was 19 years old (Millett, 2001). At that point, Berger was in the military in Würzberg, on horseback pulling heavy artillery for a military exercise. Suddenly, his horse reared, and he fell in front of the artillery. The artillery was stopped literally inches away from him. At about the same time, Berger's older sister in Coburg, more than 100 km away from Würzberg, was struck by an inexplicable sense of terror. She was convinced that the experience was linked to her younger brother's safety and urged her family to inquire about his well-being. The family sent a telegram. Berger received it but considered it a peculiar coincidence. Later, he learned the whole story, which

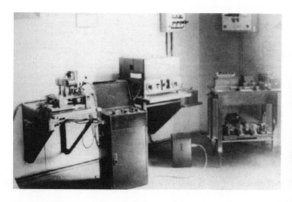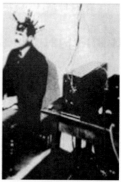

Figure 9.1 Hans Berger's EEG system.
A test participant wears scalp electrodes. Electrodes were carbon cylinders filled with saline to increase conductivity between the scalp and the electrodes. The induced current was measured by a string galvanometer, which was invented by Clément Ader in 1897 and improved by Willem Einthoven, who used it to record electrocardiograms in 1901.
Images are reproduced from Gloor, 1969, with permission

fascinated him enough to study the physical basis of psychological phenomena, including those that are somewhat mysterious.

Berger used noninvasive electrophysiological methods that had been successful in measuring cardiac activities to measure brain activity. The electrophysiological brain signals are much weaker than cardiac signals; thus, he struggled for a long time to obtain a reliable signal from the brain. In his first report in 1929, he documented two patterns – alpha waves, which are characterized by slow, high-in-amplitude oscillation, and beta waves, which are characterized by fast, low-in-amplitude activity. Moreover, he suggested that alpha waves are associated with "conscious phenomena," while beta waves reflect metabolic activity. Today, we know that beta activity also relates to conscious phenomena, e.g., planning and execution of body motion. Somewhat ironically, Berger's investigation clearly showed that electrophysiological brain activity cannot be a basis of "telepathic" communication. The signal is so weak that it is measurable only via sensors closely attached to the scalp (Fig. 9.1) – there is no way it could have traveled between Würzberg and Coburg! Nevertheless, the first scalp recording of brain activity – the **electroencephalogram (EEG)** – is a monumental event, since it broke the era of noninvasive brain function research.

9.1 Electrophysiological Activity of the Brain

9.1.1 From Neurons to Electric Field

The brain consists of neurons, glias, blood vessels, and fluids. Of these, the neurons are the main generator of electrophysiological activity. As explained in Chapter 1, action potentials, also known as "spikes," are generated near the soma, conducted on the axon, and transferred to the next neuron via the synapse. Depending on the type of presynaptic neuron, an excitatory or inhibitory **postsynaptic potential** (PSPs, EPSP and IPSP) is generated in the dendrite of the postsynaptic neuron. To record these membrane potentials of individual neurons, electrodes need to be placed in, on, or at least near the neurons. This means that an invasive procedure, such as penetrating needle electrodes into the cortex, is necessary. The application of an invasive method in humans, however, is allowed only in special cases, such as in patients who undergo brain surgery. While inserting the electrode, healthy brain tissue is inevitably damaged. Therefore, a method that measures brain activity from outside of the brain is beneficial. For nonmedical purposes, the electrode should not invade the test participants' body – the closest place for the electrode/sensors to be attached is the scalp.

The scalp electrodes, therefore, do not measure membrane potentials. Instead, the electrodes measure a physical consequence of the membrane potentials. As membrane potentials change, a weak current flows in the neuron and extracellular space. The current is further conducted in the brain tissue, and an electric field is generated. The dynamics of the field can be understood intuitively, assuming a vector that lies in the direction of the current. For example, currents that run in opposite directions cancel each other out. Each action potentially generates two opposing fields (Fig. 9.2A). Thus, the field is cancelled out no matter how many spikes are generated. Each postsynaptic potential, to the contrary, generates one field. The EPSPs and IPSPs counter each other, but they do not occur at the same synapse simultaneously. Moreover, the duration of the PSPs is long (~10 ms) relative to that of action potentials (~1 ms), which is also advantageous for the integration of the field over multiple PSPs (Nunez, 1977).

The electric field due to PSPs at one synapse is very weak. Here the structure of the cortex helps to integrate them. The pyramidal neurons have long apical dendrites that run more or less perpendicular to the cortical surface. The field of the PSPs, thus, can be considered as a vector that lies along the dendrite, changing its strength and directions constantly based on the balance between EPSPs and IPSPs. The apical dendrites of neighboring pyramidal neurons run parallel to each other; thus, the vectors are integrated in a larger field (Fig. 9.2B). The integrated field over tens of thousands of apical dendrites is strong enough to be detected by sensors placed outside of the brain. The field is represented as a dipole, which models the field as a vector (Fig. 9.2C).

Other types of neurons (e.g., basket and chandelier cells) also generate postsynaptic currents and hence could contribute to the electric field. However, their dendrites do not run in parallel as do the apical dendrite of the pyramidal cells. Thus, their currents do not integrate to form a strong field. For the same reason, synaptic currents that run through the synaptic cleft do not form a strong field. Therefore, electrophysiological signals obtained noninvasively largely reflect the postsynaptic activity of the cortical pyramidal neurons.

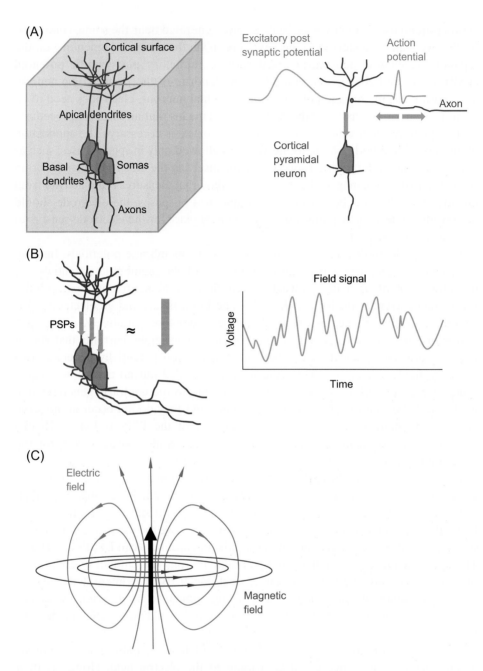

Figure 9.2 Electromagnetic field due to membrane potentials of neurons.
(A) Cortical pyramidal cells have long apical dendrites. Chemical synapse activity generates a postsynaptic potential in the dendrites. Excitatory synapse activity increases the potential (EPSP), while inhibitory synapse activity decreases it (IPSP). The PSPs integrate over time and space and generate an electromagnetic field. The synaptic activities are triggered by action potentials from other neurons.

Electrophysiological methods give various "scales" of brain signals. As discussed in Chapter 1, invasive methods, such as the patch clamp, are able to give membrane potentials from a single neuron, whereas noninvasive methods reflect the field activity of a large number of neurons. It is important to keep in mind the scale of the neural substrate for each electrophysiological signal.

9.1.2 Magnetic Field of the Neural Activity

The electrophysiological activity of a neural population generates not only an electric field but also a magnetic field. Magnetism is typically illustrated as the force that attracts or repels an object without contact. For example, two magnets facing opposite poles, N vs. S, attract, while those facing the same poles, either N vs. N, or S vs. S, repel each other. If we push the repelling magnets toward each other, resistance increases as they get closer. We see nothing between the magnets; nonetheless, we can sense the gradient of force – the magnetic field – between them. Magnetic phenomena have been known worldwide since ancient times – e.g., China, India, and Greece – and scientists in these ancient civilizations had their own descriptions of and accounts for the phenomena. For example, Plutarch wrote in 1005 BC that a magnet affects others via a tiny amount of air puffed from small holes on the surface, although this might sound absurd to us today. In his defense, we should note that Plutarch arrived at this mechanical account to refute supernatural forces, which were at the time proposed as alternatives (Yamamoto, 2003). For a long time, magnetism was studied without an explicit link to electricity – although sailors knew that a compass point is affected by thunder. The relationship between them was not understood until two British physicists, Michael Faraday and James Clerk Maxwell, established classic electromagnetism in the nineteenth century. According to electromagnetic theory, a magnetic field appears where charged particles, such as electrons, move. Electrons move as currents flow. Likewise, electrons move as neural currents flow. Therefore, a magnetic field is formed during brain activity, together with an electric field. The two fields per neural current can be imagined without confusion; they are perpendicular to each other (Fig. 9.2C). Together, they are referred to as the **electromagnetic field**.

The magnetic field is not only an interesting theoretical construct, but also quite a useful property for brain research. The magnetic field changes its strength and

---

Caption for Figure 9.2 (*cont.*) Each action potential generates two fields which cancel each other out. Thus, they contribute little to the electromagnetic field.

(B) The apical dendrites extend perpendicular to cortical layers. Postsynaptic potentials over the mass of the neurons (small arrows) are summed up (large arrows). The integrated field activity is strong enough to be recorded from the sensors outside of the brain. The integrated field is modeled as a dipole.

(C) An Illustration of the electromagnetic field: The electric field is formed as the PSPs conduct the dendrite and brain tissue. The magnetic field forms perpendicular to the currents. The field is modelled as a dipole (black arrow).

direction because of the integrated postsynaptic current, similar to the electric field. Unlike the electric field, however, the magnetic field is affected very little by brain tissue, cerebrospinal fluid, skull, scalp, or air. This high permeability allows us to measure the magnetic field activity without contacting the scalp. As we will see in Chapter 10, sensors for **magnetoencephalography (MEG)** are not attached to the scalp, unlike EEG – a test participant simply puts the head under a sensor helmet.

The magnetic field, which MEG measures, is generated by the electrophysiological brain activity. This field should not be confused with the field in MRI methods, which is generated by strong superconducting magnets. In other words, MEG does not, in contrast to magnetic resonance imaging (MRI), expose test participants to an artificial high-intensity magnetic field. Taken together with remote sensing capability, MEG is considered the least invasive brain imaging method.

9.1.3 From the Field to Sensors

Electrophysiological activity in the cortex generates an electromagnetic field that is measurable noninvasively. Signals travel between the source and the sensor. Gross anatomy of the cortex therefore affects the signal at the sensor. The cortical sheet is folded to fit into the cranium. The folding creates gyri and sulci. As a consequence, sources are arranged in various depths and orientations with respect to the sensors on the scalp. The deeper a source is, the weaker the signal becomes. Thus, activities from deep cortices (e.g., ventral and medial parts of neocortex) are under-represented in the signal relative to those from shallow areas (e.g., dorsal and lateral parts of the neocortex).

Signals from equally shallow sources could also be recorded differently. Sensitivity of the sensors varies relative to the orientation of the source current; the sensors are arranged along the scalp facing the brain. The postsynaptic current runs perpendicular to the sensors in the gyrus, whereas it runs in parallel to the sensors in the sulcus. For example, MEG sensors have higher sensitivity to the sulcus than to gyrus activity. Thus, the recorded activity contains more sulcus than gyrus activity. That is, the recorded signal is the weighted sum of source activities. The orientation sensitivity of the EEG electrode is opposite to that of MEG sensors. However, the effect of orientation is less severe in EEG than in MEG because electric signals from the gyrus and sulcus mix as they conduct. As a result, EEG sensor signals contain a good amount of both signals (cf. Section 10.3 in Chapter 10).

The electromagnetic field is the physical basis of M/EEG methods. It makes not only measurement but also modulation of neural activity possible (Box 9.1 and Chapter 14).

9.2 Electromagnetic Field Signals

The M/EEG methods sample the electromagnetic field activity in time and space. Figure 9.3 is an example of the signal, in this case, from EEG. The signal

---

Box 9.1 From the Field to Neurons

We have learned how electrophysiological activity of the brain leads to the electromagnetic field, which we can measure noninvasively. Now, let us consider the opposite: If we generate an electromagnetic field just outside of the brain, would it affect the electrophysiological activity? Yes, indeed. An artificially generated electromagnetic field has been used to bias electrophysiological activity of the brain. For example, transcranial direct current stimulation (tDCS) and transcranial alternating current stimulation (tACS) conduct electric current from scalp electrodes, and transcranial magnetic stimulation (TMS) applies a magnetic pulse from a stimulation coil placed on the scalp to the brain: A current running through the TMS coil generates a strong electromagnetic field that biases activity of cortical neurons. These methods are explained in more detail in Chapter 14.

As for the effects of spontaneous field activity on individual neuronal activity, we enter a topic that is still under debate. The neurons are immersed in ionic fluid (cerebrospinal fluid) with incomplete electric isolation. Glial cells play an important role in the insulation. Some increase insulation (e.g., Schwann cells that form myelin sheath on axons), while others decrease insulation (e.g., astrocytes that form gap junctions that are electric connections among neurons). Thus, it is theoretically possible that the spontaneous field activity would have some effect on electrophysiological activity of the individual neurons. It has been reported that field activity synchronizes spiking timing (Fries et al., 2001). Further investigation is currently under way.

---

is smooth but irregular compared with action potentials of a single neuron, which is a train of neat spikes. The smooth and irregular oscillatory behavior characterizes the field signal. The signal carries rich information about the underlying neural system, which consists of various types of neurons. Suppose a simple system is formed by mutually connected excitatory and inhibitory neuron populations. Stimulation of the excitatory neurons starts the system. The excitatory neurons then excite the inhibitory neurons, and the inhibitory neurons inhibit excitatory neurons. The activity of the system increases and decreases as long as we keep the stimulation. The field signals largely reflect dendritic activity of the pyramidal neurons, which are excitatory. However, as indicated in the model, the signal also reflects activity of the inhibitory population in a more indirect way through the effect of inhibition on the activity of excitatory neurons. From the field signals, we could estimate the dynamics of the neural system. This is only a very simple system, and many other complexities have to be added for a biologically plausible system, for example, more populations could be involved, and responses could have a delay. The resulting field signal is complex because it reflects the activity of a system that contains many neural oscillations (Lopes da Silva and Storm van Leeuwen, 1977).

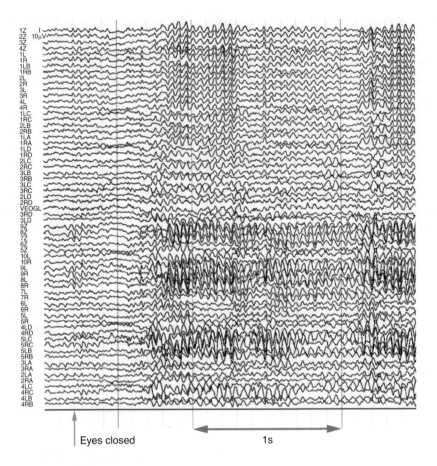

Figure 9.3 Human EEG.

EEG was recorded for 65 channels covering the whole head. Each line represents the EEG signal from an electrode. The participant, a healthy adult, was comfortably seated and relaxed. When the eyes were closed, periods with large and slow activity appeared. The slow activity is called alpha band activity. It oscillates approximately 8 to 12 times in 1 second. It is synchronized over electrodes on parietal and occipital regions.

9.2.1 Properties of the Field Signal

A time plot of the field signal is represented as a wave. A full cycle of this wave consists of a peak and a trough. The length of one full cycle is called the **wavelength**. The unit of the wavelength for M/EEG signal is usually a millisecond (ms), because one cycle of the signal is typically between 10 and 2000 ms. Thus, the wave goes up and down, again and again, for many successive cycles. The **frequency** describes the number of cycles per second, and the unit is hertz (Hz). When the signal speeds up, the wavelength decreases, thus the frequency increases (i.e., frequency is the inverse of the wavelength). The neural field signals include multiple frequencies.

The frequencies are grouped into bands. Delta (<4 Hz), theta (4–8 Hz), alpha (8–13 Hz), beta (13–30 Hz), and gamma (>30 Hz) are the most commonly used bands. The strength of the fluctuations in each of these bands changes in different situations. For example, when we close our eyes, the alpha band activity usually increases. A simple illustration of this modulation is given in Chapter 1 (Fig. 1.5).

An alternative to the time plot is a polar plot. As illustrated in Figure 9.4, the time wave can be represented as a rotating point in polar coordinates. In this representation, we show how far activity has proceeded within a cycle. This is referred to as the **phase**. The phase is expressed as the angle of rotation between 0° and 360°, or -π and π (radian). The phase tells us a lot about the state of the neural system underlying the signal: Sometimes the phase proceeds in a more or less constant angular speed, other times it changes abruptly. A sudden phase shift suggests events such as a sensory input and spontaneous phase reset. The phase also tells us about the

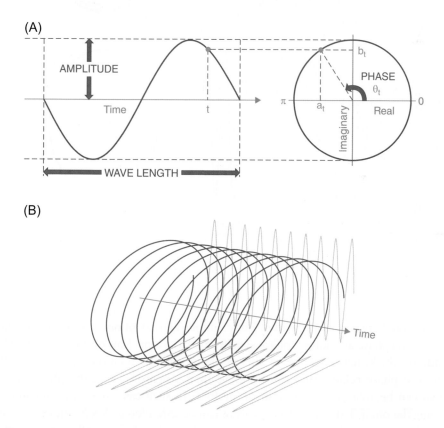

Figure 9.4 Oscillation as a wave or rotation.
(A) The signal can be represented as either a time wave or rotation. Parameters such as wavelength, frequency, phase, and amplitude characterize the signals. (B) The two representations can be considered as different views of a helix. (C) Oscillations without (*top*) and with (*middle*) amplitude change. Angular velocity of phase changes without changing amplitude (*bottom*).

(C)

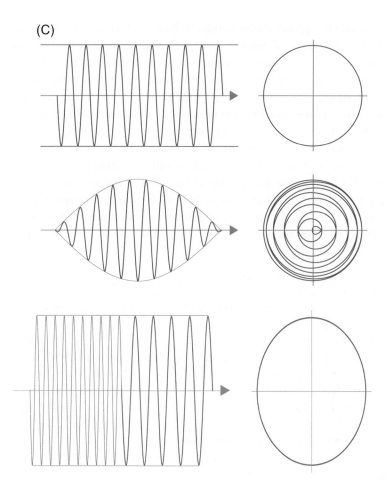

Figure 9.4 *(cont.)*

relationship between two activities. For example, activity of one sensor might rotate in the same phase as another: phase synchrony. How long, how often, and/or in what condition the synchrony appears tells us about possible relationships between the two. The phase relationship can be more than synchrony, e.g., the phase of one signal can be $1/2\pi$ faster than that of another. In such case, one activity could be leading the other. Pair-wise phase analysis can be extended to $N \times N$ sensors to draw a graph of functional connectivity. The graph changes with time, reflecting dynamics of the brain (Varela et al., 2001).

Phase at time t is θ_t. The angle can be expressed as a complex number $a_t + b_t i$, where $a_t = \cos\theta_t$ is the projection of the point on the real axis, $b_t = \sin\theta_t$ is the projection on the imaginary axes, and i is the imaginary unit (Fig. 9.4A). We could imagine phase moving in time as 'a helix' (Fig. 9.4B). The polar plot and time wave are two views of the helix.

The **amplitude** is another signal property that conveys rich information. Intuitively, it makes sense that the amplitude represents the energy of the signal; the stronger the activity, the larger the amplitude becomes. What is not so intuitive is that amplitude always has zero or positive values. This becomes clear if we see the signal in the polar plot, on the real and imaginary axes. In the plot, amplitude is the length of the vector from the origin of the plot to the data point. The length, $\sqrt{a_t^2 + b_t^2}$, cannot be negative. Therefore, amplitude is always zero or positive (see Box 9.2). In the 2D time plot on the time and real axes, signals are sometimes

---

Box 9.2 FAQ: Negative Amplitude

At this point, some readers might have a question, something like, "Isn't the amplitude of some evoked potentials (e.g., N200) negative?" Here is an answer.

First, you are not the only one who had this question. Indeed, this is one of the most frequently asked questions. Apparently, you have already read some studies using EEG measures – namely, evoked potentials. Details of evoked potentials are covered in Chapter 11 (Section 11.2.2). However, for the sake of answering the FAQ, here we sketch the outline: Evoked potentials are neural responses to a stimulus event, such as a flash of light. The evoked activity is usually buried in the ongoing oscillations. Thus, a good amount of signal processing is needed to make it observable. Once it is processed properly, we can see a beautiful complex of waves – some small and others large, some fast, others slow, rising from the baseline level of the activity with some latency from the stimulus event. The baseline level is, typically, the activity level prior to the event onset. Prominent peaks in the wave complex are often named with polarity and latency, for example, N200, a "negative" peak with latency of 200 ms. Here in the context of EEG evoked potentials, the positive or negative sign of an evoked activity simply means the peak value was higher or lower than the baseline.

For the evoked component, we cannot draw an envelope in the same way as we did for ongoing activity; the N200 appears only once after the stimulus (i.e., there is no second N200 to draw an envelope). We treat N200 as a single trough that starts from the baseline, hits the bottom at around 200 ms, and returns to baseline. Thus, the lower envelope connects the baseline, the minimum, and the baseline again, while the upper envelope is drawn between the baselines – a flat line. The half-height of the envelope is zero or larger for any time point in the component. In the radial representation (polar plot), the activity rotates in a cycle increasing the radius from zero (the baseline) to the max (the trough), and back to zero. The radius never becomes negative.

The impression of a "negative" amplitude seems to come from the appearance of the evoked component in the time domain; the activity develops in the negative direction relative to the baseline. As we learned in Section 9.2.1, in time domain, not the wave itself but the envelope should be consulted for amplitude. Thus, the short answer is, "No, the amplitude is not negative!"

plotted between negative and positive values, such as -50 to +50μV. The sign of the value simply indicates that the activity was higher or lower than the baseline value, such as mean voltage of the data. As the wave goes down from a peak to a trough, it looks as if amplitude decreases. However, in ongoing activity, this simply means that the activity is changing phase (e.g., from 90° to 270°). In a time wave, amplitude can be seen without confusion when we connect a peak to the next peak and a trough to the next trough (Fig. 9.4C). The smooth function obtained by connecting the extremes in the signal values is referred to as the envelope of the signal. We have two envelopes: the upper envelope that connects the maxima and the lower envelope that connects the minima. Half the height of the difference between the upper and lower envelopes corresponds to the amplitude. The envelope goes up and down much less than the time wave itself does; when the activity keeps peaking/dipping at the same level, the envelope does not change over time. In other words, the activity is oscillating steadily without changing its amplitude. When consecutive peaks/troughs become larger or smaller, the envelope changes accordingly, representing an amplitude change. Sleep spindles are a good example. A sleep spindle is often observed in EEG signals during sleep. For several to a few dozens of cycles, the oscillation increases and then decreases amplitude, literally drawing a spindle.

These properties are used to describe M/EEG signals. Different representations of the signal, time wave, and polar plot give us more insight about the signal (see Box 12.1 in Chapter 12). In later chapters on data analysis (Chapters 11 and 12), the different representations will be revisited.

9.2.2 Dimensions and Resolution of the Field Signal

Modern recording systems often have multiple sensors – tens, sometimes hundreds of them – covering the whole head. Simultaneously recorded signals from the multiple sensors can be plotted on the scalp or surface of an MEG helmet. The sensor-level signal map is two-dimensional because it is a projection of the brain activity on the sensor surface. A large part of data analysis is done using this 2D map. For example, the amplitude of alpha band activity can be plotted on the map. In this way, we can easily observe that the amplitude is larger in posterior than anterior sensors.

The sensor-level signal is a weighted mixture of source signals in different depths and orientations. If we wish to know where the signal comes from in three-dimensional brain space, the sensor-level signals need to be processed further. However, similar to the estimation of a 3D structure from a 2D image, the sensor-level data alone do not have enough information to specify the source location. To compensate, we need to make assumptions (e.g., where and how many sources could be in the brain). For example, when the response of the primary visual cortex to a visual stimulus is the activity of interest, we might assume a small number of dipoles in the cortex. Structural MRI images and the electrode location mapped on the image give us mathematical constraints to

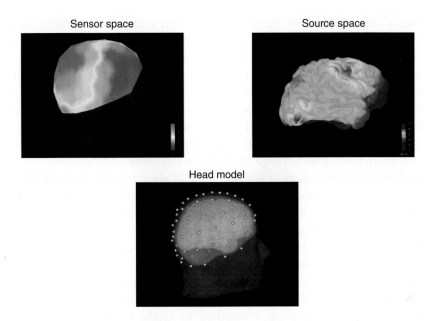

Figure 9.5 EEG in sensor space and its estimated source.
Sensor EEG-level data (*top left*) are mapped to the cortical surface (*top right*) using a head model (*bottom*). Dots on the scalp represent electrode location.

estimate activity of the sources using the sensor data. Alternatively, we could also assume a large number of dipoles covering some extent of cortex. We could also estimate source activity as activation patterns over the area. With a careful choice of assumptions and estimation methods (and meeting other conditions, such as a large enough number of electrodes), we could obtain an estimation of source activity in 3D (Fig. 9.5). More details of source localization are discussed in Section 13.3, Chapter 13.

Source estimation is one of the fastest developing branches of neural signal processing. A variety of source estimation methods have been applied and produced promising results. General limiting factors, such as sensor-source distance, affect the localization results. For instance, activity in medial and ventral cortices is difficult to estimate (Korhonen et al., 2014). In other words, with the state-of-the-art signal-processing techniques, a considerable amount of uncertainty still remains to specify where the signal comes from. Intracranial and thus invasive methods, namely, stereo EEG (sEEG) and electrocorticography (ECoG), have much less spatial uncertainty. The volume between the source and the sensors, depth electrodes for sEEG and subdural electrode for ECoG, are small. Thus, source signals are less attenuated and mixed in the ECoG and sEEG signals than in M/EEG signals (Kajikawa and Schroeder, 2011). With these invasive techniques, however, the signal is recordable from only limited regions. Electrophysiological brain imaging methods have a disadvantage in obtaining signals in

3D from a large volume of the brain, compared with other methods, namely, magnetic resonance imaging methods. By using pulse sequences, the MRI signal directly reflects the 3D location of the signal sources.

In contrast to the limited spatial resolution, the temporal resolution of the field signals is high. A typical EEG recording system can easily sample 1000 data points per second. This is much faster than that of, for example, blood-oxygenation-level dependent (BOLD) functional MRI (fMRI), which typically samples 1 data point per couple of seconds. Most important, the temporal resolution of the field signals is high enough to study a wide range of interesting dynamics of the brain.

Indeed, spatial localization of activity alone is not enough to answer all of our questions. For example, the question, When a visual stimulus is expected, does the prefrontal region activate earlier than the occipital region? could be addressed only when, besides the location, the timing of the activities is known. The brain is regarded as a system that executes a number of information processing steps. Timing, speed, and the temporal pattern of activity over many brain regions certainly need to be considered to understand the brain dynamics.

The high temporal resolution of the M/EEG signal is a clear advantage over fMRI signals. For example, the evoked response to tactile stimulation, of which the latency is around 50 ms, can easily be distinguished from activity such as that related to short-term somatosensory memory. Such temporal distinction of information processing stages is very difficult, if not impossible, using the slow hemodynamic signals of the fMRI method. Furthermore, for applications that require real-time control (e.g., brain-machine interface for driving vehicles), high temporal resolution of the field signal is crucial. Moreover, the signals can be recorded over long time periods. For example, overnight EEG monitoring is routinely done in clinical settings to assess sleep quality. The temporal range, from milliseconds to hours, covers a broad range of issues concerning the relationship between neural activity and behavioral and/or psychological phenomena.

9.3 Brain Dynamics vs. Mind Dynamics

The M/EEG signal is not only of interest to specialists but is also a source of fascination to the general public, because it correlates with our subjective experiences and mental states more than any other biological signals. For example, every night we experience immense transition between mental states: consciousness to unconsciousness. This is correlated with clear changes in the EEG signal (Fig. 9.6). As we fall asleep, the signal oscillates in slower frequency and in larger amplitude and synchronizes more over sensors. As sleep deepens, the amplitude and the synchrony increase and the peak frequency decreases further. The slow-wave sleep continues for a while, then the field signal abruptly increases frequency, combined with a decrease in amplitude and synchrony. This brain state is similar to what we experience when we are awake, yet we are still sleeping. This paradoxical sleep state is also characterized by rapid eye movements (while eyes are closed), thus, it is called rapid eye movement

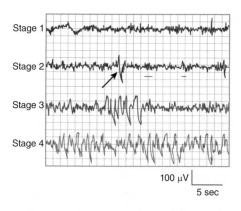
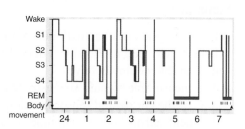

Figure 9.6 Sleep stages.

EEGs in different sleep stages (*left*). As sleep deepens from Stages 1 to 4, EEG increases in amplitude and decreases in frequency. Arrow and underbars indicate K-complex and sleep spindles, respectively. They are characteristic of Stage 2 sleep. (*right*) Sleep stages in the overnight sleep of a healthy adult.

Figures are reproduced from Carskadon and Dement, 2000, with permission

(REM) sleep (Aserinsky and Kleitman, 1953). Interestingly, the REM sleep state often correlates with dreaming. The field signal tells us that the cycle of sleep repeats several times during a full night's (6–8 hours) sleep for the healthy population. These remarkably regular brain dynamics that correlate with our subjective experience are easily derived from irregular and spatially coarse M/EEG signals.

Somewhat ironically, the membrane potential of a single neuron – the electro-physiological neural signal of the finest spatio-temporal resolution – is hardly informative enough to draw a parallel between brain and mind dynamics. When and how many times a neuron fires does not map directly to our experience at the moment. There is no doubt that the M/EEG signal is a physical consequence of membrane potentials. At the same time, the field signal has properties that the single neuron signal does not have, for example, oscillation and epileptic seizures, which emerge from a system of neurons, glias, and other supporting elements (e.g., blood vessels) and which show some correlation with mental states. A comparison between membrane potentials and M/EEG signals tells us that the appropriate level at which to search for neural correlates of our mental activity is not a single neuron but the neural system as a whole.

Correlation between the dynamics of field signals and that of our mental states, however, is moderate, for example, the brain could oscillate either slowly (slow-wave sleep) or fast (REM sleep) while we are unconscious. This may be because the field signals include variance because of non-mental activities, such as the metabolic cycle of the brain. It is still possible, however, that the result indicates that brain and mind operate differently. Such consideration revokes a millennia-old philosophical conundrum: the **mind-body (brain) problem** (Chalmers, 1996). At the same time, contemporary questions, such as the consciousness in vegetative-state patients, can be investigated using the signal (Rosanova et al., 2012). Taken together, science and applications of the field signals continue to be relevant and exciting for all of us.

Summary

- Electrophysiological activity of neurons generates an electromagnetic field. The field activity due to the apical dendritic activity of cortical pyramidal neurons is measurable noninvasively.
- The measurable signals are restricted by cytoarchitecture and large-scale anatomy of the cortex and sensor locations on/nearby the scalp.
- The field activity oscillates in time. Thus, the signal is represented as a time wave. The wave can also be represented as a rotation. Properties of oscillation, such as frequency, phase, and amplitude, are used to describe and analyze the signals.
- The field signals have high temporal resolution; thus, they carry rich information about network dynamics of the brain. Conversely, the spatial resolution is low relative to other brain imaging techniques such as fMRI.
- The field signals reflect the dynamics of the neural system. The dynamics show moderate correlation with mental states.

Review Questions

1. Explain why M/EEG signals predominantly reflect the electrophysiological signal from the cortical pyramidal neurons.
2. With which of the two statements do you agree? (A) A dipole is a super cluster of neurons that is the source of the M/EEG signal. (B) A dipole is a model to describe the electrophysiological activity of a neural population. Explain your choice.
3. Why does the M/EEG signal have a low spatial resolution compared with other neuroimaging techniques? Also, explain in words how to increase the resolution.
4. Describe three research fields or practical applications in which electrophysiological methods are used. Explain the advantages that these methods offer to these fields/domains.

Further Reading

Buzsáki, G. (2006). *Rhythms of the Brain*. New York: Oxford University Press.
Nunez, P. L. & Srinivasan, R. (2006). *Electric Fields of the Brain: The Neurophysics of EEG*. New York: Oxford University Press.

CHAPTER TEN

Electroencephalography and Magnetoencephalography

Learning Objectives

- Explaining what each electrophysiological method measures
- Following methods of signal acquisition in a research paper
- Explaining the pros and cons of the electrophysiological methods

I do not remember having ever received . . . a more dreadful shock than that which I experienced by imprudently placing both my feet on a gymnotus just taken out of the water. I was affected during the rest of the day with a violent pain in the knees, and in almost every joint. To be aware of the difference that exists between the sensation produced by the Voltaic battery and an electric fish, the latter should be touched when they are in a state of extreme weakness.

Alexander von Humboldt, 1800

From *Jaguars and Electric Eels*, selected translation of *Voyage aux régions équinoxiales du nouveau continent* by J. Wilson (2007). (The original text is available at http://dx.doi.org/10.3931/e-rara-24320.)

Friedrich Wilhelm Heinrich Alexander von Humboldt was a German (Prussian, to be precise) naturalist. His explorations to Central and South America were published as a series of books that were widely read in Europe and beyond, making him a celebrity. When Humboldt made the voyage, he was 31 years old and full of energy and curiosity. In the regions along the Orinoco River, local guides told him about the *gymnotus*, an electric eel that could grow to 2 m long. According to the guides, the eels could paralyze a horse that had come to a pond to drink water. Humbolt wanted to experience the discharge despite repeated warnings from the guides. He most likely did not exaggerate his experience, because the giant eel's discharge can reach 600 volts (V) (Catania, 2016).

Compared with the impressive power generation capacity of the eels, what our brain generates – on the order of microvolts (μV, a millionth of a volt) – is nothing. On the one hand, it is a blessing that our ongoing brain activity does not threaten others (electrically). On the other hand, however, it is a challenge to measure such weak signals. For example, a fluorescent ceiling lamp can easily emit electric activity that is 100 times higher than the brain activity. Such non-brain activity, *noise*, needs to be prevented or reduced while recording. In addition, high-fidelity sensors and amplifiers are necessary. In this chapter, two major techniques that measure the weak activity, **electroencephalography (EEG)** and **magnetoencephalography (MEG)**, are introduced.

10.1 Electroencephalography (EEG)

Electroencephalography (EEG) measures the electric signal produced by cerebral activity. As we learned in Chapter 9, the most significant contributor to the signal is the postsynaptic potential in apical dendrites of cortical pyramidal neurons. Throughout the long dendrite that runs through multiple cortical layers, hundreds of thousands of synapses – some are excitatory, and others are inhibitory – are formed. Excitatory and inhibitory postsynaptic potentials generate a complex mixture of postsynaptic currents. The current primarily runs in the apical dendrite (primary current), and also in brain tissue, cerebrospinal fluid (CSF), skull, and the scalp (return current). The conductivity of the biological tissue is not homogenous (e.g., brain tissue and CFS conduct the current better than the skull does). Thus, the current spreads along the skull, mixed with currents from other sources. As a result, a complex electric field is formed spanning the distance from the brain to the scalp. The electric signal that we obtain from a scalp electrode, therefore, reflects the activity of many different sources.

   To record the signal, we need to establish an electric circuit from the scalp to a recording device. Since most of us do not have a cable jack on the head, we use a special cable, one end of which is an electrode: The electrode is placed on the scalp using a paste, and the other end is connected to the recording device. How to induce a current from the scalp could be compared with pouring water from a water tank (Fig. 10.1). The amount of water from the tap depends on how high the water level is and how fully the tap is opened. The voltage at the scalp is very low, but we could find a yet lower point, such as the ground. The recorder is grounded. Thus, the current flows from scalp to the ground. More current runs when resistance of the circuit is lower. The highest resistance occurs at the gap between the electrode and the scalp. To keep the resistance low, the gap is filled with a conductive substance, gel or paste – the tap is opened. The recorder is placed between the scalp electrode and

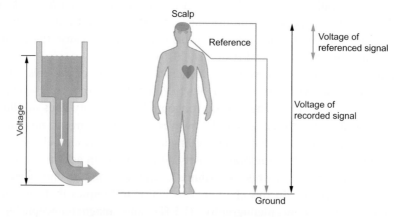

Figure 10.1 Illustration of EEG measurement.

the ground to convert the induced current to voltage, just like putting a hand in the flow of water to sense how much water is running and how high the water level is.

Note that the electrode does not apply but receives the current. The EEG technique does not inject current to the brain. A current is applied to the brain with brain stimulation techniques: transcranial direct current stimulation (tDCS) and transcranial alternating current stimulation (tACS). These brain stimulation techniques also use electrodes that apply current to the brain. Some also receive the signal (cf. Chapter 14). Both EEG and transcranial current stimulation are based on volume conduction, but electrodes with each method have different functions.

10.1.1 EEG Electrodes

Electroencephalography electrodes are placed on the scalp to register current due to brain activity. The electrodes come in a variety of shapes and sizes. Disk or button electrodes (~5 mm of diameter) are typical, but other shapes, such as pin, comb, and grid, are also used (Fig. 10.2). Bandages and/or glue are used to attach individual electrodes. To attach a large number of electrodes efficiently, an

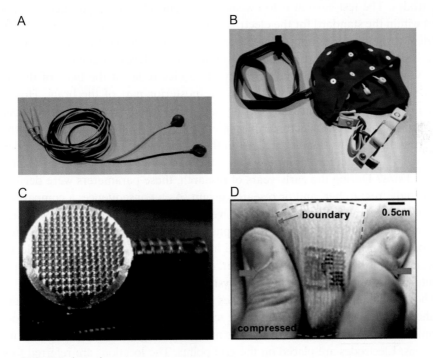

Figure 10.2 EEG electrodes.
(A) Disk electrodes. (B) An electrode cap. (C) 3D-printed, high-density dry electrodes; each pin is an electrode (Salvo et al., 2012). (D) "Tattoo sticker" electrode placed on the forehead (Kim et al., 2011).
Figures are reproduced with permission

electrode cap, to which multiple electrodes are set, is often used. Materials such as silver (chemical symbol Ag), tin (Sn), and sintered silver and silver chloride (Ag/AgCl) are used for the electrode. These materials are conductive and safe to attach to the scalp. The signal quality differs slightly depending on the material used (Tallgren et al., 2005). Thus, materials are chosen based on the purpose of the recording. For example, evoked brain responses to external stimulation often contain slow activity. The Ag/AgCl electrodes provide a stable slow signal; thus, they are often preferred in recordings of evoked responses.

The small gap between the scalp and the EEG electrodes is filled with a conductive substance: paste, gel, or saline that contains ions, such as chlorite ions (Cl⁻). The filler is used to decrease electric resistance, known as contact impedance, between the scalp and the electrode. As the contact impedance decreases, the current from the scalp to the electrode increases. The impedance affects high- more so than low-frequency activity (Kappenman and Luck, 2010). To have a good **signal-to-noise ratio** (SNR or S/N) for a wide frequency band, the impedance needs to be kept as low as possible – less than 5 kΩ has been recommended (Picton et al. 2000). Commercial EEG recording systems offer an impedance check function: The contact impedance is measured by running a weak alternating current of 10 Hz to the electrodes. The test current is too weak to be noticeable to test participants and is kept within the standard for the electrical safety of medical devices (ICNIRP, 2010).

Ideally, the locations and the number of electrodes should be determined based on the aim of each study. For example, when we are interested in the brain response to a visual stimulus, we would certainly place electrodes at the back of the head, near visual cortices that are located in the posterior part of the brain. However, when we are interested in EEG during, say, mind wandering, it is not so straightforward to decide *the* electrode placement. We could place multiple electrodes covering the head to sample EEG from the whole head. How many electrodes do we need in this situation? Is it okay to use the same number for everyone regardless of head size? During the early years of research, these parameters were decided in each study, researcher, and/or research group. As a consequence, a comparison of results of several studies was, at the very least, cumbersome. In 1947, at the International Congress of Electroencephalography and Clinical Neurophysiology in London, an initiative to establish the international standard for EEG electrode placement was begun. Eleven years later, combining several major electrode placement systems, the **international 10–20 system** was established (Jasper, 1958).

The international 10–20 system specifies electrode locations based on a grid drawn on the scalp. The grid lines segment of the scalp is based on 10% and 20% points on the perimeter of the head (see Box 10.1). The name "10–20 system" stands for this ratio of divisions. Electrodes are placed on the grid points. The locations are referred to with abbreviations: frontal-polar (Fp), frontal (F), central (C), parietal (P), occipital (O), and temporal (T). Locations on the left hemisphere are given an odd number, while those on the right hemisphere are given an even number, e.g., F3 and F4. Locations on the midsagittal line are marked with "z" for Zentrum, e.g., Fz. The system specifies

Box 10.1 The International 10–20 System in Five Steps

Step 1

The electrode locations are decided based on four skeletal landmarks: **nasion**, **inion**, and left and right **preauricular points** (Box Figure 10.1). The frontal nasal bone suture crosses the midsagittal line at the nasion. On the scalp, it corresponds to the

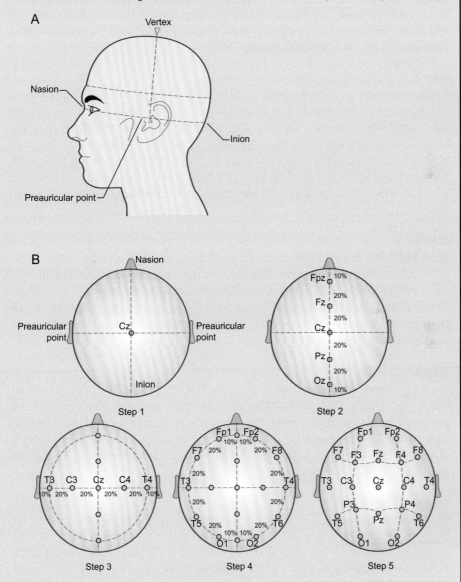

Box Figure 10.1 Anatomical landmarks for the international 10–20 system (A). The five steps for specifying the electrode locations on the scalp (B).

lowest point of the nose ridge. The point at which the external occipital protuberance crosses the midsagittal line is the inion. It corresponds to the point just below the highest point on the back of the head on the midsagittal line. The preauricular point is above the intertragal notch, roughly in front of the earhole. Most of the brain, the neocortex in particular, is located above these landmarks. Now, draw an arc from nasion to inion via the vertex of the head, and another from left and right preauricular points via the **vertex**. The front-back and left-right arcs cross at their midpoints. The first electrode is placed at the crossing point. The location is called the central-midline and noted as Cz (i.e., Central-Zentrum).

Step 2
Divide the nasion-Cz-inion arc in 10%, 20%, 20%, 20%, 20%, and 10% segments of the arc length. This gives us five dividing points between nasion and inion. The first point, the 10% point, from the nasion is called the frontal-polar-midline (Fpz). The second point, the 30% point from the nasion is the frontal-midline (Fz). The third point is the 50% point from nasion or inion, i.e., Cz. The fourth point, the 70% point, is the parietal-midline (Pz). The fifth point, the 90% point, is the occipital-midline (Oz), which is 10% above the inion. All electrodes on the midsagittal line are indexed with "z."

Step 3
Likewise, divide the left preauricular–Cz–right preauricular arc in 10%, 20%, 20%, 20%, 20%, and 10% segments. This gives us five electrode locations: From left to right, the five locations are referred to as left temporal (T3), left central (C3), Cz, right central (C4), and right temporal (T4), respectively. Note that electrodes on the left hemisphere are indexed with odd numbers, while those on the right hemisphere are indexed with even numbers.

Step 4
Draw a perimeter connecting four 10% points, Fpz, T3, Oz, and T4. Divide the left arc (Fpz-T3-Oz) in 10%, 20%, 20%, 20%, 20%, and 10% segments. The electrodes are placed on the sedimentation points: The electrode locations are called, from front to back, Fp1, F7, T3, T5, and O1, respectively. Likewise, the right arc (Fpz-T4-Oz) is divided in 10% and 20% segments. This gives electrode locations Fp2, F8, T4, T6, and O2.

Step 5
The last four locations are decided by adjacent electrode locations. Draw a short arc between F7 and Fz and another between Fp1 and C3. The arcs cross at their midpoints. Location F3 is placed at the crossing point. Location F4 is defined in the same manner using F8, Fz, Fp2, and C4. Likewise, P3 is defined by T5, Pz, O1, and C3. Location P4 is defined by T6, Pz, O2, and C4.

In the 10–20 system, two out of the 21 scalp locations, Fpz and Oz, are not used in order to avoid uneven electrode density, e.g., O1, Oz, and O2 electrodes would become closer than C3, Cz, and C4. Thus, the total number of electrodes is 19. Location Fpz is sometimes used as a ground location. In higher density systems, e.g., the 10–10 system, Fpz and Oz are included as valid scalp electrode locations.

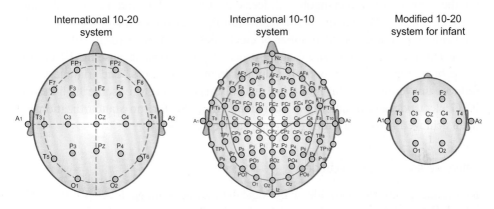

Figure 10.3 The international 10–20 system, the international 10–10 system, and the 10–20 system for infants.

19 electrode locations that cover the whole head (Fig. 10.3). The locations are roughly equally spaced, suitable for monitoring activity from the whole brain. The locations are determined by the ratio; thus, the same number of electrodes is used regardless of head size, which made inter-individual comparison easy. The system also specifies six possible reference electrode locations (cf. reference and ground electrodes).

Based on the 10–20 system, a few more systems were developed. The **international 10–10 system** (AES, 1994) divides the arcs in 10% segments. Thus, more electrode locations, more specifically, 73 scalp locations, are specified. Four rows of electrodes are added to the electrodes in the 10–20 system: anterior-frontal (AF), fronto-central (FC), fronto-temporal (FT), centro-parietal (CP), temporo-parietal (TP), and parieto-occipital (PO). Nasion, inion, and lateral positions on the perimeter are also included as electrode locations. The electrode notation differs slightly between the 10–10 and 10–20 systems; electrodes on the 10% perimeter are noted as T7, T8, P7, and P8 in the 10–10 system, which correspond to T3, T4, T5, and T6 in the 10–20 system, respectively.

For neonatal infants, a modified 10–20 system with nine electrodes was proposed (Kellaway and Crawley, 1964). The neonatal system replaces Fp1 and F3 with F1, which is on the 20% perimeter and 10% left of the midsagittal line. Likewise, Fp2 and F4 are replaced by F2. In addition to F1 and F2, T3, C3, Cz, C4, T4, O1 and O2 are included.

The 10–20 system also serves as a frame of reference on the scalp. An electrode location that is unique to a study is often reported, referring to the 10–20 system, e.g., "... the electrode is placed between C3 and Cz locations." Likewise, an electric or magnetic brain stimulation location is often specified using this system (Herwig et al., 2003).

Alternatives to the 10–20 system have been developed to cope with ever-increasing numbers of electrodes. In the 10–20 system, the electrodes are placed on the vertices of a rectangular lattice, e.g., Cz, C4, P4, and Pz. The distance between Cz and P4 (diagonal) is longer than that between Cz and C4 (side). The unevenness increases as the number of electrodes increases to 10–10, 10–5, and so forth. This is a problem for some signal-processing methods, because the EEG from some brain regions is less densely sampled than from others. The triangle lattice reduces unevenness of the inter-electrode distance. Therefore, some high-density EEG electrode arrays employ a triangular lattice. So far, no standardization has been achieved across different triangular-lattice systems.

Reference and Ground Electrodes

Reference electrodes provide a biological baseline voltage level for the EEG signal. Why do we want to have such a baseline? In addition to the brain, organs such as the heart and muscles also show electrophysiological activity. The non-brain electrophysiological activity is often stronger than the brain activity. The non-brain activity is conducted through the body up to the scalp and is added to the brain activity. In other words, the voltage between the scalp and ground is inflated by the non-brain activity. Reference electrodes measure the biological noise. A reference electrode is attached, for example, to the earlobes and nose tip, which are close to the scalp, but there is no brain beneath. Therefore, the signal from the reference electrode could be regarded as noise. When preprocessing the EEG signal, the reference signal is subtracted from that of a scalp electrode (see Fig. 10.1).

The 10–20 system specifies six reference locations; the left and right **earlobes** are noted as A1 and A2, respectively. Materials for earlobe electrodes are the same as those for scalp electrodes, but the shape might vary, e.g., a clip for an earlobe. The designations M1 and M2 stand for the left and right **mastoids** and reference electrode locations behind the ears, where the temporal bone is thick and thus is distanced from the brain. Electrodes of the same type as those for the scalp are usually used for the mastoids. Nasopharyngeal electrodes are denoted by Pg1 and Pg2 and are placed in the left and right **nasal cavity**, respectively. The nasopharyngeal references are used in clinical settings, such as in a diagnosis for brain death. The electrodes are rod shaped so they can be placed in the nose cavity. Reference locations are chosen according to the aim of each study. In addition to the six locations of the 10–20 system, other locations, e.g., nose tip and a combination of electrodes, could also be used. How do we decide what reference to use?

This issue closely relates to artifact removal, which is discussed in Chapter 11 (Section 11.1.2).

The ground electrode is attached to protect participants from accidental electrical leakage. The material and type of ground electrode are usually the same as those used for scalp electrodes. The electrode is placed on the head, e.g., Fpz, an unused location in the 10–20 system. Different locations may be used in different recording systems. The signal from the ground electrode is sometimes used to compute the ground voltage level. The ground level is near zero, but it fluctuates. Environmental noise, e.g., power supply to electric appliances, affects the baseline level. The signal from the electrode is used to compute an adequate ground level. Therefore, the ground electrode is sometimes called the "recording reference."

EOG Electrodes

Electrooculography (EOG) measures the electric activity caused by eye movements. The eyeballs are statically charged. As the eyes move, the electric field changes around the eyes, forehead, and scalp. Thus, the charge is added to the EEG signals. In fact, the electrooculogram (also abbreviated EOG) is one of the major artifacts in the EEG recording. To remove the artifact, EOG needs to be monitored simultaneously with EEG.

Four electrodes are placed around the eyes (Fig. 10.4). The electrodes at the left of the left orbita and right of the right orbita measure the horizontal EOG (HEOG). The electrodes above the eyebrow of the non-dominant eye and below the infra-orbital border measure the vertical EOG signal (VEOG). The materials used for the electrodes are the same as those used for EEG electrodes. The recording ground is usually shared with EEG. Most commercial EEG recording systems provide an EOG interface. EOG artifact removal is described in Chapter 11 together with other preprocessing techniques.

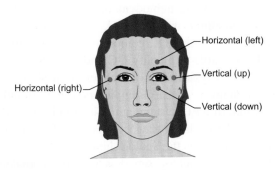

Figure 10.4 EOG electrode placement.
Four electrodes are placed. Electrodes for vertical EOG are often placed around the non-dominant eye.

Box 10.2 Dry Electrodes

Dry electrodes refer to EEG electrodes that do not require conductive filler, such as gel and paste. Dry electrodes are used, for example, for ultra-high-density recording. As the density of the electrode increases, inter-electrode distance decreases, e.g., 2 mm (see Fig. 10.2C). The electrodes record similar signals, but each signal varies slightly among them. In the high-density recording, even a small leakage of gel could cause a short circuit among the electrodes. This so-called gel-bridge makes signals of the bridged electrodes identical, thus ruining the recording. Gel-bridges do not occur with dry electrodes. Another advantage of dry electrodes is convenience. The time and effort it would take to apply gel to multiple electrodes are saved. Moreover, electrodes without wet and sticky gel are comfortable for test participants.

Impedance of dry electrodes is often higher than it is with wet ones. To compensate for the high impedance, a special amplifier is often required. At this time, the signal quality is worse and special amplifiers tend to be more expensive than those of conventional systems with wet electrodes. However, the potential of the dry electrode method is clear: Imagine a high-density electrode array worn like a headphone or hair ornament.

10.1.2 EEG Amplifier

The electric activity measured from the scalp is weak; the voltage – on the order of μV, i.e., one-millionth volt – is too weak to drive any recording devices that typically require an input signal of 5 V or more. Thus, amplification is essential for EEG recordings. In fact, it is so essential that "EEG amplifier" is often used as a synonym for "EEG recording system." An EEG amplifier amplifies the weak signals with little distortion. The frequency range of amplification is set typically between 0.1 and 500 Hz. The lowest frequency is determined by a parameter called the **time constant**. The longer the time constant becomes, the slower the lowest frequency becomes. To obtain "ultra-slow" activity, e.g., 0.1–0.03 Hz, which corresponds to the dominant frequency range in the hemodynamic response fMRI signal, a special amplifier, called a **DC amplifier**, is often used. The letters DC stands for "direct current" and the frequency of this DC component is 0 Hz; thus, it is *the* slowest activity. A DC amplifier is able to amplify DC and very slow components without distortion. In this regard, a typical EEG amplifier is an **alternating current (AC) amplifier**. Because the majority of EEG amplifiers are AC amplifiers, we tend to skip the "AC." In a modern EEG system, amplification is applied more than once, first using an analog signal, then later using a digital signal. A preamplifier refers to a device that amplifies and rectifies the analog signal.

After preamplification, the analog signal is fed to an **analog-to-digital (AD) converter**. The AD converter samples the analog voltage signal in a short time interval, e.g., every 2 ms. The number of samplings per second is called the **sampling**

frequency or **sampling rate**. For example, if we sample data every 2 ms, the data are sampled 500 times per second. Thus, the sampling frequency is 500 Hz. If the sampling frequency is too low relative to the signal frequency, the samples do not represent the original signal properly: A slow component that does not exist in the original signal is generated. This problem is called aliasing (Fig. 10.5A). According to the **sampling theorem** (also known as the **Nyquist theorem** as introduced in Chapter 1), the sampling frequency should be more than twice the frequency of the signal. The theorem could be understood intuitively by imagining how to code one cycle of a sine wave. At least a point at the peak and another at the trough, i.e., *two* points, are needed to code *one* cycle. In the case of EEG, often the frequency range of interest is 0.1–50 Hz. Thus, the sampling frequency needs to be 100 Hz or higher.

For signal processing on a computer, the sampled values are binarized. In 1-bit coding, each value is coded 0 or 1 relative to a single threshold, e.g., the mean voltage value. In 2-bit coding, the value is coded in $2^2 = 4$ levels: 00, 01, 10, and 11 (Fig. 10.5B). Similarly, 3-bit encoding has $2^3 = 8$ levels: 000, 001, 010, 011, 100, 101, 110, and 111; 4-bit encoding would be $2^4 = 16$ levels: 0000, 0001, 0010, and so on. The level of binarization is called the **AD level**. The higher the level, the more details of the signal are encoded. For EEG recording, AD level is typically 8 bit: $2^8 = 256$ levels, or higher.

The digitized EEG is a large matrix of data points; M data points in time by N electrodes. Together with the EEG data matrix, recording information, e.g., sampling frequency, channel labels, and participant information, is saved. When a task is applied, event markers, e.g., stimulus onset and response button press, are also saved. Some EEG file formats save EEG and recording information in one file, while other formats save them in separate files. Most EEG recording systems and analysis packages support multiple output file formats.

10.1.3 Procedure for Data Acquisition

The last element of the EEG recording involves the test participants. Without their cooperation, no good signal is acquired. Therefore, it is important to keep them happy and relaxed as much as possible. When electrodes are attached, it takes some minutes for the conductive gel to stabilize the contact impedance between the electrodes and the scalp. Other sensors, such as EOG electrodes, are also attached to monitor artifacts. Cables from the electrodes and the sensors are secured to prevent drift artifacts caused by motion of the cables. The participant is seated in a chair or lies on a bench in an **electrically shielded room**. The shielded room is covered by conductive materials. The materials capture and drain environmental electric noise activity (cf. a **Faraday cage**). Thus, the space inside of the room is not affected by the noise. It is also possible to measure EEG without a shielded room; recent EEG recording systems often offer effective noise reduction functions with

A

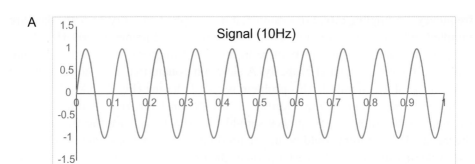

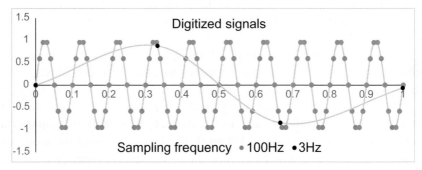

B

AD in 1bit

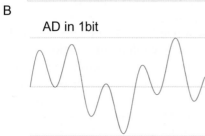

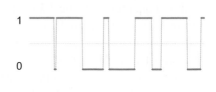

AD in 2bit

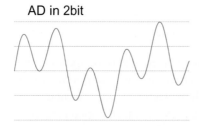

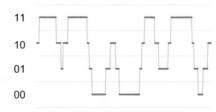

AD in 3bit

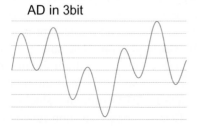

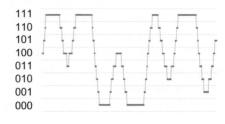

which a reasonable signal can be obtained. Also, a test room is usually sound attenuated, and the lighting is adjusted to control background sensory inputs.

During the recording, the participant is instructed to minimize body motion. Chin-, head-, and/or armrests could be used to help the participants to keep the same posture comfortably, which in turn helps to reduce noise. At the beginning of the recording session, a rest or baseline period is recorded. Blocks of specific task manipulations follow. Often, the rest/baseline period is repeated after the task. After a recording session, electrodes are removed, and gel is wiped or washed off.

The methods section in an EEG paper is rather uninviting; it is filled with technical terms and abbreviations. That "jargon," however, tells us what was done concisely and precisely. By now, we have learned enough details to understand a typical section of recording information. Here is an excerpt from an EEG paper (Bruggemann et al., 2013) in which recording information is described. Let's try to read it!

Electrocortical data were recorded from 30 Ag/AgCl sintered electrodes, arranged according to the international 10–10 system, and referenced to the nose tip. Only data from fronto-central electrodes (i.e., F3, Fz, F4, FC3, FCz, FC4, C3, Cz, C4) are reported here. ... Horizontal and vertical electro-oculograms were recorded from tin electrodes positioned adjacent to the outer canthus of each eye, and above and below the left eye, respectively. The electrical impedance of each electrode was maintained at less than 10 kilo-ohms. These data were acquired continuously via NeuroScan SynAmps hardware with Scan 4.3 software. ... The sampling rate was 500 Hz.

10.2 Magnetoencephalography (MEG)

Magnetoencephalography (MEG)measures the magnetic field resulting from brain activity. In Section 9.1.2 in Chapter 9, we learned how a magnetic field emerges as a result of electrophysiological activity of neurons: As postsynaptic currents run in the apical dendrites of cortical pyramidal cells, a magnetic field is formed perpendicular to the direction of the current. Magnetoencephalography measures the strength of the magnetic field. The source of the MEG signal is the same as that of the EEG signal. In this sense, MEG could be considered as the twin of EEG. However, the MEG signal is not identical to the EEG signal. For example, the magnetic field permeates brain tissue, cerebrospinal fluid (CSF), skull, scalp, and air with little distortion. This is a big difference from the electric field, which is bent and mixed as

Figure 10.5 Sampling frequency and AD level.
(A) A 10 Hz sine wave (blue line) is sampled in two different sampling frequencies, 100 Hz (orange dots) and 3 Hz (black dots). The 100 Hz sampling represents the original signal adequately, while the 3 Hz sampling does not. The 3 Hz sampling is not sufficient and created a low-frequency artifact. This phenomenon is called *aliasing*. (B) The signal (blue line) is encoded at different AD levels, 1, 2, or 3 bits. As the level increases (2, 2^2, and 2^3 levels), more information from the original signal is encoded.

it conducts the mass between the source and electrodes. We could imagine the magnetic field as a bundle of **magnetic flux** that exits the brain, goes through CSF, skull, scalp, into the air, and returns to the brain. The magnetic flux is caught by MEG sensors outside of the scalp.

Where the flux is dense, the field is strong. However, field strength due to brain activity is on the order of 10^{-15} to 10^{-12} T (i.e., 1 fT – 1 pT, femto- to pico-tesla). To put this into perspective, the Earth's magnetic field has a strength around 10^{-6} T (μT), and the field strength of a typical refrigerator magnet is on the order of 10^{-3} T (mT). To measure such a weak signal, MEG requires a super-high-fidelity measurement device *and* a magnetically shielded room.

10.2.1 MEG Sensors

As the magnetic flux passes through a metal **coil**, such as a copper coil, a current is induced in the wire. The strength of the current is proportional to the magnetic field strength (cf. Faraday's law of induction). A MEG sensor has an induction coil. As the magnetic flux due to the postsynaptic current passes through the coil, a current is induced. Because the field is very weak, the current is also very weak. At room temperature, the current disappears quickly because of the resistance of the coil itself. However, when the coil is cooled close to absolute zero, superconductivity, in which resistance is effectively zero, occurs. Under super conductivity, the current survives and runs through a coil. The pick-up coil is connected to an input coil to a **Superconducting QUantum Interference Device (SQUID)** (Fig. 10.6). As the current runs through multiple turns of the input coil, the flux is intensified and rectified (thus, the input coil is also called a flex fixing loop) and passed to the SQUID. The SQUID amplifies the flux virtually without noise and with high gain based on the Josephson effect in superconductivity.

To achieve superconductivity, liquid helium (-269°C) is used to cool the SQUID sensors. The sensors are placed in a dewar, with coils facing down. The dewar is a huge vacuum flask made of fiberglass, the bottom of which is concave to fit a participant's head (Fig. 10.6). Liquid helium is poured into the dewar to cool the sensors so that they are superconductive. The dewar is attached to a supporting frame to place the bottom of the dewar on a participant's head. The dewar is highly insulated to maintain the high-level cooling. Because of the insulation, the outside surface of the dewar, especially the bottom, which touches the head, is kept at a comfortable temperature for the participant. Note that pick-up coils are not in contact with the scalp. They are inside the dewar, but receive the signal because magnetic flux permeates tissues, air, and materials.

Pick-up coils come in different configurations. To understand the functional difference between the coils, we need to pay attention to the direction of flux and current. Magnetic flux always comes out from N pole and returns to the S pole. According to Fleming's right-hand rule, the right thumb represents the direction. As the flux goes through a coil, current is induced in the direction of the right fingers.

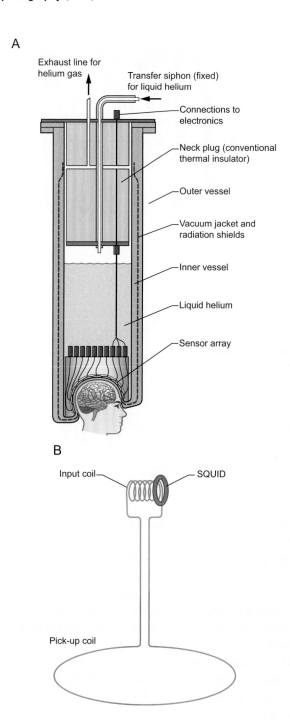

Figure 10.6 Schematic illustration of an MEG system.
(A) The dewar keeps MEG sensors in liquid helium. (B) The MEG sensors consist of pick-up coil, input coil, and SQUID.
The figure (A) is reproduced from Hansen et al., 2010, with permission

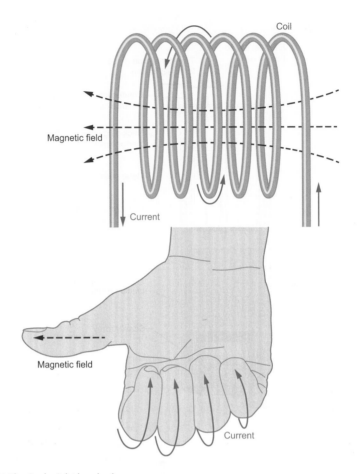

Figure 10.7 Fleming's right-hand rule.

(Fig. 10.7). As the field strengthens (thus, the density of the magnetic flux increases), the current increases.

Now let's suppose there is a single-loop coil on the scalp. Magnetic flux from the brain activity goes through the coil and induces current in the coil. The strength of the current measures the strength of the magnetic field, and the direction of the induced current indicates the direction of the magnetic flux – coming out of or sinking into the brain. The single-loop coil is called a **magnetometer** (Fig. 10.8). The term "magnetometer" literary means a device to measure a magnetic field. In the context of MEG, it refers to a single-loop pick-up coil. The diameter of the coil is typically 10–20 mm. The magnetometer picks up fluctuations of the field strength, which reflect dynamic changes in cortical activity. The coil, however, also picks up magnetic flux noise.

To increase the signal-to-noise ratio, multiple loops are configured in a specific pattern. The multi-loop coil is called a **gradiometer**. In a **planar gradiometer**, loops are shaped into a figure 8. The coils turn opposite to each other. Now, let's suppose

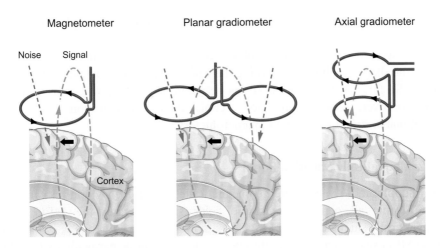

Figure 10.8 MEG coil configuration.
Illustration of magnetometer, planer gradiometer, and axial gradiometer. Black arrows indicate the direction of current induced by the brain activity.

a source current in a sulcus beneath the center of the figure 8 coil. A magnetic field forms and magnetic flux runs around the current. As the flux comes out of the brain to the air, it goes through one loop. As the flux returns from the air to the brain, it goes through the other loop. The coils turn opposite to each other; thus, the two currents add up. Signals from off-center sources are spatially subtracted from each other. However, the activities are not likely to be identical; thus, the differentiated signals remain. The planer gradiometer therefore has the highest sensitivity to the sources beneath the center of the figure 8 coil and also picks up signals from off-center sources.

Another type of gradiometer is the **axial gradiometer**, in which two opposing loops are arranged on an axis. The lower loop is closer to the brain than is the upper loop. Therefore, the lower loop picks up a stronger field, thus generating a stronger current than the upper loop does. The two currents subtract from each other; however, the result would be non-zero. Relative to the signal sources, noise sources are farther away from both coils. For example, the distance between the lower coil and an environmental noise source is approximately the same as that between the upper coil and the noise source. In other words, the strength of the noise current in the lower and upper coils is approximately the same. The currents run in opposite directions; thus, they cancel out or at least are reduced more than those of the brain signal. Typically, the upper and lower loops are 50 mm apart, which is reported to provide sensitivity for the whole brain (Dössel et al., 1991). The axial gradiometer has the best sensitivity to the tangential sources beneath the coils, and it picks up more focal activity than the planer gradiometer does.

Some systems incorporate **reference coils** to measure environmental field strength. Unlike EEG, reference sensors in MEG measure the environmental baseline instead of the biological baseline. Thus, they are not placed close to the head.

Recent systems have had up to 300 sensors. Such a large number of sensors are fixed in the shape of a helmet, covering the whole head. Sensor layouts differ across systems. So far, no standardization has occurred across major systems, unlike in EEG. Moreover, some systems allow a choice in coil configuration, e.g., combination of planar gradiometers and magnetometers.

10.2.2 Magnetically Shielded Room

Power supply, radio waves, the geomagnetic field, and even vibration caused by remote traffic all generate magnetic fields stronger than the MEG signal. A magnetically shielded room blocks these noises; thus, having one is essential for a good MEG signal. Layers of materials with high magnetic permeability (Ni-alloy, called Mumetal or Permalloy) and electrical conductivity (e.g., aluminum) cover the room. The environmental magnetic flux and electric fields run through the permeable and conductive walls and frames, but not inside the room. Active noise cancellation could be added to this passive shielding. An active noise cancellation system consists of magnetometers to monitor environmental noise and magnetic field generators to generate counter fields to cancel out the noise. The magnetically shielded room is not merely a room but is also a device critical for MEG recording and thus an inherent part of the MEG system.

The American physicist David Cohen, who reported the first human MEG in 1968, knew the importance of the shielded room in obtaining a good signal. Without the room, for example, the magnetic signal due to cardiac activity, a magnetocardiogram (MCG), was recognizable; however, the MEG signal was buried in noise. Extensive signal processing was necessary to make the signal recognizable (Cohen, 1968). The first MEG was recorded without SQUID, because superconductive instrumentation had just begun to be developed. Soon, Cohen started to collaborate with Jim Zimmerman, the inventor of SQUID, and combined it with a high-quality, magnetically shielded room at the Massachusetts Institute of Technology (MIT). The result was a remarkably clear signal (Fig. 10.9).

The MEG signal from the sensor goes through a few more subsystems to be rectified, amplified, and digitized. The instantaneous field strength is computed from the digitized signal. Then, finally, the sensor-level MEG signal, the time series of the field strength, is saved in a data file. The MEG signal is also described in frequency (Hz), phase (° or π), and amplitude. The unit of amplitude can differ between studies, ampere-per-meter (A/m), tesla (T), gauss (G), and oersted (Oe). Magnetic field strength is measured in A/m and G. density of magnetic flux is measured in T and Oe (used in the same way that some people use meters while others use feet). In all units, higher values correspond to higher magnetic activity. Because the activity is very small, the units are often prefixed with "n" for nano (10^{-9}), "p" for pico (10^{-12}), or "f" for femto (10^{-15}).

A

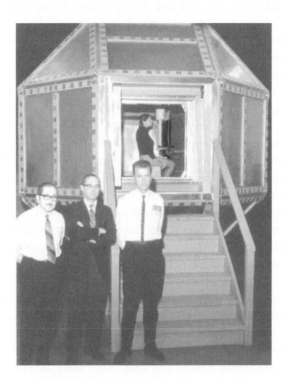

B

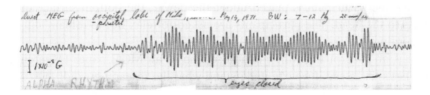

Figure 10.9 The first MEG recorded with SQUID in the MIT shielded room in 1971.
(A) Magnetically shielded room at MIT. The dewar (cylinder inside of the shielded room) is placed next to the participant for display. Front from left: Ed Edelsack, another pioneer of medical magnetic sensing, David Cohen, and Jim Zimmerman. (B) MEG recorded in the facility. The activity during the "eyes closed" period is alpha band activity.
Figures courtesy of Prof. David Cohen

10.2.3 Procedure for MEG Data Acquisition

Prior to measurement, sensors are calibrated, and the environmental noise level is measured. All equipment (e.g., stimulus display) is turned on without a test participant, and the baseline noise level is measured for a few minutes (Gross et al., 2013).

Participants need to be as metal free as is possible. Metal objects, e.g., earrings, piercings in the head, eye glasses, a wrist watch, are removed. Individuals with medical implants – a heart pacemaker, for example – are often excluded from voluntary participation, because the device could cause magnetic noise. Demagnetization is performed to neutralize remaining metals such as dental fillings.

Similar to EEG, electrodes to monitor EOG, EMG, and/or ECG artifacts are attached to the participant. The electrodes are made of materials without ferromagnetic components (e.g., high-purity silver). Thus, MRI-compatible electrodes work well. In addition, **head position indicator (HPI) coils** are attached to the participant's head. Head motion is a major source of noise in MEG. During the measurement, participants are instructed to minimize body motion; however, small head motion is inevitable. Because MEG sensors are not affixed to the head, relative position of the head and sensors changes. As a result, the magnetic field signals appear to be changing; however, the fluctuation is not due to a change in the field strength, but instead to motion. To identify the motion noise components, at least three HPI coils (e.g., detecting yaw, pitch, and roll of the head) are attached to the participant's head. The HPI coils are not superconductive. Before and after a MEG data recording, a weak current is induced in the coils. This generates a magnetic field at the scalp coil locations. The location relative to the helmet is recorded by MEG sensors.

Moreover, fiducial points, such as nasion, left and right preauricular points, are sampled by a magnetic pen digitizer to record their 3D locations. The points are used to coregister the sensor helmet and anatomical MRI data of the participants or of a standardized head/brain model. For a higher quality of coregistration, more points (~100) might be sampled from the whole head.

Finally, the participant is placed under the dewar, the bottom surface of which contacts to the head. The participants are asked to relax but to remain still during the recording.

Here is an excerpt from the method section of an MGE paper (Meeren et al., 2008). Let's try to see if we can understand what the researchers did!

MEG data were acquired with a 306-channel Neuromag VectorView system (Elekta-Neuromag Oy, Helsinki, Finland), which combines the focal sensitivity of 204 first-order planar gradiometers with the widespread sensitivity of 102 magnetometers. Eye movements and blinks were monitored with vertical and horizontal electro-oculogram. The location of the head with respect to the sensors was determined using four head-position indicator coils attached to the scalp. A head-based MEG coordinate frame was established by locating fiduciary landmarks (nasion and preauricular points) with a Fastrak 3D digitizer (Polhemus, Colchester, VT). The data were digitized at 600 samples/second with an anti-aliasing low-pass filter set at 200 Hz.

10.3 Comparison between EEG and MEG

The EEG and MEG measure different aspects of the electromagnetic field due to the postsynaptic current of cortical pyramidal neurons. Therefore, it is not surprising that the signals are similar to each other. In particular, temporal characteristics of the signals, such as frequency and response latency to a sensory stimulus, are very similar between the two.

However, the signals are not identical. The signals reflect gyri and sulci activity differently. Electroencephalography electrodes are most sensitive to the electric field perpendicular to them, i.e., radial dipoles such as gyrus activity. However, due to **volume conduction**, currents from sulci are also mixed, and picked up by the electrodes. Magnetoencephalography coils are most sensitive to the magnetic field perpendicular to them. Given that the magnetic field forms perpendicular to the current, the coils are sensitive to tangential dipoles, such as sulcus activity. The magnetic signal **permeates** volume between the source and the sensor with little mixture. This is a big advantage in estimating source locations (cf. Section 13.3 in Chapter 13). However, the high permeability also has a disadvantage; coils pick up primarily sulcus activity. In other words, the effect of dipole direction and location is more severe in MEG than in EEG (Hillebrand and Barnes, 2002; Malmivuo, 2012).

The power of the frequency components also differs between the two: In the EEG signal, high-frequency activity, namely, the gamma band (>30 Hz), is attenuated as it conducts. In particular, the skull attenuates the current severely. For example, one of Hans Berger's test participants had a hole in his skull (Berger is one of the pioneers of the EEG method; cf. Chapter 9). The participant had undergone two craniotomies for the removal of a brain tumor, leaving him with a large cranial defect (Millet, 2001). Surely, Berger observed a much stronger EEG signal from the electrode on the scalp above the hole than from the electrodes on other scalp locations. To the contrary, the magnetic flux permeates the skull as well as other tissues and masses. Therefore, MEG signals contain more high-frequency signals, such as high gamma band activity (80–200 Hz).

These differences exist; however, EEG and MEG signals are still similar to each other. The signals are similar enough for the same analysis methods to be applied, as we will see in Chapters 11 and 12.

The most significant difference exists at the practical level: MEG is significantly more expensive than EEG. The SQUID and the magnetic shielding room cost more than the EEG amplifier. Liquid helium is costly and needs to be refilled more or less weekly. The whole facility occupies a large space. A lab technician may be needed for management and maintenance of the system. Overall, the running cost of an MEG lab is (much) higher than an EEG lab, as costly as MRI. As a result, the number of MEG facilities is (much) less than that of EEG labs.

Unarguably, MEG is more advanced than EEG. Technologies advanced in the late twentieth century are combined to detect tiny electromagnetic field activity from the brain. On the one hand, together with source localization, MEG offers brain signals with high temporal *and* spatial resolution. On the other hand, the size and complexity of a current MEG recording system prevent the technique from being used with some applications, such as mobile, real-life, and/or long-duration recording. For these applications, EEG has an advantage over MEG. Small/wearable

EEG devices are available commercially. With further development of the dry electrode technique, EEG applications might be incorporated into our daily lives. In the twenty-first century, EEG and MEG techniques might develop into different niches.

Summary

- Electroencephalography measures the electric field activity due to the postsynaptic current, of which the major contributor is the cortical pyramidal neuron.
- An EEG system consists of electrodes, amplifiers, and AD converters. The system converts the neural current to voltage signal, and the signal is amplified, digitized, and saved as a data file.
- Magnetoencephalography measures magnetic field activity due to the postsynaptic current.
- An MEG system consists of SQUID sensors, amplifiers, AD converters, and a magnetically shielded room. The magnetic field strength is measured, amplified, digitized, and saved as a data file.
- EEG and MEG measure different aspects of the electromagnetic field in the brain. Thus, signals are not identical but very similar. Both signals have rich information, especially in time. Frequency, phase, and amplitude of the signals allow us to investigate brain dynamics in detail. Conversely, spatial resolution of the signals is low. Moreover, the sensor-level signals are not three dimensional but two dimensional.
- Both are low risk/low intervention methods (cf. MRI in which test participants are exposed to a high magnetic field).

Review Questions

1. Name three key components for EEG recording and explain how the components are used to record the signal.
2. What is the contact impedance? Why does it need to be low?
3. Name three key components for MEG recording and explain how the components are used to record the signal.
4. List three similarities between EEG and MEG. List three dissimilarities.

Further Reading

Hansen, P. C., Kringelbach, M. L. & Salmelin, R. (2010). *MEG: An Introduction to Methods*. New York: Oxford University Press.

Schomer, D. L. & Da Silva, F. L. (2012). *Niedermeyer's Electroencephalography: Basic Principles, Clinical Applications, and Related Fields*. Philadelphia: Lippincott Williams & Wilkins. (The reference book for EEG technique.)

CHAPTER ELEVEN

Basic Analysis of Electrophysiological Signals

Learning Objectives

- Naming major artifacts in magnetoencephalography/electroencephalography (M/EEG) signals
- Understanding signal processing procedures as reported in the M/EEG literature
- Becoming familiar with the idea of the transformation of M/EEG signals, in particular time and frequency domain representations

I am no longer surprised that in hieroglyphic texts it is so difficult to differentiate the jackal from a dog. . . . A dog is defined only by a tail curled up like a trumpet. This distinction is taken from nature: all Egyptian dogs carry their tail pointing upward in this way.

Jean-François Champollion, 1828
Adopted from a translation by Rynja, 2009

What we really want to know is not always written in our native language. Data analysis is somewhat similar to deciphering. Data sit quietly, much like an ancient script on a stone, inviting us to figure out their meaning. One decipherer was Jean-François Champollion, a nineteenth-century French Egyptologist who successfully decoded Egyptian hieroglyphs. One of his basic texts was the inscription on the Rosetta Stone. There, an ancient Egyptian text was etched in a hieroglyphic script and repeated in demotic script. Moreover, translation in ancient Greek was added. After its excavation, the Rosetta Stone was considered the key to decoding the hieroglyphs. Because of complex European politics, the stone was moved around Egypt, England, and France. Because the stone was seldom displayed in public, numerous copies of the inscription were made. However, in an unconfirmed anecdote, Champollion had an opportunity to see the real stone when he was 11 years old at the salon of Jean-Baptiste Joseph Fourier, a governor of Isère province in France and at the time the custodian of the Rosetta Stone. Fourier is known today not as a politician but as a mathematician who established the foundation for signal processing. He proved that a complex oscillatory signal can be described as a sum of simple oscillatory functions, sines and cosines. Fourier analysis is *the* analysis for oscillatory signals, including those in magnetoencephalography/electroencephalography (M/EEG).

The complexity and dimensionality of M/EEG signals are often daunting. Hundreds of thousands of data points show a complex pattern of activity, changing in frequency and amplitude. The oscillations synchronize and desynchronize, thus making an intricate spatio-temporal pattern. Like any real data, M/EEG data contains **noise**. Signal processing is first applied to remove, or, at least, to reduce, noise in the data. We then face the fact that the brain is a multi-tasking/ multi-functional organ. The signal reflects not only the brain activity of interest but also those that are "irrelevant." To make things worse, the relevant signal is often (much) weaker than irrelevant signals. Here, signal processing is applied to enhance the brain signal of interest relative to those that are irrelevant. For example, when we are interested in brain response to a visual stimulus, we apply a method to enhance the visually evoked response and depress spontaneous ongoing brain activity. The method, however, will not be applied when we are interested in spontaneous activity during sleep. Thus, different methods are used for different purposes. Various signal-processing techniques have been applied in M/EEG data analysis. Tacitly or not, we often make assumptions when applying a method, e.g., that the brain response to a visual stimulus is the same over repetition. Heuristics are also frequently incorporated. In other words, we have been using everything we know to decode the complex brain signal, somewhat in the same manner that Champollion used everything, from his polyglot genius to the shape of the dog's tail, to decode the hieroglyphs. In this chapter, we introduce basic M/EEG signal analysis methods, which might seem to be a bit of a hodge-podge.

11.1 Preprocessing

The M/EEG signal analysis consists of two parts, preprocessing and main signal processing. Where one ends and the other begins is not always clear. Both processes aim to increase the signal-to-noise ratio. Roughly speaking, in preprocessing, the brain signal is increased relative to non-brain signals, such as eye movement artifacts and environmental noise, while in main signal processing, the brain signal of interest is selected or enhanced relative to irrelevant brain signals.

11.1.1 Noise

Noise comes from biological, artifactual, and/or environmental sources. For example, muscular activity generates large potentials. Muscle cells generate action potentials. When the action potential spreads over muscle fibers, the muscle starts to contract. Contraction cascades through bundles of muscle fibers, generating a complex spatio-temporal pattern of electrophysiological activity, the **electromyogram (EMG)**, which shows a wide frequency band, the peak power of which is around 60–80 Hz. The number of muscles in the head, face, and neck is not large, but these muscles are close to the M/EEG sensors. Thus, their EMG is sufficient to contaminate M/EEG signal. The frontalis muscle covers the frontal upper part of the skull. This muscle moves when the forehead is wrinkled or the eyebrows are raised. These movements affect frontal sensors especially. The temporalis muscles cover right and left sides of the skull. They move when the jaw is clenched and unclenched. The temporal electrodes are often affected by these movements. The occipitalis muscle, which covers the lower back of the skull, moves with the frontalis muscle. The movements affect the occipital electrodes. The activity of neck muscles, which move and hold the head, affect the occipital electrodes. The muscular artifacts can be reduced by instructing test participants to relax the forehead, jaw, and neck. It is also helpful to adjust their seating position for them to maintain a comfortable posture during recording.

Eye movements generate complex artifact components; the cornea is charged positively relative to the retina. As the eyeballs move, the electric potential gradient around the eyes changes. The **electrooculogram (EOG)** is recorded by electrodes around the eyes, but the activity spreads to a wider area, contaminating the M/EEG signal. The ocular artifacts often exhibit a specific shape; a step-like waveform appears during saccadic eye movements, which occur, e.g., during reading and looking for something. A slow wave appears when the eyes are drifting. A wedge-shaped component appears during an eye blink. The eye blink artifact is generated when eyelids slide over the eyeballs, which are charged. It is sometimes misunderstood that eyeballs rotate upward during an eye blink. However, this is not the case for the normal population (Picton et al., 2000). Electrooculogram artifacts are prominent in frontal polar and frontal electrodes but could spread widely. Because the eyeballs are moved by six extraocular muscles, their muscular artifacts also exist, e.g., as a saccadic spike potential. To reduce eye-movement artifacts, a test participant is often instructed to maintain fixation at a specific point and to suppress blinks.

The activity of cardiac and vascular muscles generates pulsatile electrophysiological activity, represented in the **electrocardiogram (ECG)**. Blood vessels cover the entire scalp; thus, the noise could appear in the M/EEG from any of the electrode/sensors. The noise could be significant if an electrode is placed on a large blood vessel. It could be more disruptive if a reference electrode were affected. In this case, all EEG channels would show a prominent cardiovascular artifact. Adjustment of the electrode location is effective to avoid contamination of the whole recording.

At rest, the respiratory rate is slower than 0.1 Hz. **Respiration** could generate a slow artifact. To measure it, an elastic band respiration sensor is attached around a participant's chest. Alternatively, a small flow meter can be attached below the nose. Monitoring of such slow activity is important when ultra-slow M/EEG activity is the frequency band of interest.

Sweat gland activity also affects the EEG. The state of the sweat glands changes skin conductance. **Galvanic skin response (GSR)**, which was named for Luigi Galvani who conducted the frog experiment (p.191) is slow activity (<0.1 Hz). This adds a slow drifting noise to the EEG signal. The temperature of the test room should be adjusted to prevent participants' sweating.

Head motion affects MEG more severely than it does EEG. The MEG coils are not attached to the scalp; thus, small head movements could create pseudo-signals. At least three head position indicators are attached to monitor head movements. The motion signals are used to identify head motion–related artifacts.

In addition to biological noise, recording and environmental noises also exist. Typical recording noise is due to **high electrode impedance**. A bad/old sensor exhibits a similar noisy pattern. **Environmental noise** could be reduced by

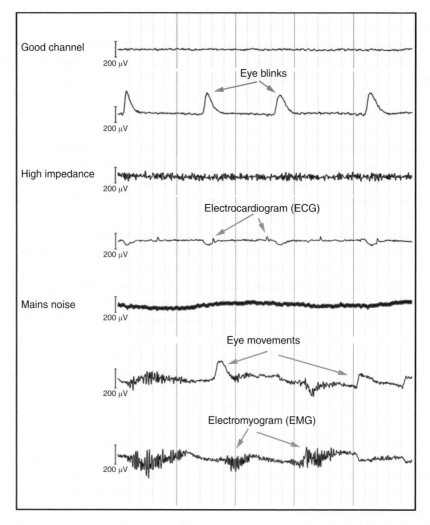

Figure 11.1 Major noises in M/EEG.
EEG segments contaminated by typical artifacts are shown. The horizontal axis represents time (s). Note that the scale of the vertical axis is 200 μV, which is several times larger than the typical scale of raw EEG (~50 μV). As a result, EEG waveform of the good channel appears flattened. These artifacts appear similarly in MEG records.

recording M/EEG inside of an electrically/magnetically shielded room. The shielded room is critical for MEG in particular. The room, however, cannot prevent noise generated within the room, e.g., the power supply (alternating current of 50 Hz or 60 Hz, also known as AC noise) of a computer display or a florescent lamp generates activity with the frequency that will be included in the M/EEG. The noise could be reduced by increasing the distance between electric devices and the test participant, properly grounding the equipment, and electrical isolation of the test participant.

No matter what we do, however, it is obvious that we cannot completely prevent all these noises. The noises are removed offline using signal-processing techniques. For identification and removal of the artifacts, EMG, EOG, ECG, respiration, and/ or head motion are recorded simultaneously with M/EEG. Most recording systems support such polygraphic functions.

11.1.2 Montage

Montage rereferences the voltage level of the EEG signal to a biological baseline. As we saw in Chapter 10, EEG is measured relative to a low voltage level, typically ground level. The recording signal is a mixture of brain and non-brain electric activities, such as muscle activity and environmental charges. As a result, the baseline level of the recording signal is inflated. In the inflated signal, we see a miniature fluctuation of big voltage values, such as 1 000 212, 1 000 227, 1 000 219, 1 000 200, . . . , and 1 000 103 µV. The recording signal alone cannot tell us how much of it is the brain signal. For this purpose, we use a reference signal. Suppose the reference signal from the left earlobe, which is recorded simultaneously with the scalp signal, gives values such as 1 000 150, 1 000 152, 1 000 148, 1 000 150, . . . , and 1 000 100 µV. The signal shows that the earlobe is charged due to (primarily) non-brain activities. Given the location, we could assume that a similar level of non-brain activity is added to the scalp recording. Based on this assumption, the reference signal is subtracted from the scalp signal. This yields a new time series of 62, 75, 71, 50, . . . , and 3 µV. A large portion of voltage that is (presumably) of non-brain origin is removed. As a result, the fluctuation becomes easy to observe. This montage puts the signal at the right level but does not remove all artifact components. As we will see, further artifact removal is necessary. Montage is not applied to the MEG signal. This is because the MEG method measures not the relative but the absolute level of magnetic field strength.

The international 10–20 system specifies six reference locations: left and right earlobes, left and right mastoids, and left and right nasopharynges. In addition to these, locations close to the scalp and without brain tissue and muscles beneath, e.g., tip of the nose, are often used as a reference location. When a single reference is applied to all the scalp electrode signals, the montage is called a **monopolar derivation**. In the monopolar derivation, the distance between the reference and each scalp electrode affects the derived signal. For example, if the left earlobe is chosen as the reference, amplitude of the signal will be smaller in the left than in the right hemisphere.

To reduce such imbalance, an average over electrodes, e.g., all scalp electrodes, is often used as a reference. The average over scalp electrodes could be a good baseline if the electrodes are distributed evenly over the scalp and the number of electrodes is not too small. In the EEG literature, "average reference" often refers to the average over all scalp electrodes. Because the **average reference** does not depend on one electrode, derived EEG signals do not show the location bias found in monopolar derivation. The average reference method, however, is not suitable for measuring large-scale activity that is distributed over many electrodes. Such activity would be removed by applying the average reference.

In **bipolar derivation**, baseline activity does not come from a reference, but another scalp electrode. When one scalp signal is subtracted from another, brain signals that are common to both loci are also removed. Bipolar derivation therefore can be seen as a more aggressive method than monopolar derivation. It gives a signal that is specific to the particular scalp electrode.

How to reference the signal, therefore, is decided according to the purpose of a research study. Most of the recent EEG recording systems offer real-time montage functions that allow flexible rereferencing. Montage can also be performed offline.

11.1.3 Segmentation and Visual Inspection

The M/EEG signal is often recorded continuously over multiple trials or runs. The continuous record is broken down into segments and inspected visually. Some segments are apparently "bad," e.g., the signal reached 500 μV. If such an artifact appeared in most of the channels, we could simply exclude the segment from the data analysis. Similarly, if one channel was noisy throughout the recording, we could omit that channel. Visual inspection is a simple but effective way to remove artifacts.

11.1.4 Independent Component Analysis for Preprocessing

Some noises, such as ECG, spread over sensors and segments cannot be removed by segment rejection. To remove, or, at least, to reduce, the noises, we apply signal processing to the data. **Independent component analysis (ICA)** is often used for that purpose (and beyond). In the analysis, N channels of EEG are transformed to N independent components. The transformation is intuitively understood as rotation. Figure 11.2 illustrates how ICA works. For the sake of illustration, N is set at 2. The two channels of the signal are plotted as a two-dimensional scatterplot. Now, we rotate the axes slightly and project each data point onto the new horizontal and vertical axes. This gives us two sets of values, components, which are a weighted sum of the original signals. As illustrated, if we keep adjusting the angle of rotation, by chance and with luck, we might find a "correct" angle by which to separate the

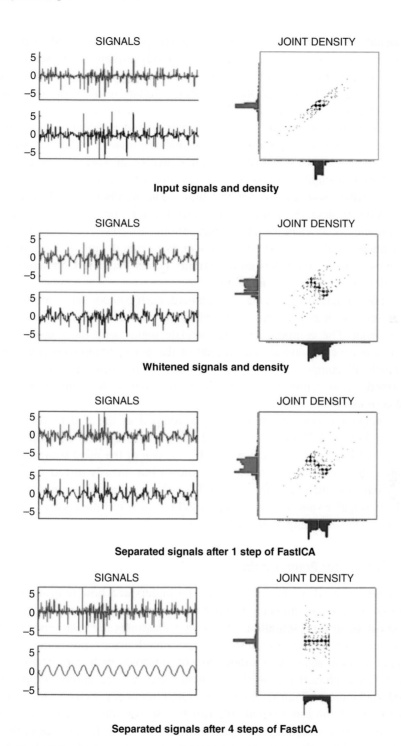

Figure 11.2 ICA steps.
Two simulated time signals (*left*) are represented in a scattergram collapsing time (*right*). The FastICA algorithm searches for a set of weights that transforms the data into the independent components. The transform can be understood as a rotation of the data.
Figures are courtesy of Patrik Hoyer

mixed signals into source signals. Independent component analysis algorithms, such as InfoMax (Makeig et al., 1996) and FastICA (Hyvarinen, 1999), search for the angle to obtain the independent components. These algorithms are slightly different from each other. However, they provide similar results for the sake of preprocessing.

The algorithms assume that (1) source signals are independent of each other, (2) the number of sources is the same as or less than the number of EEG channels, (3) the distribution of source signal values is non-Gaussian, and (4) the time delay of the signal mixing is negligible. These assumptions are met for the artifact removal: By definition, artifact sources are not the brain. The number of artifact sources is typically smaller than the number of electrodes, e.g., one heart, two eyes, and several muscles vs. 19 channels in the international 10–20 system. The distributions of the artifact signals are often non-Gaussian. For example, the distribution of data points during an eye blink has more extreme points than the Gaussian (i.e., it is leptokurtic). And the delay is negligible.

Once independent components are obtained, each component is compared with artifact signals, such as EOG and ECG, which are recorded simultaneously with the M/EEG signal. The components that correlate highly with the noise signals are considered noise components. The weight of the noise components is set to zero, after which all components are rotated back to the original axes. The back-transformed signal represents the EEG in the original N channels without the artifact components.

Independent component analysis was developed at the end of the twentieth century (Jutten and Herault, 1991) and was rapidly applied to various signals, including M/EEG. In the bigger picture, ICA is one of the blind source separation techniques that are suited to separate unknown but linearly mixed signals. Blind source separation includes other methods, such as **principal component analysis (PCA)** and **singular value decomposition (SVD)**. These techniques are also used for signal preprocessing (Jung et al., 2000).

11.1.5 Filtering for Preprocessing

Another widely used method is filtering. To understand how filtering works, we need to spend a few minutes on another representation of the M/EEG signal, the **frequency-domain representation**. Figure 11.3 illustrates the relationship between the frequency-domain representation and the time-domain representation. The M/EEG-like periodic signal is a summation of sinusoids with various frequencies, amplitudes, and phase lags. On the frequency axis, we see the amplitude of each sinusoid. As Figure 11.3 illustrates, the time- and frequency-domain representations are two views of the same signal. We can switch from one representation to the other without losing anything. Joseph Fourier came up with this idea in the nineteenth century. Since that time, mathematicians have developed a family of Fourier transforms. The **discrete Fourier transform (DFT)** transforms a discrete signal, such

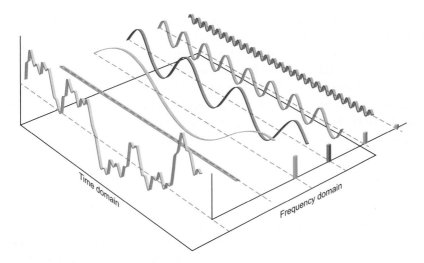

Figure 11.3 Time and frequency representations of waves.

as a digital M/EEG signal, into a discrete frequency domain signal, which is the sum of the frequency components. The inverse of the DFT transforms the frequency-domain signal back to the original time-domain signal. The DFT and inverse DFT are the theoretical bases for various M/EEG signal analysis methods.

A related (and somewhat confusing) term is the **fast Fourier transform (FFT)**, which is a computer algorithm that performs the DFT efficiently. It was introduced by American mathematicians James Cooley and John Wilder Tukey in 1965 (Cooley and Tukey, 1965). They showed that the computation for the DFT is efficiently performed when the number of data points is an exponent of 2 (2^n). The fast Fourier transform implements the efficient, thus fast, DFT algorithm. It turns out that the algorithm had already been discovered in the early nineteenth century by Carl Friedrich Gauss, one of the great German mathematicians. Cooley and Tukey re-discovered the algorithm at the right time. Helped by the dramatic increase of digital computational resources, the FFT has become the de facto standard algorithm for the DFT. A sentence such as "FFT was applied to the data" in an M/EEG paper means that digital M/EEG data was DFTed using the FFT algorithm. More details of the algorithm are discussed in Section 11.2.1.

As we know by now, some artifacts are localized in particular frequencies, e.g., AC noise at 50 or 60 Hz. To remove such noise, we could apply the DFT to the contaminated M/EEG data. In the frequency domain, the signal at the noise frequency, e.g., 50 Hz, is set to zero. Then, the signal is transformed back to the time domain via the inverse DFT. Cutting a narrow frequency band, e.g., 45–55 Hz for 50 Hz AC noise, is called **notch (band-cut) filtering. High-cut filtering** removes components higher than a threshold frequency. Thus, it is also called **low-pass filtering**. A high-cut filter is applied, for example, to remove muscular artifacts that typically have a power higher than 50 Hz. Conversely, a low-cut **(high-pass)** filter removes components lower than a threshold frequency. A low-cut filter is applied, for example, to remove slow drift due to respiration, the frequency of which is lower than 0.3 Hz at rest. The threshold needs to be adjusted carefully. For example, some event-related potentials are slow. In such cases, the low-cut threshold is set to 0.1 Hz or even lower (Tanner et al., 2015). It is interesting to compare these values with the filter settings employed in other methods such as functional magnetic resonance imaging (fMRI). For example, in resting-state fMRI the signal retained after filtering is the part below 0.1 Hz (cf. Chapter 8), which is not considered interesting for most EEG work.

11.1.6 Resampling

Magnetoencephalography/electroencephalography data have a large number of time samples, e.g., a 10-s data epoch with a sampling rate of 1000 Hz contains 10 000 data points per channel. As we know from the sampling (Nyquist) theorem (cf. Chapters 1 and 10), we could analyze the signal up to 500 Hz. The theorem also tells us that a lower sampling rate is sufficient if we are interested in lower frequency bands only. For example, when the bandwidth of interest is 1–50 Hz, a sampling rate of 100 Hz (twice as fast as this highest frequency of interest) is theoretically sufficient. In other words, we could use 1 out of every 10 data points to obtain results equivalent to those of full data point analysis. To reduce the computational cost, **down-sampling** is often applied. In practice, a somewhat higher sampling rate than the theoretical rate, such as 200 Hz for up to 50 Hz, is used as a safety margin. With this conservative criterion, we could use 1 out of every 5 data points, which means data analysis can be completed five times faster than with the original data (at least on paper). Subsampling the original data points, e.g., selecting 1 every 5 data points, is one way to down-sample the data. Alternatively, we can interpolate the original data and then resample with a slower sampling rate. The resampling is handy when the ratio of the original and the new sampling rates is not an integer (e.g., down-sampling from 1000 Hz to 256 Hz). Let us also point out the relationship between the down-sampling and low-pass filtering. The down-sampling reduces the highest frequency of the signal. Thus, it is low-pass filtering (without using the DFT).

Conversely, **up-sampling** increases the number of data points. The original data points are interpolated and resampled with a shorter sampling interval than the original. Up-sampling is applied, for example, to make the number of data points an exponent of 2 for the FFT. For example, if the number of data points is 250, it can be changed to $2^8 = 256$ using up-sampling without changing the data length in time. This is a better solution than "zero padding," which appends six zeros to the original data and introduces artifacts.

After proper preprocessing, artifacts are removed or reduced, and the M/EEG data are properly formatted for the main signal processing. Improper preprocessing does not increase signal-to-noise ratio and could even generate noise. Although preprocessing is often reported inconspicuously in an M/EEG paper, it is a very important stage in data analysis.

11.2 Main Signal Processing

The brain does a lot of things at the same time, and not all of these events are relevant to a specific research question that we are asking. Regardless of the question, the irrelevant brain activities exist in M/EEG data. The aim of the main signal analysis is, therefore, to separate relevant signals from irrelevant ones. This is significantly more difficult than preprocessing; unlike noise, we know little about target brain activity a priori, what it looks like, when it appears in what frequency, and so forth. Previous findings and heuristics are incorporated to reduce the uncertainty. Moreover, various assumptions are made to bridge the gap between the actual properties of the M/EEG signal and the requirements of mathematics behind each signal analysis technique. In this section, we introduce basic analysis methods. More advanced methods are covered in Chapter 12.

11.2.1 Spectral Analysis

In M/EEG data, we often spot changes in amplitude. For example, in Figure 9.3 in Chapter 9, when the eyes were closed, the amplitude of the signal increased. However, the exact frequency of the modulated component is hard to see in the time wave. A plot of amplitude against spectrum of frequency would be a better representation. Earlier in this chapter, we learned that the DFT converts the data from the time to the frequency domain. We would therefore use the DFT to obtain a frequency-amplitude representation of the data.

The DFT converts N time samples to N frequency data points. To compute the contribution of each frequency component from each time sample, the computation is repeated N^2 times. The total number of computations is a lot, because M/EEG data have many time samples, e.g., for 8 s of data with 512 Hz of sampling frequency (f_s), $N = 4096$, $N^2 = 16\,777\,216$. The FFT reduces the number of computations to $N\log_2 N$: $49\,152$ times per channel in this example. You could imagine that the FFT makes a huge difference in terms of computational cost. FFT is also widely accessible; even a spreadsheet package, such as Excel and Open Office, has it as a function. For the FFT to work, N needs to be exponent of two, e.g., $N = 2^{12} = 4096$. The number could be made to 2^n by padding zeros in each end. The zero padding is often used as a default in various FFT functions. Alternatively, data can be resampled during preprocessing.

Prior to an application of the FFT, the edges of the segment are smoothed. The DFT assumes that a signal is periodic, and the period repeats infinitely. Clearly, this does not hold for a segment. At both ends of the segment, the signal strength drops to zero: edges. The edges generate false frequency components over a wide range of frequencies. To reduce the spill-over, the edges are tamed. The segment is multiplied by a smooth function called a window function, e.g., Hanning, Hamming, and Gaussian functions.

The typical output of an FFT function has N complex numbers. As we learned in Chapter 9, a time wave can be represented in the polar coordinate with real and imaginary axes (cf. Fig. 9.4). Each complex number of the output represents a frequency component. Of the output, for the sake of spectrum analysis, we are concerned only with the first half of the N complex numbers. (The second half contains negative frequency components, which are mathematical and do not exist physically.) The first complex number corresponds to the $(1 * f_s/N)$ Hz component. The second complex number corresponds to $(2 * f_s/N)$ Hz, and so forth. For example, for 8 s of data with $f_s = 512$ Hz, $N = 4096$. Thus, the frequency components are 0.125, 0.250, 0.375, . . . , 256 Hz. The lowest frequency makes sense, because we cannot estimate an activity slower than 8 s, i.e., the lowest frequency is $1/8 = 0.125$ Hz. The highest frequency also makes sense according to the Nyquist theorem, 512/ 2 = 256 Hz.

The amplitude of each frequency component is computed from the complex number. In the polar plot, amplitude is the length of the vector. The length is $\sqrt{a^2 + b^2}$, where a and b corresponds to the real and imaginary parts of the components. The relationship is obvious if we imagine the vector in the polar plot and its projection to real and imaginary axes.

The amplitude is the coefficient that determines the contribution of the frequency component to the original signal, also referred to as the Fourier coefficient. The larger the coefficient, the higher the contribution becomes. The amplitude of the 0 Hz component is zero, because the signal is baselined to its mean value in an FFT. (The contribution of the direct current component can be computed by simply taking the average of the time data points.)

We are ready to plot the results. Data are often band-passed during preprocessing, e.g., 1–50 Hz. Components outside of the range are not meaningful, thus they are usually omitted from the plot. The **amplitude spectrum** plots the coefficients against the frequency. In an amplitude spectrum, we can see which frequency is dominant relative to others. A **power spectrum** shows the power of the amplitude, $a^2 + b^2$. Thus, the power spectrum is another way to show the the contribution of each frequency component to the original signal. The **amplitude spectral density (ASD)** and the **power spectral density (PSD)** are standardized spectra, in which each coefficient is divided by the sum of the coefficients over all frequency components. Thus, the unit of the standardized spectra is arbitrary. The standardized spectra are used, for example, for group data analysis.

Figure 11.4 shows a PSD of an EEG while a participant closed the eyes and relaxed. A peak is observed around 10 Hz. The activity is called **alpha (α) band** activity, the range of which is about 8–13 Hz. The name, *Alpha-Wellen* in German, was given by Hans Berger in the first human EEG in 1929. The power of the α band activity reduces when the participant is alert and performing a task. On a scalp map, the activity appears strongly over parietal and occipital electrodes/sensors. It is known, however, that not only parietal and occipital but also other cortical and subcortical regions, e.g., the thalamus, can generate alpha band activity. The alpha band activity is the most prominent oscillatory component in M/EEG signals, and

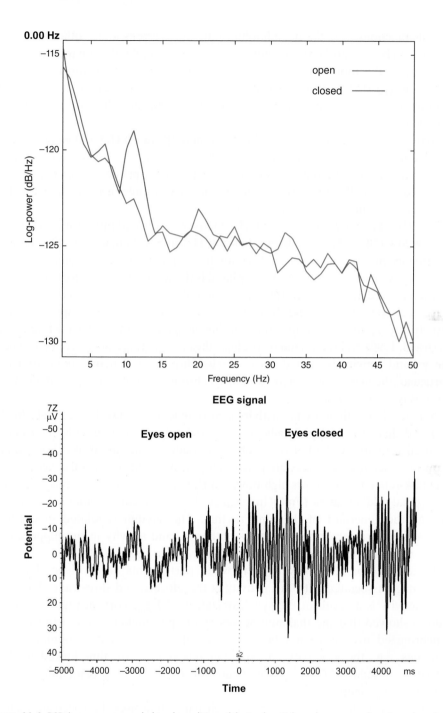

Figure 11.4 PSD in eyes open and closed conditions (electrode ~O_2), and corresponding time domain signal (*bottom*).

various functions, e.g., the default/idling state and suppression of other bands, are suggested (Başar, 2012). In the motor cortex, for example, the α band activity will occur while the motor system is idling. The motor-related rhythm is sometimes called mu (μ) rhythm to distinguish it from other α band activity. The μ rhythm is observed in EEG from the central electrodes that are close to motor-related cortical regions.

Activity faster than α band is divided into **beta (β, 13–30 Hz)** and **gamma (γ, >30 Hz) bands**. As a test participant emerges from rest and is prepared for an experimental task, the α band reduces and the β band activity appears. For example, in the motor cortex, the β band activity appears when a movement is planned, performed, or imagined (Pfurtscheller et al., 1996).

The γ band activity extends to 200 Hz, and is often divided further into sub-bands, such as **low (30–60 Hz)** and **high γ (60–200 Hz) bands**. Magnetoencephalography/electroencephalography data analysis for the γ activity is challenging for several reasons. As we can see on a PSD, the γ band is the weakest signal. Moreover, micro-saccade-related artifacts (~40 Hz), AC noise (50 or 60 Hz), and EMG (~60–80 Hz) noise overlap with the γ band. Nevertheless, various functions are implicated in the activity, e.g., feature integration and working memory retention (Tallon-Baudry and Bertrand, 1999). In intracranial recordings, these artifacts are of less concern. There, the γ band activity is related to the excitability of local neural populations. In particular, the high γ has been related to synchronization of action potentials (Fries, 2009; Ray et al., 2008).

Activity slower than α band activity is also divided into two bands, **theta (θ, 4–8 Hz)** and **delta (δ, <4 Hz) bands**. The θ band activity is commonly seen among children who are awake but is not obvious in adults who are awake. Some adults show the θ activity while they are performing a task requiring mental concentration. The task-related theta shows high power in Fpz and Fz electrodes. Thus, it is called the **frontal midline theta (Fmθ)**(Inanaga, 1998). The medial frontal cortex is considered the generator of the Fmθ rhythm. The rhythm is related to cognitive functions such as error monitoring. Another θ band activity in the hippocampus has been related to memory functions (Raghavachari et al., 2001).

Typically, δ band activity appears when participants are in deep sleep; the sleep stage associated with this activity is therefore called **slow-wave sleep**. The slow activity is a result of the synchronization of large cortical regions. Animal studies showed that the thalamus serves as the pacemaker of the activity that is synchronized over large numbers of electrodes. The activity modulates other activities, e.g., the γ activity and spontaneous spiking are time-locked to the δ activity (Steriade, 1997). A possible function of the activity is memory consolidation during sleep.

Now, let's try to read part of a research paper that uses the spectrum analysis technique. This example study investigates whether slow-wave sleep consolidates what we learned during the day (Yordanova et al., 2012). Volunteers learned a complex problem-solving task. Then, they slept overnight in an EEG lab, while

EEGs were recorded. Sleep was classified as Stage 2 (S2) sleep, which is considered shallow sleep; slow-wave sleep (SWS); and rapid eye movement (REM) sleep. The EEGs in each sleep stage were analyzed using a spectrum analysis. Figure 11.5 and its caption are reproduced from the study. What do they tell us about the role of slow-wave sleep and consolidation of learning?

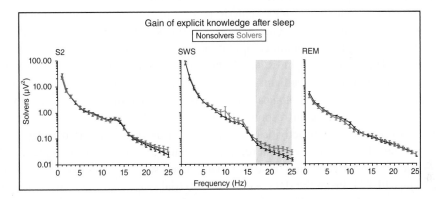

Figure 11.5 Example of a spectrum analysis.
"... Depicted is the grand average power spectrum (across electrodes C3 and C4) for three sleep stages: S2, SWS, and REM. The shaded area in SWS indicates the frequency range of significant differences between non-solvers and solvers. Standard error bars are presented for each frequency bin."
Excerpt from Yordanova et al., 2012. Figures are reproduced from with permission

Box 11.1 Phase Spectrum

Using the output of an FFT, we could compute not only the amplitude spectrum, but also the phase spectrum. The relationship among phase θ, the real part a, and the imaginary part b is $\tan\theta = b/a$ (cf. Fig. 9.4 in Chapter 9). The inverse of tangent (i.e., arctangent) of the ratio gives us the phase. The phase represents a shift of the sinusoidal component. For example, a 90° phase shift of the 10 Hz component shifts the signal 25 ms in time. To recover the original waveform from the amplitude spectrum, each frequency component is shifted according to the phase shift before summing the components. The phase shift is different from the instantaneous phase. The moment-by-moment phase change cannot be observed in the FFT(DFT)ed signal, because it does not have the time dimension. We will learn how to compute and use the instantaneous phase in Section 12.2 in Chapter 12.

The phase spectrum is a representation used less frequently than the amplitude spectrum in M/EEG data analysis. The phase spectrum is always computed in MRI signal processing: To obtain the k-space, the MR signal is DFTed, and the amplitude and the phase spectra are computed (cf. Box 2.1 in Chapter 2).

11.2.2 Event-Related Potential Analysis

In everyday life, we often recognize objects and external events quickly. For example, it takes less than a second to judge whether we are looking at a face or a house. If we want to know *when* the information processing for a face differs from that for a house, we need to analyze a brain signal with sub-second time resolution, such as M/EEG signals, from the onset of the stimulus.

Event-related potential (ERP) analysis is able to tell millisecond-by-millisecond changes of the brain activity. The method is probably the most popular method of M/EEG data analysis. The main computation is averaging of M/EEG data segments over trials. The trial averaging is simple but efficiently increases the signal-to-noise ratio in the **event-related paradigm**. In the paradigm, an event of interest is defined not only in physical and/or psychological dimensions, but also in time, e.g., a flash of visual stimulus at time t. The brain response to the event is the signal, while ongoing and stimulus-irrelevant neural activities are considered as noise in this paradigm. The signal is mixed with the noise; therefore, it is hard to observe in a single-trial M/EEG. Now consider repeating the event many times, say 200 trials every 2–3 s, while recording M/EEG. From the data, we obtain 200 trial segments, which are segmented around the stimulus, e.g., -200 to +1500 ms from the stimulus onset. Because the event is the same, we could assume that the neural response is the same, or at least similar, in waveform and latency over the trials. Conversely, ongoing activity is not time-locked to the event, and there is no a priori reason to assume similarity among them across the trials. When all trials are aligned with the event and averaged over trials, non-evoked components cancel out and only evoked responses remain. The average waveforms are called **evoked potentials (EPs)** (Fig. 11.6).

Evoked potentials to sensory stimulation are prefixed by modality: **VEP** (visual), **AEP** (auditory), **SEP** (somatosensory), **OEP** (olfactory), and **GEP** (gastric). Not only an external stimulus but also an internal state modulate potentials. For example, when a beep is presented repeatedly in 1 Hz, a participant starts expecting the beep. If the expected beep was skipped, the lack of event evokes a component. In this case, the activity occurred not due to a stimulus/exogenous event, but due to an endogenous event. **Event–related potential (ERP)** is the collective term for brain activities elicited by exogenous and endogenous events. Psychological factors, e.g., attention and memory load, modulate ERPs.

Event-related potentials are evaluated relative to baseline activity, which is the activity during a no- or neutral stimulus period. Often a prestimulus period, e.g., -200 to 0 ms, is taken as the baseline. **Amplitude** and **polarity** (negative or positive) of major components are determined relative to the baseline (cf. Box 9.1 in Chapter 9). Also, from the onset/offset of the stimulus, the **order** or **latency** is specified. For example, P3 is the third positive component. The same component is sometimes referred to as "P300," a positive component that appears around 300 ms from the event. **Scalp distribution** is also important in specifying a component, e.g., the maximum peak of P3 is often found in parietal electrodes (Fig. 11.6). The P3 is

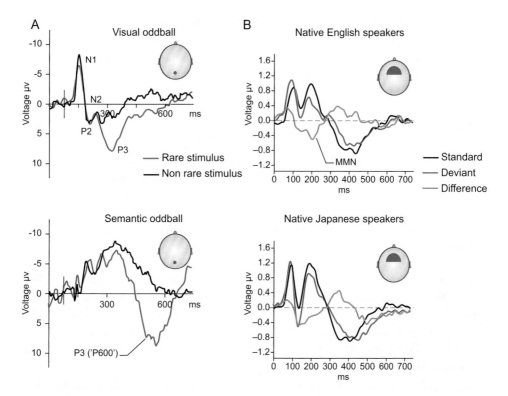

Figure 11.6 ERP components.

(A) In response to a stimulus, a sequence of ERP components appears. Note that the Y-axis is reversed. This "upward-negative" style is common in the ERP literature. The ERPs to a rare stimulus (red) show larger late components (P3) than do those to non-rare stimuli (black). Latency of P3 depends on task conditions (Kotchoubey et al., 2002). (B) Difference waves (orange): Native Japanese speakers do not distinguish /r/ and /l/ sounds. Difference between ERPs to /r/ and /l/ sounds are computed for the Japanese and native English speakers. The native English speakers show larger mismatch negativity around 200 ms than the Japanese speakers (Zevin et al., 2010).

The figures are reproduced with permission

one of the first components discovered to show sensitivity to endogenous factors, such as stimulus uncertainties, attention, and semantic processing. For example, the amplitude of the P3 after a rarely presented tone will be higher than that after frequently presented tones. The effect does not depend on sensory modalities (Sutton et al., 1965).

Difference waveforms between conditions are also useful in identifying a component. For example, in a difference wave between ERPs of rare and frequent tones, we can spot a negative component around 200 ms in centro-frontal electrodes. This component is called mismatch negativity (MMN) (Näätänen et al., 1978). The component tells us that stimulus probability information is processed within 200 ms from the stimulus onset.

Even-related potentials also show that **selective attention** starts affecting information processing in its early stages. For example, the amplitude of ERP components P1 and N1 (latency 80–150 ms) is larger for the components of attended than an unattended stimuli (Hillyard et al., 1973) (see also Fig. 11.7). An MEG ERP study showed an even earlier effect (Poghosyan and Ioannides, 2008).

The ERPs earlier than P1 reflect activity due to early sensory processes. For example, in response to a click tone, there is a complex of components that appear within 15 ms. The **auditory brainstem response (ABR)** reflects the activity of auditory nuclei in the brainstem. The response is modality specific and insensitive to endogenous factors, such as attention. The auditory brainstem response readily shows the power of the ERP method. Such early activity that originates from a deep brain structure, and therefore is faintly present in the recording, can be observed in this method.

The ERP analysis assumes that (1) the event evokes the signal consistently over trials, (2) the timing of the signal is also consistent over the trials, (3) signal and noise are uncorrelated, and (4) the noise is random with zero mean. Violation of these assumptions results in poor signal quality. For example, if the latency jitters from trial to trial, the averaging cancels out the activity, and thus the amplitude of the EP will be small. Note that the small average amplitude does not mean small single trial amplitude in this case (cf. Section 12.2.5. in Chapter 12). Instead of the mean, the median can be used to ease the effect of outliers.

A variant of the ERP method is the **steady-state evoked potentials (ssEPs) method**, which is the brain response to repeated stimulation. For example, when a visual stimulus is presented at 12 Hz, the tail of one evoked response overlaps with the head of the next. Averaging of the segments gives the sequence of the peaks. When the data are DFTed, the PSD shows a peak at 12 Hz, which reflects the 12 Hz stimulation. The peak changes not only with exogenous but also with endogenous factors, similar to ERP amplitude. For example, the PSD peak was higher when observers attended to the flashing stimulus than when they did not (Morgan et al., 1996). The DFT collapses the time dimension. Thus, on the one hand, we lose time information. On the other hand, however, it is more robust against latency jitters than trial averaging. Therefore, the signal-to-noise ratio of ssEP is typically better than ERP.

Now, let's take a look at part of an ERP paper (Clark and Hillyard, 1996). This paper reports when the effect of visuo-spatial attention appears in EEG signals. Participants focused on the left or right side of the visual field. Brain responses to visual targets that appeared in the attended and nonattended side are shown in the ERP measure. In all waveforms, ERPs recorded before 100 ms did not show any difference between the attended and nonattended conditions.

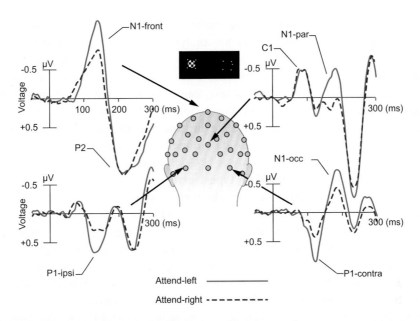

Figure 11.7 Example of an ERP analysis (grand average of VEPs).
"Grand average visual ERPs over 17 subjects recorded from four scalp sites in response to small circular checkerboard stimuli in a spatial attention task. Stimuli were flashed in a rapid, randomized sequence to the left and right visual fields while subjects attended to one visual field at a time. ERPs shown are in response to left field flashes, with waveforms superimposed for attend-left (solid lines) and attend-right (dotted lines) conditions. Note that attending to the stimulus location produces an increased amplitude of the P1 components (80–130 ms) over the contra- and ipsilateral occipital scalp, as well as of multiple N1 components (120–200 ms) over frontal (front), parietal (par), and occipital (occ) scalp areas. In contrast, the earlier C1 component (50–90 ms), which was localized to primary visual cortex, did not change as a function of attention. Abscissa, time base in milliseconds."
Excerpt from Hillyard and Anllo-Vento, 1998. The figures were originally published in Clark and Hillyard, 1996. The figures are reproduced with permission

11.3 Statistical Tests

As a result of M/EEG analysis, we have multivariate results; for example, 2 s of ERP in a 500 Hz sampling rate has 1000 data points, which may be computed for each of the 128 channels, in 2 task conditions for each of 20 participants. This yields a matrix of 1000 x 128 x 2 x 20 data points. To find where in time and in what channels a difference exists between conditions, a multivariate analysis, e.g., multivariate analysis of covariance (MANCOVA), can be applied (Friston,

Stephan, Heather, et al., 1996). The analysis fits a linear model to the multidimensional data. This is similar to an analysis of covariance (ANCOVA) for univariate data, which have one data point per condition per participant, e.g. a mean error rate. Univariate methods, e.g., ANCOVA, analysis of variance (ANOVA), and Mann–Whitney U test, can also be applied with **type-I error correction**, e.g., family-wise error correction (FWE). The error correction is necessary, because the results correlate in time and in sensor space (cf. Chapter 7). Prior to a univariate test, the data dimensions could also be reduced. For example, principal component analysis (PCA) could reduce the 128 channels to several principle components. The type-I error correction is less harsh for the several components than for the 128 channels of data.

Previous findings and heuristics are important for the data analysis. They tell us a priori which aspect of the results becomes relevant, e.g., by predicting whether the amplitude of the P300 ERP in parietal regions would differ between two conditions. Such heuristics, on the one hand, could reduce the dimensionality of the results dramatically. For example, if we select the peak amplitude of P3 of the Pz electrode, the multivariate ERP result is reduced to a univariate result, a 2×20 matrix. On the other hand, subsetting results requires careful consideration, e.g., why peak value is used instead of the area under the curve, why other parietal electrodes were not included, and other arguments for the subsetting need to be sound and clear. This is important to avoid a circular analysis (Kriegeskorte et al., 2009), as was explained in Chapter 7.

Box 11.2 ANOVA and Power Spectrum

It may be useful to know that spectral analysis is closely related to ANOVA. To obtain a power spectrum, a time domain signal is DFTed to frequency components, then the amplitude is *squared*. In a way, each power value represents the variance of the analyzed signal that is explained by oscillatory activity at that frequency. Thus, power is a kind of variance. Now we remind ourselves how variance is computed given N data points: Difference between the mean and each data point is *squared*. Then the squares are summed and divided by N. Thus, variance is a kind of power. Mathematically, variance of the original signal equals half of the total spectrum power. Therefore, variance due to a certain frequency band, such as alpha band activity, can be obtained by summing power values within the band (e.g., 8–13 Hz) and halving the sum. If we wish to know whether the alpha band power differs between two conditions, we could compute the power spectrum, derive the variance, and take the ratio of variances between the two conditions. The ratio is an *F*-statistic that we consult in ANOVA.

Summary

- Magnetoencephalography/electroencephalography (M/EEG) signals are processed using digital signal-processing techniques. Roughly, we could consider two stages: Preprocessing reduces/removes artifacts in M/EEG signals. Main signal processing selects the brain signal of interest from the non-interesting part of signal.
- Via Fourier transform, M/EEG signals can be represented in time or frequency domains.
- Artifacts can be identified by their characteristics in time and/or frequency domain signals.
- A large number of signal-processing methods are applicable to M/EEG signals. Usually more than one signal-processing method is applied.
- Statistics are often multivariate. Dependence between the variables is dealt with in ways similar to other brain imaging data.

Review Questions

1. Name five major artifacts in EEG recordings. How can they be identified?
2. Suppose you have an EEG record that is contaminated by eye blinks. Describe two methods for the removal of the artifacts.
3. Explain what spectrum analysis is. Describe in words how to obtain power spectral density (PSD) from M/EEG data. Name two research fields or application domains in which PSD analysis is frequently used.
4. Explain what the evoked potential (EP) is. Describe how to identify a component in an EP. List two examples of an EP used in psychological studies.

Further Reading

Delorme, A. & Makeig, S. (2004). EEGLAB: an open source toolbox for analysis of single-trial EEG dynamics including independent component analysis. *Journal of Neuroscience Methods*, **134**, 9–21. (This is a concise introduction to the ICA method in M/EEG analysis.)

Hyvärinen, A., Karhunen, J. & Oja, E. (2004). *Independent Component Analysis*. New York: John Wiley & Sons.

Luck, S. J. (2014). *An Introduction to the Event-Related Potential Technique*. Cambridge, MA: MIT Press.

Van Drongelen, W. (2006). *Signal Processing for Neuroscientists: An Introduction to the Analysis of Physiological Signals*, Cambridge, MA: Academic Press. (This textbook includes a chapter that explains the FFT in detail.).

CHAPTER TWELVE

Advanced Data Analysis

Learning Objectives

- Understanding M/EEG data in different representations, namely, time plot, frequency plot, time-frequency plot, and correlogram
- Understanding the relationship between discreet Fourier transform and short time Fourier transform
- Understanding the key ideas behind wavelet transform
- Understanding the basics of phase analysis
- Understanding the relationship between autoregressive analysis and Grainger causality

The verb "advance" means moving forward in a purposeful manner. Advanced analysis on M/EEG signals, therefore, should move us closer to what we want to know from the data. So far, we've learned that the M/EEG time series can be transformed to the frequency domain applying the discrete Fourier transform (DFT). In the frequency domain, contributions of each frequency component are clearly observed. However, in the frequency domain, we cannot tell whether the contributions changed with time. What should we do if we want to know, for example, whether the alpha band activity increased before or after a stimulus presentation? We've also learned that M/EEG signals have a fine time resolution. Taking advantage of the resolution, we can observe moment-by-moment interactions between brain regions, such as synchrony and desynchrony between frontal and parietal signals. In this chapter, we introduce some advanced data analysis methods to observe such fascinating aspects in the signal.

12.1 Short Time Fourier Transform and Wavelet Transform

12.1.1 Short Time Fourier Transform

The M/EEG data can be represented in either a time or frequency domain via the DFT. However, neither of the representations is sufficient if we wish to know when and which frequency component changed its activity. In such a case, we need to represent the signal in time *and* frequency. A possible strategy is to apply the DFT not to the whole data, but to short segments one after another. As a result, we obtain a time series of the DFT. Figure 12.1 shows a time series of a power spectral

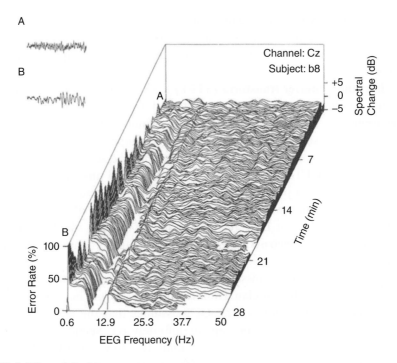

Figure 12.1 PSD stuck in time.
The figure is taken from Makeig and Inlow (1993). EEG spectral power was computed from 4 s EEG segments of a 28 min session of a subject performing a task. Performance error at each segment was plotted on the vertical axis. Activity around 10 Hz activity is high when the error rate is low (the error rate is projected on the long wall), while the opposite relation is seen in activity around 4 Hz. (A) and (B) show a representative time-domain signal of the low and high error trials, respectively.
The figure was reproduced with permission

density (PSD) computed from the results of a DFT applied to such short segments (420 4 s segments). The time series of the PSD gives us a **time-frequency representation** of the signal, in which we can observe when and which frequency component changed in amplitude.

The temporal and frequency resolution of the spectrogram is determined by the length of the data segment. For example, if the length is 100 ms, a spectrum is obtained every 100 ms. To increase time resolution, the segment length may be decreased, e.g., to 25 ms. This, however, creates another problem; a 100 ms segment could include about one cycle of alpha activity, while a 25 ms segment cannot, i.e., we cannot obtain a reliable estimation of alpha band activity using a 25 ms segment. If we increase the length, for example, to 200 ms, the reliability of the estimation for alpha band activity (8–13 Hz) would increase, but the time resolution of faster activity will decrease; for example, beta band activity (13–30 Hz) has about 10 cycles in the 200 ms segment. The DFT collapses time; therefore, we cannot tell which of the cycles changed its activity. The dilemma is clear: When we increase resolution in time, we decrease that in frequency, and vice versa. This trade-off is fundamental to time-frequency analysis, Thus, it is called the uncertainty principle of the Fourier transform.

The **short time Fourier transform (STFT)** eases the problem by incorporating a "moving window" technique. The window slides over the data in time. The DFT is applied to a data segment within the window. The window has a fixed length and smooth shape, e.g., 200 ms and a bell shape (Gaussian). The window function is applied to tame the edges of a segment; the segment is multiplied by the window and is DFTed. Then, the window of a small time step is shifted, e.g., 2 ms, which is one data point in a 500 Hz sampling rate, and the DFT is applied again. The moving window technique gives us a time series of the DFT results in small time steps. Adjacent DFT results are similar but not identical. The result is represented by a **spectrogram**, which plots amplitude/power in time and frequency.

The STFT using the Gaussian moving window was introduced by the Hungarian-British mathematician Dennis Gabor (1946). The window function is used to tame segment edges. The DFT assumes that the signal is stationary and periodic and that the period repeats infinitely (cf. Section 11.2.1 in Chapter 11). No real M/EEG data continue infinitely. However, the DFT sees the signal not as a segment but as an infinite concatenation of the segment. The concatenation of the data segments often adds sharp edges in the signal. These pseudoedges add noise to the DFT results. To tame the pseudoedges, the signal is attenuated toward the ends of the segment. A tapered window function is applied to each data epoch prior to DFT. Intuitively, we could understand that the problem of the edges worsen as the segment shortens. Thus, the window function is particularly important in STFT. In addition to the Gaussian, other window functions, e.g., Kaiser-Bessel, Hamming, and Hunning functions, are also used depending on the specific purpose of the STFT analysis (Gao and Yan, 2010).

Back-transform from the spectrogram to the time-domain signal is seldom performed in M/EEG analysis because it is rather complex due to the moving window; segments are weighted and overlapped in the STFT (strictly speaking, the spectrogram is not equal to the original time-domain data), which makes the inverse of the STFT more complex than the inverse DFT of an entire segment.

In a spectrogram, we wish to see time-resolved frequency activity. For the best result, prior knowledge of the activity of interest needs to be incorporated into the analysis. For example, when we expect to see a transient amplitude change in alpha band (8–13 Hz), the segment length would be set to 125 ms, i.e., a period of an 8 Hz sinusoid or longer. In an exploratory analysis, however, such parameters are not available. Using a fixed length window, there is the possibility of missing interesting activity because the segment is too short or the activity is smeared, thus being hard to localize in time because the segment was too long. In other words, the problem in using the STFT is the fixed segment that forces a single time-frequency resolution to the signal, the resolution of which trades off between time and frequency.

How the STFT was developed from the DFT is a good example of how our predecessors advanced the analysis. Not all problems were solved, but at least they managed to see what they wanted to see.

12.1.2 Wavelet Transform

The wavelet transform is another way to obtain a time-frequency representation of the signal. The method is derived from a different line of thinking from that involved in Fourier transforms. Fourier took ever-repeating sinusoids as the basis of signal decomposition. We could, however, think of other basis functions. Consider a pattern: a short positive pulse followed by a negative pulse. The repetition of this pattern in time makes a continuous oscillation. Scaling and shifting of the pattern make more complex patterns possible. Let's stretch and shrink the pattern, shift the scaled patterns in time, and sum over the patterns. As a result, a complex temporal wave appears, which might look like M/EEG signals. The example here shows that such a pattern, a **wavelet**, can be a basis function of signal decomposition that is an alternative to sinusoids. Sinusoidal basis functions are stationary and repeat infinitely. Conversely, wavelet functions are local. The M/EEG signal is often not stationary. Moreover, transient activity, e.g., an evoked response to a face stimulus, is often the activity of interest. In other words, wavelet transform is an attractive alternative to the DFT in M/EEG signal analysis.

In principle, any short time pattern could be a basis function of the wavelet transform if the pattern is scaled and shifted freely. In fact, some popular wavelets are pretty bizarre looking. In M/EEG signal processing, wavelets such as Morlet, Gaussian, and Mexican hat are often used. Of these, probably the most widely used is the **Morlet wavelet**, named after Jean Morlet, a French geophysicist and one of the founders of wavelet analysis. The Morlet wavelet function is the product of two time functions, sinusoid and Gaussian (Fig. 12.2). It resembles a piece of cosine wave. The number of cycles in the Morlet wavelet is called the wavenumber. Typically, the wavenumber, c, is set to 5 or more, which works well for most of the M/EEG frequency range. The "mother" wavelet is scaled: compressed for faster or expanded for slower frequencies. All "children" have the same number of cycles, but the length is different. For example, given $c = 5$, the wavelet for 10 Hz has the five cycles in 500 ms, while that for 5 Hz extends to 1000 ms.

To compute a 10 Hz amplitude at time t, the center of the 10 Hz Morlet wavelet is placed at t. The wavelet and M/EEG data are multiplied, and the products are summed over the length of the wavelet, in this case, 500 ms. The sum is called the **wavelet coefficient**. The meaning of the wavelet coefficient is clear if we remind ourselves what the Fourier coefficient meant in the DFT:

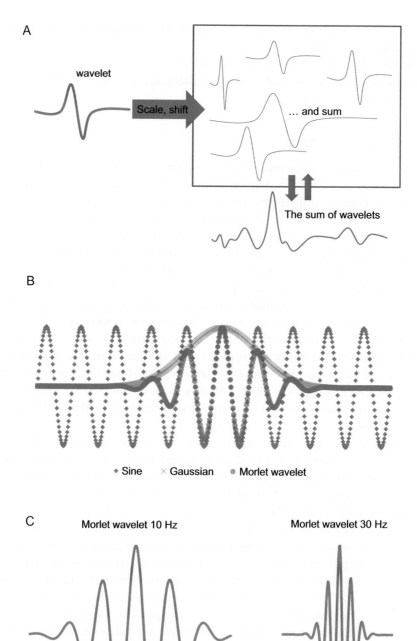

Figure 12.2 Illustration of wavelet analysis.
(A) From a wavelet to wave, vise versa. (B) The Morlet wavelet is the product of a sinusoid and the Gaussian function. The example contains 5 cycles. (C) Scaling of the wavelet. (D) Result of the convolution between the 10 Hz Morlet wavelet and the EEG signal.

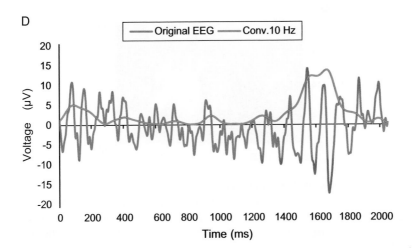

Figure 12.2 (*cont.*)

The Fourier coefficient shows the contribution of each sinusoidal component to an M/EEG signal, collapsed over all time points. The coefficient is the amplitude of the sinusoid. Likewise, the wavelet coefficient shows the contribution of the wavelet to the M/EEG signal at time t. Thus, the coefficient is the amplitude of 10 Hz oscillations at time t. The wavelet is shifted one data point in time, and the computation is repeated. The sweep of computation is equivalent to computing the convolution between the wavelet and the data, which gives a time series of wavelet coefficients. In this example, it gives a series of **instantaneous amplitudes** of 10 Hz oscillations. The convolution is repeated for other scales of wavelets, e.g., 2 Hz, 4 Hz, 6 Hz, 8 Hz, 12 Hz, 14 Hz, and so forth. The instantaneous amplitude is plotted on the time and frequency axes. The time-frequency representation of the signal is called a **scalogram** (Fig. 12.3). The scalogram looks similar to the spectrogram of the STFT, but it is different. Unlike a spectrogram, the time-frequency resolution of the scalogram is not fixed because the length of the wavelet is scaled to each frequency.

The following is an example of a scalogram taken from an EEG study (Pfurtscheller and Da Silva, 1999). The study investigated timing and frequency of the motor-control-related EEG signal. The cortical regions on the front bank of the central sulcus and pre-central gyrus play a critical role in motor control. The motor cortex controls the limbs contralaterally, the reason a trauma to the left motor cortex often results in a paralysis of the right limbs. Figure 12.3 is a scalogram of EEG data from the C3 electrode during right index finger tapping (Pfurtscheller and Da Silva, 1999). We can see when and in what frequency the motor-related brain activity occurred in the time-frequency plot.

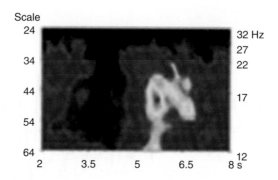

Figure 12.3 Example of wavelet analysis (scalogram during finger tapping).
"Scalogram displaying the squared and over all trials averaged wavelet coefficients for the time
interval 2 to 8 s (x axis). Scale (left axis) running from 24 to 64 corresponds to a frequency range
(right axis) from 12 to 32 Hz. Color-scale from 'black' (minimum) to 'red' (maximum): The maximum
is marked by a cross."
Excerpt from caption of figure 5 in Pfurtscheller and Da Silva, 1999. The figure was reproduced with permission

12.1.3 STFT or Wavelet?

In the 1960s, Jean Morlet was working as an oil exploration engineer in a French oil
company, Elf-Aquitaine. To search an underground oil reserve, an artificial seismic
activity is induced. Hundreds of underground formations reflect the activity, and the
mixture of the reflections is recorded by probes on the ground. Morlet applied the
STFT to the data; however, the results were not promising. The data had many
transient activities – in other words, the data were not stationary enough for the
DFT to work. He finally shortened the sinusoidal basis functions to "wavelets." The
results allowed him to track transient changes in the data that could indicate
qualitative differences in the formations, signaling borders with a potential oil
reserve. Most of his colleagues initially believed neither the method nor the results
(Hubbard, 1996). Interestingly, more or less the same idea was simultaneously
developed in different fields of science in different parts of the world. We can still
see traces of this parallel evolution, e.g., Morlet wavelet and Gabor wavelet are
practically the same function. The different names come from the different schools
of the analysis, French or British.

Unlike wavelet, the STFT assumes the signal to be stationary and infinite.
These assumptions may not fit the reality of the M/EEG signal, which often
includes nonstationary segments and always has finite length. The wavelet transform adjusts the window length according to the frequency. Thus, it provides a
multi-resolution time-frequency representation. Such an adjustment of the time-
frequency resolution works well as long as slow components always change slowly
and fast components always change quickly. However, in real data, a slow component could increase in amplitude suddenly. In such a case, the STFT may still
perform better, e.g., an STFT with 100 ms segment would locate a sudden change

of a 10 Hz amplitude in time better than a 10 Hz Morlet with $c = 5$ would. Prior knowledge about the target phenomenon, such as its frequency and timing, matters for the choice of one over the other method.

There are more differences between the two methods. Let us list one more, which is about the inverse function. The wavelet method has an inverse wavelet transform. The wavelet transform and its inverse are frequently used to band-pass the M/EEG signal. Taking the inverse of the STFT is possible but significantly more complex than that for the wavelet. Thus, the inverse is seldom used in M/EEG analysis.

Finally, there are a couple of naming conventions that often cause slight confusion. The STFT uses DFT, because M/EEG data are discrete (digitized). In this respect, the wavelet transform of the M/EEG signal could also be called a "discrete" wavelet transform. However, the term **discrete wavelet transform (DWT)** often refers to something very different. It means that scaling and translation of a wavelet is not continuous, e.g., a wavelet is shifted on data with a step size of 2^n samples (cf. multi-resolution analysis). The wavelet transform with continuous scaling and translation, including the Morlet wavelet, is therefore called **continuous wavelet transform (CWT)**. If you are looking for the Morlet wavelet function in a signal-processing package, instead of the DWT menu, try the CWT menu.

12.2 Phase Analysis

12.2.1 Computation of the Phase

As we learned in Chapter 9, the phase is an angle between 0° and 360°. However, the unit of time domain signal is μV. Apparently, we need to do something to obtain the phase from the data. The DFT lets us compute a phase spectrum; however, the transform collapses time (cf. Box 11.1 in Chapter 11). To obtain phase angles, which are changing moment by moment, i.e., **instantaneous phase**, we need to process the signal differently. One way to compute the instantaneous phase is to apply the **Hilbert transform**. The function transforms the time "wave" to a "helix" (cf. Fig. 9.4B in Chapter 9). The transformation is necessary to obtain a unique phase for each time point. For example, consider a cosine time wave that oscillates between -1 and 1. When the cosine is 0.50 at time t, trigonometry tells us that two angles, 60° and 300°, correspond to the single cosine value. Which one should we take? To disambiguate, we need to check the cosine *and* the sine of the wave at t; if the cosine and sine are 0.50 and 0.87, then the phase is 60°. If the values are 0.50, and -0.87, then the phase is 300°. The Hilbert transform of the cosine wave gives a wave 90° apart, i.e., the sine wave. When the cosine and the sine waves are plotted in 3D, we see a helix. There is no ambiguity of phase in a helix. The M/EEG signals are not sinusoid; however, the Hilbert transform computes a signal with a phase shift of 90° from the original signal. The pair of signals is called an **analytic signal**. The phase is not ambiguous in the analytic signal.

Each time point in the analytic signal is therefore expressed as a complex number, $a_t + b_t i$, where i is the imaginary unit (cf. Fig. 9.4A in Chapter 9 and Box 12.1). The real part is $a_t = \cos \theta_t$ and the imaginary part is $b_t = \sin \theta_t$, where t is time. Trigonometry tells us that the relationship among θ_t, a_t, and b_t is $\tan \theta_t = {b_t}/{a_t}$. Therefore, the instantaneous phase is given by the inverse of the tangent, i.e., the arctangent of the ratio.

Accuracy of the phase estimation increases as the band width of the signal decreases, because the narrower the band, the closer the band-passed signal to a sinusoid. Thus, often the signal is band-passed prior to the application of the Hilbert transform.

Another way to compute the phase is to use the complex Morlet wavelet transform. The wavelet is a pair of Morlet wavelets that are shifted relative to each other in 90°, i.e., a piece of cosine and sine waves in a Gaussian envelope. Application of the wavelet gives a pair of time series, one real and the other imaginary. From the complex time series, the phase is computed in the same way as we did for the analytical signal of the Hilbert transform. The results of the two methods of phase computation do not have much difference in the practice of M/ EEG phase analysis (Le Van Quyen et al., 2001). Both the Hilbert transform and complex Morlet are available in various signal analysis libraries, e.g., the scipy. signal library of Python.

12.2.2 Phase Synchrony

A concrete example may help us to understand how phase analysis works: Let's suppose that we want to know whether left and right motor cortices synchronize their activity during a bimanual motor task. To find out, we measure EEG during the task and at rest. The electrodes C3 and C4 are approximately on the left and right motor cortices. To check to see whether the EEG from these electrodes synchronize, we could simply correlate the signals. The results of the correlation primarily reflect alpha band and slower activity, because the slow components have a large contribution to the signal (cf. lopsided PSD in Fig. 11.4 in Chapter 11). However, it is known that the motor-related activity appears around 20 Hz in the beta band (Conway et al., 1995). The correlation in the beta band is overshadowed by that of the slow activities: The coherence analysis of the full signal could miss the synchrony of interest.

We could band-pass the signal for the beta band prior to computing the correlation. This yields better results than the full-signal coherence, but they are not perfect. Even if the signals go up and down in exactly the same timing, the correlation coefficient does not become 1 because of differences in amplitude. For example, if the reference is on the left ear, the amplitude of C3 is smaller than that of C4. To eliminate the effect of amplitude, it is better to use the phase than the band-passed signal.

To estimate the beta band synchrony between the motor cortices, we compare the phase of 20 Hz activity between C3 and C4. For a reliable synchrony estimation, the signals are compared for at least several cycles (Lachaux et al., 1999). For example, for a 20 Hz oscillation, a 200 ms segment contains 10 cycles. For each time point, we take the difference between the two phases. The difference, or relative phase, is yet another angle. So, we consider the relative phase as a vector on a circle with radius 1 (Fig. 12.4). We can plot all the relative phases from the segment as vectors on the unit circle. When the two signals are not synchronized, the vectors point in different directions on the unit circle. When the vectors are averaged, the length of the mean vector is close to 0 (Fig. 12.4A). Conversely, while the two signals are synchronized, their relative phase stays around the same angle over time. Thus, the length of the mean vector becomes close to 1 (Fig. 12.4B). That is, the length of mean vector takes a value between 0 and 1. Zero indicates that the phase relation of the pair is random, while 1 means perfect phase synchrony. The length of the mean vector has several labels: **phase coherence**, **synchrony index (SI)**, **phase-locking index (PLI)**, and **single-trial phase-locking value (S-PLV)**.

Phase coherence can be computed with a moving window. The results show dynamic changes of synchrony between the two signals. The time resolution of synchrony estimation is determined by the length of the window.

When the difference between the two stays close to 0°, we could consider that the signals are synchronized. Sometimes, the difference constantly shows a

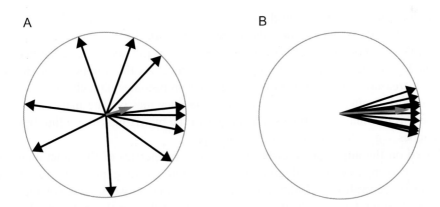

Figure 12.4 Averaging phases.
The phases are represented as unit vectors (length = 1). When the vectors are pointing to various directions (A), they cancel each other out; thus, the length of the mean vector (red) becomes close to 0. In such a case, the mean phase (angle) is not reliable. Conversely, when the vectors are pointing in a similar direction (B), the length of the mean vector is closer to 1, and the mean phase is reliable.

non-zero angle, e.g., 72°. For the 20 Hz activity, the phase difference corresponds to 10 ms. That is, the signals have a constant time lag of 10 ms. Such phase locking with time lag, lagged synchrony, is also an interesting relationship between the two activities.

Figure 12.5 shows an example of phase synchrony analysis (Nikouline et al., 2001). In this MEG study, the synchrony between bilateral motor cortices in beta band activity was investigated. The MEG signal was obtained while the test participants were relaxed and awake. As expected, the PSD of the signal from the sensors above the bilateral motor cortices shows a peak around 20 Hz in addition to a peak in the alpha band. The beta signal is extracted via a complex Morlet transform from which the phase was computed. The phase difference between the two is computed for each time point. The histogram of the phase lag shows a peak at around 0°. The result suggests that left and right motor cortices were synchronized in the beta band activity in the rest condition.

The example also illustrates the issue of signal power in phase analysis. Figure 12.5D has three histograms of a phase lag that are computed from sensor pairs that showed strong, medium, and weak beta activity. Phase concentration is less apparent for the weaker beta activity. The result, however, does not necessarily mean that the weaker beta activity is less synchronized. It is likely that the result is confounded with signal strength; A weak signal is a noisy signal. Any estimation using a weak signal is less clear than that with strong signals. This example tells us that signal should have sufficient power for a reliable phase estimation.

12.2.3 Network Analysis

Once we compute phase synchrony, network analysis is just one step away. A network is defined by **nodes** and **edges**, which are the link between a pair of nodes. For example, we could consider the sensors as the nodes. An edge between two nodes can be drawn based on phase coherence. As the number of nodes and edges increases, a graph drawn on a head diagram becomes difficult to read. Thus, the network is often represented with the adjacency matrix. The matrix is $N \times N$, where N is the number of nodes. Each entry of the matrix indicates a link between two nodes, e.g., 1 for an edge, or 0 for no edge.

Based on the **adjacency matrix**, the network properties of the functional network are computed, e.g., degree of distribution, average path length, cluster coefficient, centrality, and network motif. Numerous network indices have been proposed. Some have implications for information flow in the network (Fornito et al., 2016). The relationship between these network properties and brain function in the context of cognitive neuroscience is currently under investigation. Therefore, we do not investigate functional implications of the properties but simply present an example (Fig. 12.6). In the study, the structure of a synchrony-based functional network was compared between dyslexic and control group

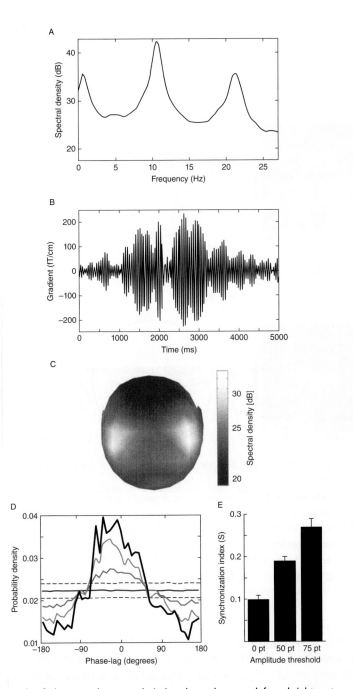

Figure 12.5 Example of phase synchrony analysis (synchrony between left and right motor cortices). "An example of beta oscillations (right hemisphere, subject N5). (a) Spectrum of the MEG signal. Note the prominent peak at ~21 Hz. (b) Band-pass filtered (17–23 Hz) beta oscillations (5 s). (c) Spatial distribution of beta activity in the two hemispheres (top view).

"Phase synchrony between beta oscillations in the two hemispheres. (d) Phase-lag distribution for: no amplitude-threshold (pink line) calculations, 50th percentile amplitude threshold (blue line) and 75th percentile amplitude threshold (black line) calculations. The solid horizontal line and the dashed lines represent mean and 3 s.d. of 1000 simulations, respectively. Data from subject N7. (e) S index for the conditions mentioned in (d) (grand-average across the subjects)."

Excerpt from Nikoulin et al., 2001. Figures are reproduced with permission

Control (N = 15)

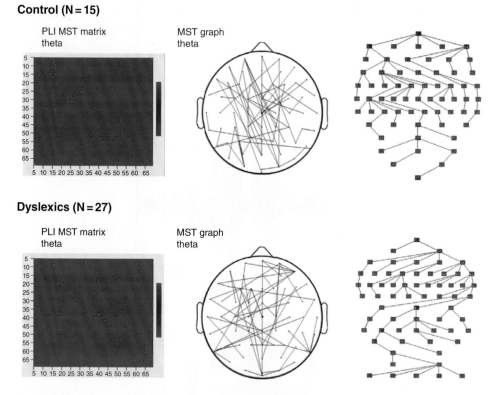

Dyslexics (N = 27)

Figure 12.6. Example of a network analysis (functional network of theta band activity in control group and dyslexic children).

The network was defined by a phase-locking index. A specific type of graph, the minimum spanning tree (MST), was extracted from the network.

"[Adjacency] matrices (left panels) and MST graph in scalp view (center panel) and tree view (right panel) for the theta band for controls (above) and dyslexics (below). For illustrative purposes the MST algorithm was performed on the averaged PLI matrices."

Excerpt from Fraga González et al., 2016. Figures are reproduced with permission

children who were eight and nine years old (Fraga González et al., 2016). The EEG was recorded while they closed their eyes and were relaxed. The resting-state EEG data could reflect fundamental network activity for all mental activity. The data were band-passed to delta, theta, and alpha bands. In each band, phase coherence was computed for all the electrode pairs. Based on phase coherence, the functional network was constructed, simplified, and represented as a finite graph. The graph was compared between the two groups of participants in various network properties. Two of the network properties showed group difference: leaf fraction, which has been related to information integration in a tree graph, and the inverse of diameter, which has been related to the efficiency of communication between nodes. The properties in the theta band network were lower in the dyslexic than in the age-matched control children.

12.2.4. Inter-trial Phase Coherence

One of the assumptions of event-related potential (ERP) analysis is consistency in signal timing; the evoked response should occur over trials more or less in the same timing as in the event of interest (cf. Section 11.2.2 in Chapter 11). The violation of the assumption results in weak or no signal in the trial average. With phase analysis we can directly compute the consistency of the timing over trials. Let's suppose we want to know whether the alpha band activity changed in phase consistency after a visual stimulus onset. Thus, we compute the alpha band phase, cut it into trial segments, align the segments from the stimulus, and average. The procedure is the same as in ERP analysis, except that the average is performed over unit phase vectors. A unit phase vector has a length of 1. Also, the amplitude of the alpha band activity may change in the segment. This means that the vector of the alpha band activity changes its length. Changes in amplitude add noise to the estimation of the timing. Therefore, we set the length of the vector to 1 to eliminate the effect of amplitude. We take the vector mean over trials at each time point. Because the vectors were unitized, the length of the mean vector takes a value between 0 and 1. The length indicates the variance of the phases. If the phase at a given time point is random across trials, the vectors are pointing in random directions. Therefore, the length is close to 0. Conversely, if the phase is consistent, the length becomes closer to 1. The mean vector length has different names, such as **inter-trial phase coherence (ITPC or ITC)**, and **phase-locking factor (PLF)** (Makeig et al., 2002, Tallon-Baudry et al., 1996).

An example of an ITPC result is shown in Figure 12.7. In the study, a visually evoked MEG response was recorded from healthy and schizophrenic young adults (Grützner et al., 2013). The ITPC was computed in multiple bands and shown in a time-frequency plot. Phase-coherent activities are localized in two poststimulus periods at a frequency lower than 40 Hz. For a comparison, the scalogram of the same data is shown.

The two figures show the visually evoked activity from different perspectives, in timing and in energy level. It is important to keep in mind that red in a figure does not always mean high amplitude.

The phase is a **circular value**. A vector operation is applied to compute mean, variance, and higher order statistics over circular values. Directional statistics (also known as circular or spherical statistics) is an established branch of statistics that offers various ways to represent and test circular valued data, e.g., the Rayleigh test of non-uniformity of phase for ITPC. These tests are implemented in statistical software such as an R package 'Circular'.

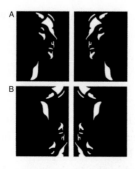

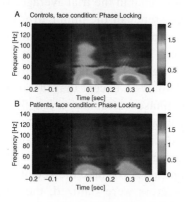

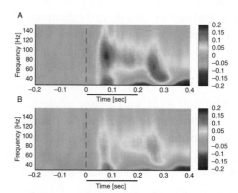

Figure 12.7 Example of an inter-trial phase coherence (ITPC) plot (MEG response time-locked to a visual image in control and schizophrenic groups).

ITPC across all sensor groups in both controls (left top) and patients with schizophrenia (left bottom). The colored scale (0–2) indicates change in ITPC relative to baseline. Corresponding scalograms are also listed (right top for the control, and right bottom for the patients).

"The analysis of ITPC-values revealed prominent increases in the low gamma-band range during an early (5–120 ms) and a later time window (220–320 ms), which likely reflected transient activity related to the onset and offset response of the stimulus. Accordingly, we defined three time windows: (1) an early evoked time window (onset-response: 5–105 ms); (2) an induced period (105–220 ms); and (3) a second evoked window (offset-response: 220–320 ms)."

Excerpt from Grützner et al., 2013. Figures are reproduced with permission

---

Box 12.1 Mathematical Expressions for Oscillation

In Chapters 9–12, we have been using complex notation to represent various aspects of oscillatory signals. For example, in Chapter 9, we used a formula to refer a time point on an oscillation:

$$a_t + b_t i$$

where i is the imaginary unit, and t is time.

In a sinusoid of unitary amplitude (1), the real part is $a_t = \cos\theta_t$ and the imaginary part is $b_t = \sin\theta_t$. Substituting the items of the first formula, we get the second formula:

$$\cos\theta_t + \sin\theta_t i$$

This refers to a time point on the helix (cf. Fig. 9.4 in Chapter 9). To represent all time points on the helix, no specification of time is needed. Thus, the oscillatory component is represented as:

$$\cos\theta + \sin\theta i$$

The third formula is a half of Euler's equation:

$$\cos\theta + \sin\theta i = e^{i\theta}$$

Either side of the equation represents the helix. Here, θ is no longer an angle at a specific time point. It represents frequency and phase shift of the oscillation: $\theta = \omega t + \alpha$, where ω is frequency, t is time, and α is phase shift. We also know that amplitude is not always 1. The amplitude can be expressed as a coefficient, A. If we put frequency, phase shift, and amplitude in the Euler's equation, we get:

$$A\cos(\omega t + \alpha) + A\sin(\omega t + \alpha)i = Ae^{i(\omega t + \alpha)}$$

Either side can be used to express an oscillatory activity. Which side to use is our choice. For some reason, the exponential form seems less popular in the classroom. Outside of the classroom, however, it is preferred, because some computations become much simpler using the exponential form. Therefore, the exponential expression often appears in research papers. It is handy to remember what part of the formula corresponds to which property of the signal: The coefficient A represents amplitude, and the exponent represents frequency and phase shift.

12.2.5 Trial Averaging Revisited

Trial averaging in phase gives us ITPC, while the averaging of the original time signal gives us ERPs. Figure 12.8 illustrates the relationship between the phase in single trials and the ERP waveform. Where phase consistency is high across trials, the ERP amplitude is large. Conversely, where the consistency is low, ERP amplitude is small. Note that the difference in ERP amplitude is *not* because the single trial signal changed in amplitude, but because the phase – timing – of activity varied across trials. Pure amplitude difference can be observed in averaging only the amplitude signal, e.g., a scalogram. In the average of the amplitude, time-shifted activity is smeared in time but does not cancel out (because amplitude is always positively valued).

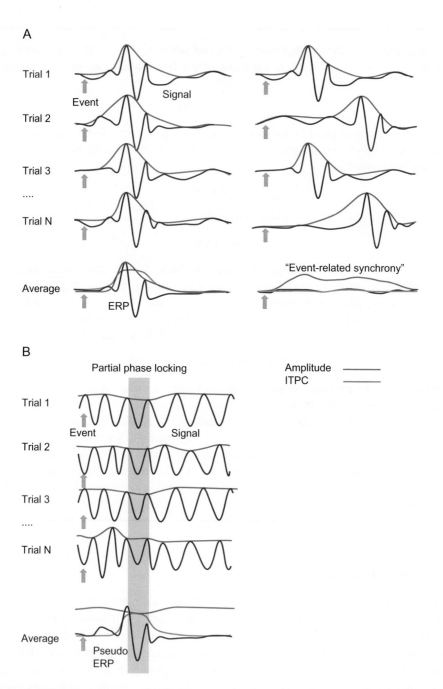

Figure 12.8 Phase and ERPs.
(A) Single trials and average waveforms with consistent or inconsistent activity timings. (B) Single trials with the partial phase locking and their average. Inter-trial phase coherence (ITPC) is indicated in light blue (note that the unit of ITPC is arbitrary).

A slightly confusing naming convention is **event-related synchrony**. In spite of the name, it has little to do with phase synchrony (Pfurtscheller and Da Silva, 1999). It refers to event time-locked changes in *amplitude*. For the amplitude to increase in response to an event, it is assumed that many neurons start firing together at some time. Thus, the increase in average amplitude relative to the baseline level is sometimes referred as event-related synchrony. Likewise, an event-related desynchrony means that the average amplitude decreased relative to the baseline.

An event could change not the amplitude, but the phase. The phase reset causes transient phase synchrony across trials, **partial phase locking (PPL)** (Fig. 12.8B). Averaging over the PPL trials generates pseudo-ERP components. The pseudo-ERPs can be distinguished from veridical ones checking the ITPC and the average amplitude; the ITPC would be high, while the average amplitude would show little change.

Trial averaging in the original, amplitude, and phase signals show different aspects of an event-related brain responses. Thus, they increase our understanding of brain responses around the event (Makeig et al., 2004).

12.3 Autoregression and Granger Causality

So far, we have extended our data analysis by incorporating properties of waves, such as amplitude and phase. In this section, we pay more attention to the fact that M/EEG data are a series of data points sampled in *time*.

12.3.1 Autoregression

Time has a direction. The past can explain, at least in part, the present and the future, but not the other way around. To know how much the past predicts the present state in time series data, we usually compute the **autocorrelation**: The data are shifted in time, e.g., $t - 1$, then the correlation is computed between the original and the shifted time series. For example, if the sampling interval of the data is 5 ms (i.e., a 200 Hz sampling frequency), the autocorrelation coefficient indicates how similar the current state is to itself 5 ms ago. As we repeat the autocorrelation but changing the time lag, we can obtain series of correlation coefficients. The **autocorrelation function (ACF)** is a plot of the coefficients as a function of the time lag (Fig. 12.9). Trivially, autocorrelation at lag 0 is 1. The autocorrelation decreases initially as the lag increases. As the lag increases further, the correlation could increase again, showing peaks in the ACF. Each peak means that the past states at the time lag are similar to the present state. Suppose there is a peak at lag 20 in ACF computed from M/EEG data with sampling intervals of 5 ms. The peak means that the time series is similar to

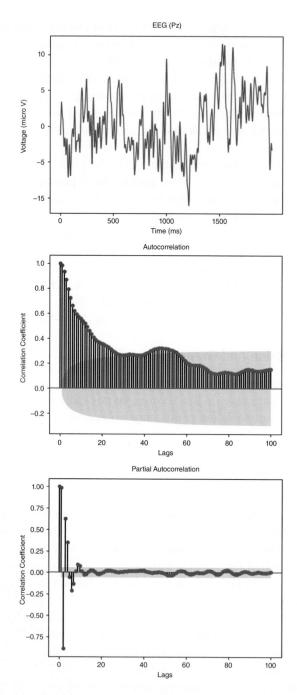

Figure 12.9 Autocorrelation function and partial autocorrelation function.
EEG: In the eyes open/relaxed condition, the electrode placement is at Pz. Sampling frequency is 512 Hz.
ACF: Shaded area indicates the confidence interval (95%). A peak around lag 50 corresponds to the alpha band activity.

itself 100 ms ago. In other words, the signal comes to a similar state every 100 ms: oscillation in 10 Hz. We could obtain frequency information of the signal form of the ACF without using the DFT.

An autocorrelation coefficient combines the effect of all past states, e.g., in the case of lag 3, the effect of states at t - 1, t - 2, and t - 3 are combined. Sometimes we want to know the effect of a specific past state, e.g., t - 3, on the current states. In such a case, a multiple regression technique is applied to remove variance due to t - 1 and t - 2. The adjusted function is the **partial autocorrelation function (PACF)**, which indicates the effect of each past state.

The ACF and PACF are yet another representation of M/EEG data. The representation could be considered as a model in which past states predict the present and the future states. For the model to work, the past states should not be very different from the current states, i.e., the signal needs to be more or less stationary. When the lag is large, distant past states are included in the model. The model takes into account a slower activity as the lag increases. The assumption of stationarity, and the relationship between the lag and frequency remind us of the STFT. Indeed, the two analyses are mathematically related (Brillinger, 2001). In practice, the computation of the autocorrelation is simpler thus faster than that of the spectrum. Thus, the autoregressive method is a powerful tool in real-time signal processing such as in the brain-machine interface. The stationarity assumption tells us, however, that the **autoregressive (AR) model** does not fit well with a non-stationary signal. Moreover, effects of events from the distant past, e.g., long-term memory, cannot be studied using the model derived from a short epoch of signal.

Models related to the AR model are the **moving average (MA)**, the **autoregressive moving average (ARMA)**, and the **autoregressive integrated moving average (ARIMA) models**. Just like the AR model, they model the current and future states based on a combination of statistics of past states, e.g., sum and average. The models provide an insight into different stochastic processes that could explain the data (Box et al., 2015).

12.3.2 Granger Causality

Based on the idea of autoregression, we could consider causality between two activities. As we know, the past states of Signal 1 are a good predictor of the present state of Signal 1. The same applies to Signal 2. Then, could the past states of Signal 1 predict the present state of Signal 2? If the two are independent, the answer is no. If the signals are correlated, the answer is yes. Then, what if the combined past states of Signals 1 and 2 explain the present of Signal 2 *better* than its own past does? This means that Signal 2 is in the present state as a result of the past states of itself *and* Signal 1. Thus, Signal 1 has a causal influence on Signal 2. Such causal relationship is known as the **Granger causality** (Granger, 1969). Granger causality can be computed to test whether the activity of Region 1 modulates that of Region 2, which is referred to as effective connectivity.

Granger causality and related measures, such as **Granger–Geweke (GG) causality**, have been applied not only to M/EEG but also to functional MRI (fMRI) and other time series data in neuroscience. These methods share the same assumption: that the system is approximately linear and time invariant, a so-called **LTI system**. The validity of a functional structure estimated by the method and its interpretation are also discussed in detail by Stokes and Purdon (2017).

We have come a long way. In raw M/EEG data, it was difficult to know which aspects of the signal represent actual brain signals. Preprocessing is applied to remove or reduce artifacts. For that purpose, we needed to know the characteristics of noise signals as well. The brain signal is then represented in time, frequency, or time-frequency. The representation allows us to test our hypothesis on the relationships between brain activity and the behavioral and psychological phenomena.

There seems to be no end to the list of data analysis methods available. We are able to cover only a handful in this book. However, it might be worthwhile to keep in mind that advanced methods begin with basic methods, and new methods often combine known methods. Thus, to some extent, we can always understand an advanced method based on what we learned here.

Summary

- Each signal-processing method gives results in a specific format, e.g., power spectral density (PSD), event-related potentials (ERPs), scalogram, phase synchrony matrix, inter-trial phase coherence plot (ITPC), and autocorrelation function (ACF).
- Short time Fourier transform and wavelet transform give time-frequency representation of data. Results are constrained by the uncertainty principle of the Fourier transform.
- Temporal order decides causality, assigned in Granger causality.

Review Questions

1. Explain what the time-frequency representation of a magnetoencephalography/ electroencephalography (M/EEG) signal is. Describe in words how to obtain the representation. Explain two examples in which the time-frequency representation is more suitable than time or frequency representation.
2. Describe the difference between phase synchrony and inter-trial phase coherence.
3. Suppose that you averaged single-trial segments of EEG data to compute ERPs. How can you assure that the ERP waveforms are veridical?

Further Reading

Cohen, M. X. (2014). *Analyzing Neural Time Series Data: Theory and Practice.* Cambridge, MA: MIT Press. (This book provides a thorough and comprehensive explanation for wavelet analysis and more.)

Fornito, A., Zalesky, A. & Bullmore, E. T. (2016). *Fundamentals of Brain Network Analysis.* Amsterdam: Elsevier/Academic Press.

Palva, S. (2016). *Multimodal Oscillation-Based Connectivity Theory.* Berlin: Springer.

Stam, C. J. (2005). Nonlinear dynamical analysis of EEG and MEG: review of an emerging field. *Clinical Neurophysiology,* **116**, 2266–2301.

Van Drongelen, W. (2006). *Signal Processing for Neuroscientists: An Introduction to the Analysis of Physiological Signals.* Cambridge, MA: Academic Press. (This textbook includes LTI analysis.)

PART IV
Complementary Methods

By this point, the reader of this book has learned about an overwhelming diversity of human brain imaging techniques. None of them is perfect. Each method has drawbacks and depends on important assumptions that might be invalid. For example, going back to the diagram in Figure 1.8, it is obvious that there is no noninvasive method that provides us with a high spatial and a high temporal resolution.

How should human neuroscientists deal with this problem? A particularly unproductive response would be that the experts on the individual methods would spend their time trying to prove that their method of preference is better than the other methods. In addition, the researchers could proclaim that the questions that can be answered with this method are the most important questions, ignoring other questions. Electroencephalogram (EEG) researchers really do not understand why anybody could be interested in a method like functional magnetic resonance imaging (fMRI) with such a poor temporal resolution. Functional MRI researchers dismiss EEG as an old-school, outdated method with a spatial resolution that is oh-so 1980s. We are exaggerating, of course, and luckily most colleagues look at these matters with more nuance. Nevertheless, scientists are human, and thus are subject to all the cognitive biases that exist. It is unavoidable that they will have preferences for particular methods simply because of how they were trained and what they know best. Many EEG researchers might believe that temporal resolution is more important than spatial resolution, and vice versa for fMRI researchers. Because, after all, how can you study cortical dynamics with fMRI and how can you understand the organization of the brain with EEG?

A more fruitful approach is to combine multiple methods, use one technique to compensate for the flaws of another technique, and search for converging evidence across multiple techniques. Despite their individual biases, human neuroscientists can achieve a consensus that no single method can answer all questions. United we stand! In Chapter 13, we describe a few case studies of questions that have been targeted by a combination of multiple methods.

There are also some limitations that all imaging methods share. One major limitation is the reliance on correlations between brain activity and behavior. We manipulate a particular cognitive process X, and we observe increased brain activity in cortical area A and event-related potential (ERP) component P. We can conclude that brain activity in A and at the time of P is correlated with the execution of process X. However, we have not yet proved that changes in brain activity in A at the time of P have a causal effect on the execution of process X. Here we need methods that allow us to change and perturb brain activity. In most cases these methods are applied in combination with imaging techniques. These causal methods are the topic of interest in Chapter 14.

CHAPTER THIRTEEN

Multi-modal Imaging

Learning Objectives

- Being able to articulate the benefits and challenges when combining different imaging and analysis methods
- Understanding how functional magnetic resonance imaging (fMRI) and magnetoencephalography/electroencephalography (M/EEG) can be combined to overcome their limitations in, respectively, temporal and spatial resolution
- Knowing how structural MRI can aid source localization for M/EEG
- Understanding the potential offered by combining multiple methods such as multi-voxel pattern analysis and connectivity analysis

In this book, we have introduced many imaging techniques. We covered three groups of techniques, structural, hemodynamic, and electrophysiological imaging, each with two or three example methods that were highlighted, with even a further subdivision within each of these examples (e.g., T2- versus T2*-weighted fMRI; resting-state versus task-based fMRI). In Chapter 1 we touched briefly on the strengths and weaknesses of different types of methods. For example, hemodynamic methods typically have a better spatial resolution and a poorer temporal resolution compared with electrophysiological methods. The description of the methods in the later chapters gives the reader an insight into the causes of the strengths and weaknesses of each of these methods.

Here we will discuss how these methods can be combined in so-called **multi-modal imaging**. Multi-modal imaging allows us to combine the strengths of different approaches and overcome the weaknesses that each method has when used in isolation. There are many combinations possible, with a combinatorial explosion of the possible number of hybrid approaches. It is impossible to provide a comprehensive overview of all the multi-modal options that are available. Instead, we will present a small number of case studies centered on research questions that have been addressed by different combinations of methodological approaches. We hope that these examples will set the stage for a multi-modal and interdisciplinary way of thinking.

There are five case studies in this chapter. First, we provide a recent example of the combination of fMRI and MEG with multi-voxel pattern analysis (MVPA), illustrated in the context of visual category representations. This example showcases the usefulness of combining the high spatial resolution of fMRI with the high temporal resolution of MEG in the context of a condition-rich experimental design. Second, we discuss the development of simultaneous measurements of fMRI and EEG, here specifically applied to the study of visual face representations. This example highlights the benefits but also the challenges that come with the simultaneous combination of these methods. Third, we discuss the combination of structural and functional MRI with M/EEG for the purpose of source localization, which showcases how the input of one method can impact the information gained from another method. Fourth, we give an example of the combination of fMRI diffusion tensor imaging (DTI), functional connectivity, and MVPA in the context of neurodevelopmental disorders. This last example illustrates how a comprehensive understanding of disorders necessitates a combination of methods. Finally, we briefly touch on how a combination of multiple methods together with advanced statistical tools that integrate the information coming from the different methods might be a promising approach to aid the use of imaging for individual diagnostics.

13.1 The Spatial and Temporal Unfolding of Visual Category Representations

An obvious application of multi-modal imaging is to combine fMRI, with its relatively high spatial resolution, with EEG or MEG, with their high temporal resolution. Through this combination we obtain information about both where and when a particular cognitive process is implemented. Here we illustrate the power of this approach with an example that in addition capitalizes on the ability of representational similarity analysis (Chapter 8) to combine data across different methods. These advanced statistical tools touch upon the domain of artificial intelligence, which is also a promising add-on to the toolkit of a human imager (see Box 13.1).

A series of human imaging studies have used the same experimental design with 92 stimulus conditions, which is a subset of the images of an earlier study using single-unit recordings in monkeys by Kiani and colleagues (2007). The 92 images span many different object categories, equally divided over animate and inanimate objects, with animate objects including human and nonhuman body and face stimuli, and inanimate objects including natural and artificial objects.

The condition-rich fMRI experiment of Kriegeskorte (Kriegeskorte, Mur and Bandettini, 2008; Kriegeskorte, Mur, Ruff, et al., 2008) was introduced briefly in Chapter 8. The data were analyzed through MVPA. The authors extracted the multi-voxel activity patterns in several regions of interest. The multi-voxel patterns were correlated between all 92 conditions, resulting in a 92x92 correlation matrix. The values were inverted to create dissimilarity matrices. These matrices are displayed in Figure 13.1A for four regions of interest (ROIs): the early visual cortex (EVC), including primary visual cortex and nearby regions; right parahippocampal place area (rPPA), defined by higher activation for images of scenes than other

Box 13.1 From Biological to Artificial Brains

In recent years there has been an increased interaction between researchers investigating the brains of humans and other animals on the one hand and scientists working on artificial intelligence on the other hand. Computational models and artificial neural networks have a long history—almost as long as human brain imaging—and so research at the intersection of these two fields has been around for some time. However, in the past, the neural network models tended to be toy models that were unable to mimic the full complexity of human information processing. And they could not reach human performance on complex tasks. Recently, the increased computing power and memory capacities of computers and some clever modifications in the architecture and learning rules of neural networks have resulted in a revolution in this field (LeCun et al., 2015). For example, networks referred to as deep neural networks have been shown to be able to categorize objects in complex pictures with human-like performance (Krizhevsky et al., 2012).

The relevance of these developments for behavioral sciences in general and human brain imaging in particular was illustrated in a series of papers showing similarities between networks and humans in the representations that emerge in the network layers and in brain areas and behavior (Khaligh-Razavi and Kriegeskorte, 2014; Kubilius et al., 2016). Based on this research, it seems that cutting-edge artificial neural networks have the potential to help refine and quantify the hypotheses that drive human imaging research.

The comparison between biological and artificial brains is facilitated by the ability to apply a similar analysis approach to the two. In biological brains we have neurons at the smallest scale and voxels or sensors at the imaging scale, while a neural network consists of units with mathematically defined inputs and outputs. Just as a neurophysiologist can measure the action potential activity of a single neuron and a neuroimager can measure the blood-oxygenation-level dependent (BOLD) signal in a single voxel, a computational neuroscientist can compute the output of single units in an artificial network. Often researchers apply more complicated methods that consider the pattern of output across multiple neurons, voxels, or units. By now, this approach must ring a bell, as this is exactly what is done in an MVPA representational similarity analysis. By replacing voxels with network units, one can apply the same methods to an artificial neural network (also see Fig. 8.10).

images; right fusiform face area (FFA) (see Chapter 5); and the human inferotemporal cortex (IT), a large ROI including the ventral part of the temporal lobe.

The four matrices in Figure 13.1A illustrate the power given by the spatial resolution of fMRI, namely, to identify regions with meaningfully different representations of object images. The dissimilarities in EVC do not reveal a clear clustering of conditions. In rPPA and rFFA, we see some pattern emerging. In rPPA there is a clustering of inanimate objects (blue values in the lower right of the matrix = low dissimilarity), whereas in rFFA there is primarily a clustering of

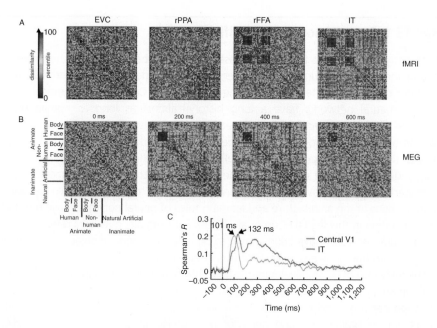

Figure 13.1 The application of multi-voxel/sensor pattern analyses to fMRI and MEG data from a condition-rich design with 92 object conditions. (A) Dissimilarity matrices from fMRI in four regions of interest: early visual cortex (EVC), right parahippocampal place area (rPPA), right fusiform face area (rFFA), and a large inferior temporal (IT) region. To calculate dissimilarity, correlations between multi-voxel patterns were first transformed into dissimilarities by subtracting the correlations from one and expressed as percentiles (lowest correlation = highest dissimilarity = percentile 100). Matrices reproduced with permission from Kriegeskorte, Mur and Bandettini, 2008, Kriegeskorte, Mur, Ruff, et al., 2008. (B) Dissimilarity matrices from MEG at four different time points after stimulus onset. Colors express percentiles based on decoding performances. (C) Correlations, as a function of time after stimulus onset, between fMRI dissimilarity in two regions of interest, the central part of EVC and IT, and MEG dissimilarity. Images in B and C reproduced with permission from Cichy et al., 2014

animate objects. The clearest structure emerges in IT, with a clear separation between animate and inanimate objects.

Based on knowledge of the structure of the visual system in primates, we can assume that information processing flows from EVC to IT. First, neurons in EVC respond, and then they provide input to further regions, until this input eventually reaches the occipitotemporal cortex (rPPA and rFFA) and temporal cortex. In primates, responses in EVC are known to appear 40–50 ms after stimulus onset. In the temporal cortex, the response latency is 80–100 ms, thus about 40 ms later than in EVC. However, fMRI does not have the temporal resolution to show this flow of information. The fMRI results do not pinpoint when the animate/inanimate distinction emerges in the IT cortex, nor how long it lasts. It could start at around 70 ms after stimulus onset, or later. It could stay for a long time, hundreds of milliseconds or even seconds, or disappear relatively rapidly.

To resolve these uncertainties, Cichy and colleagues (2014) designed an MEG experiment with the same 92 conditions. In contrast to the tens of thousands of voxels measured through fMRI, this MEG dataset is composed of 306 MEG channels. Nevertheless, the dataset lends itself to analyses similar to MVPA. Instead of investigating multi-voxel patterns in a specific region of interest, the MEG data can be analyzed by performing pattern analyses on multi-channel MEG data. These data contain signals coming from all of the brain. However, in contrast to fMRI, where we have a signal pooled across the full stimulus event, MEG offers us a high sampling rate of one measurement per millisecond.

Given this very high temporal resolution combined with a low spatial resolution, the focus is no longer on different brain regions, but on different time points. For each time point, a 92x92 dissimilarity matrix is constructed. In this study, dissimilarity was measured for each pair-wise comparison through a decoding approach. Figure 13.1B shows matrices for four different time points after stimulus onset: 0 ms, 200 ms, 400 ms, and 600 ms. The color scale is defined in terms of percentiles, which results in a similar distribution of colors (including the same average color) in all four matrices. However, the overall decoding performance became significant only after about 50 ms; thus, the matrix at 0 ms only represents noise and no signal. At later time points, there is a clear blue square in the matrices, which shows a very low dissimilarity (high similarity) for faces.

An important potential of these MEG findings comes from the fact that we also have fMRI data available. One possible analysis is to take an fMRI matrix from Figure 13.1A and correlate it with the MEG matrices of all the different time points. The results are shown in Figure 13.1C for EVC/V1 and IT. The V1-MEG correlation peaks around 100 ms after stimulus onset, while the IT-MEG correlation finds its maximum 30 ms later. In addition, the IT-MEG correlation is more sustained and remains at higher levels in the later parts of the response. In this way, fMRI and MEG provide information about the neural basis of object recognition with high spatial and high temporal resolution.

13.2 Simultaneous Application of EEG and fMRI

Here we go even further with the integration of methods. Whereas in the previous section the data from different modalities were obtained in separate sessions, we now turn to the combination of different imaging modalities that are acquired simultaneously. This is a difficult goal to achieve, and researchers should always carefully consider whether the drawbacks are overruled by the benefits of new potential insights and analyses that require simultaneous imaging.

Typically, simultaneous multi-modal imaging is cumbersome, because it is very difficult to acquire good data for two imaging modalities at once. Some combinations are even impossible. In particular, fMRI and MEG cannot be combined. Magnetoencephalography is already challenging with typical ambient magnetic field strengths, and it would not work in the presence of a strong and time-varying MRI field.

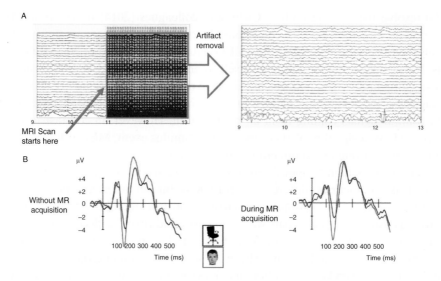

Figure 13.2 Simultaneous fMRI-EEG shows face-selective ERP responses. (A) The effect of fMRI data acquisition on the simultaneously measured EEG signal, before (*left*) and after (*right*) artifact removal. (B) The face-selective N170 as measured in event-related potentials without (*left*) and during (*right*) fMRI acquisition.

Images reproduced with permission from Sadeh et al., 2008

Other combinations are difficult but not impossible. Around the year 2000, monkey researchers had already combined fMRI with invasive electrical measurements (e.g., Logothetis et al., 2001). Around 2005–2010, researchers started experimenting with the combination of fMRI and EEG in human research. One study by Yovel and colleagues (Sadeh et al., 2008) is illustrated in Figure 13.2. The combined measurement requires specific hardware and software for the EEG. It is reasonably straightforward to acquire EEG data in the presence of the static magnetic field. However, as soon as fMRI data acquisition starts with its typical fast variations in magnetic gradients, the EEG signal is flooded with artifacts (top left panel). EEG researchers are used to artifact removal (see Chapter 11), but the fMRI-related artifacts are of a different order of magnitude and require special routines to be resolved. Nevertheless, it is possible to clean up the signal substantially, resulting in EEG tracks with typical spatio-temporal characteristics (Fig. 13.2A). Quantitative event-related analyses of these EEG tracks show very similar event-related potentials in the absence and presence of MRI acquisition, with specific differences between conditions such as a larger N170 for face images compared with object images (Fig. 13.2B).

Nevertheless, we should be realistic about the practical aspects of simultaneous imaging. The signal in the separate image modalities is often compromised to a certain extent. Even in very experienced facilities, the data quality will on average be lower in multi-modal imaging than if each technique had been acquired separately. The MRI acquisition will frequently increase the noise in the EEG tracks,

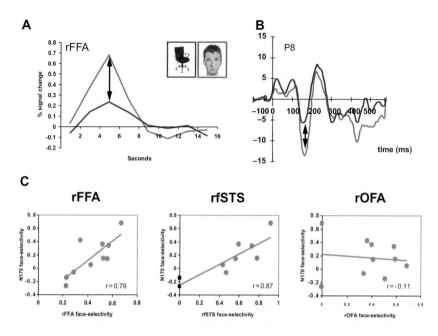

Figure 13.3 Correlations between fMRI-derived and EEG-derived face selectivity in simultaneous fMRI-EEG. (A) fMRI signal changes after the presentation of faces and objects in rFFA. (B) The event-related potential after the presentation of faces and objects in electrode P8, with clearly face selective N170. (C) Correlation across participants between N170 face selectivity and face selectivity in the fMRI signal in rFFA, rfSTS (right face-selective superior temporal sulcus), and right occipital face area (rOFA). Reproduced with permission from Sadeh et al. (2010).

despite apparently successful artifact removal. The EEG apparatus will have an impact on the quality of the MRI data, despite the use of scanner-compatible EEG hardware. In addition, the odds that something goes wrong with at least one of the methods is higher. For all these reasons, acquiring the two datasets separately might in the end result in better data with less trouble.

Because of the foregoing challenges, simultaneous fMRI-EEG acquisition is most often reserved for experimental questions that require simultaneous imaging and would be hard to answer using separate datasets. One such question was made in a follow-up study by Sadeh and colleagues (2010). The researchers investigated the fMRI signal in three independently defined regions of interest: occipital face area (OFA), fusiform face area (FFA), and the face-selective region in the superior temporal sulcus (STS). The fMRI and EEG signals were acquired while subjects were presented with face and object images. For each subject, the researchers calculated the fMRI face selectivity (faces–objects) in the three regions of interest, and the EEG face selectivity at several time points, including the peak of the N170 (Fig. 13.3B). There was a correlation across subjects between the fMRI face selectivity in FFA and STS and the N170 face selectivity (Fig. 13.3C). This was interpreted as evidence that the N170 is probably related to activity in FFA and STS.

The authors suggest that the sensitivity to pick up such across-subject correlations is much higher in simultaneous fMRI-EEG measurements. Apart from this example, one can expect simultaneous imaging to be highly relevant to investigating trial-by-trial correlations in the activity in the different methods and to understand the neural basis of and similarities between the different imaging methods.

13.3 M/EEG Source Localization

The M/EEG sensors pick up a rich mixture of field signals. Even though researchers are aware that the choice of M/EEG brings with it a serious limitation in terms of spatial resolution, they still try to pinpoint as much as possible the sources of measured signal components. For this purpose, the sensor signals need not only to be decomposed, but also to be related to brain regions. Unlike MRI data, M/EEG sensor data do not have the depth dimension. How then can we "recover" this third dimension from the data? Figure 13.4 illustrates the problem. Any of these combinations of sources gives the same sensor signal. In fact, there are infinite combinations of sources that can give rise to the signal. We need restrictions to further constrain the subspace of possible combinations. Some of these restrictions are relatively simple. A first restriction is that locations outside of the brain are not considered as possible source locations. In addition, general limiting factors of the M/EEG sensor signal (cf. Chapter 9) are good to start with, such as the knowledge that M/EEG signal primarily comes from cortex. Deeper activity contributes less to the signal. Relative orientation between sensors and the cortical sheet also affects the signal, and this information is available when we coregister sensor location in a brain space, e.g., using a T1-weighted MRI. We could try source estimation without an individual structural MRI, e.g., taking a sphere as a volume conductor model.

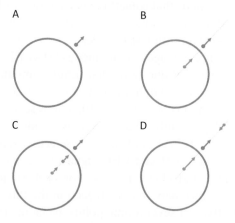

Figure 13.4 Source localization as an ill-posed problem. A sensor-level activity (green vector in A) could be given by combinations of source activities (B and C). A source outside of the brain (D) is irrelevant. However, such a restriction needs to be given to an estimation algorithm.

Needless to say, estimation of source locations restricted by anatomical information is better than that without it. Thus, here, we discuss the multi-modal method of M/EEG source estimation with MRI data.

Source estimation has two stages. The first stage is building a head model, which tells us the theoretical sensor signal level given a source activity. The M/EEG sensors and the brain need to be placed in the real 3D coordinates for a realistic head model, so M/EEG sensor locations are coregistered with anatomical MRI using marker positions and anatomical fiducial points. The marker positions could be recorded during MRI acquisition or sampled using a separate 3D position recording system. Dipole is used as the model of local source activity. Source current decays as it conducts through tissues. Moreover, conductivity differs among tissues, e.g., it is higher in brain tissue and cerebrospinal fluid (CSF) than in the skull and scalp. The anatomical distribution of different tissue types is also computed from MRI. A head model of volume conduction is computed by, for example, the boundary element method (BEM) and the finite element method (FEM). These methods give us a lead-field matrix that maps the activity of M sources to N sensors: a forward model.

The second stage is "backward"; data from N sensors are mapped to M sources. Suppose that we have visual evoked potential (VEP) data. We want to know which region contributed to the activity at a particular point in time. Antecedently, we expect that activity from visual cortices and ventral temporal regions would contribute to the evoked response. This heuristic is incorporated in the source localization: A small number of dipoles are provisionally placed at the possible source locations, e.g., bilateral V1/V2, V4, and lateral occipital sulcus. Using the forward model, we compute theoretical activity at each sensor, assuming all dipoles have the same strength. Of course, the theoretical values are different from those of the real data. Then, we adjust the direction, magnitude, and location of the dipole to reduce the error. We repeat the comparison and adjustment until the error does not decrease further. This method is referred to as the equivalent current dipole (ECD) method, which generates dipole location, direction, and time series for the dipole activity (Salmelin, 2010). The estimated activity is the source current; thus, the unit of current density, such as [A/m], applies to the results from EEG data as well.

Sometimes, however, we have reason to believe that target activity is not focal but spread in the volume. In such a case, dipoles distributed over the cortex may be a better model than sparse dipoles, as in the ECD model. In a distributed dipole model, the number of dipoles often becomes larger than that of the sensors. Thus, we need additional constraints to decide how the sensor signal is distributed over the sources. We first choose the source space, such as gray matter computed from the MRI image. Estimation methods, such as minimum-norm estimates (MNE), minimum-current estimates (MCE) and low-resolution brain electromagnetic tomography (LORETA) distribute sensor activity over the large number of dipoles. For example, MNE selects the current distribution that has the minimum overall power (Hamalainen and Ilmoniemi, 1994). The results of a distributed source modeling give a representation of M/EEG activity projected on the 3D brain space, which is a dipole image. This dipole image could be considered the best of two worlds: a representation of the M/EEG signal with high time and spatial resolutions. However, it is important to keep in mind that any focal activity will be smeared in space.

In sum, ECD is useful for representing brain activity in terms of a small number of focal activity points, e.g., from 128 electrode data to several dipoles, $M << N$. In contrast, distributed dipole models give a large number of sources (e.g. 10 000 dipoles), which cover the entire neocortex in approximately 5 mm intervals; thus, $M >> N$. In other words, the method can be applied without knowing where relevant source activity could be. The result of a distributed dipole modeling can be represented as a movie in which we can observe the evolution of a spatial pattern of the activity on the brain.

The two approaches share a number of problems. First, activity in the medial and ventral cortices is difficult to estimate (Korhonen et al., 2014). Second, field activities close to each other are difficult to estimate separately. (Some techniques, e.g., beamformer, are reported to be better in the estimation of such sources.) And third, field activities that face each other are difficult to detect, because they cancel each other. Thus, field activities in banks of a sulcus – close and opposing activities – are significantly more difficult to localize than those in a gyrus.

Source estimate libraries have become accessible to the wider scientific community, and packages such as Brainstorm and MNE-Python offer source localization options. However, overall, source level analysis is still costly and cumbersome. Often more than 100 sensors are recommended for quality localization. This means that we need to have high-density M/EEG data. Moreover, MRI images need to be acquired from each individual and transformed from voxels to a surface mesh to specify dipole locations and boundary elements. The image processing alone takes a considerable amount of time and care. Forward and backward modeling is computationally costly, and results could contain considerable errors, such as dipoles located outside of the brain and ghost activity.

Nevertheless, the potential of the MRI informed source estimation technique is large. For example, it could change M/EEG signal processing significantly in other steps that discussed in previous chapters: In the near future, we might place dipoles in eyes, muscles, and other tissues of the head to separate artifact components from brain signals.

13.4 Differentiating between Representational and Access Theories of Disorders

Brain disorders might have many different causes at many different levels. In the early days of human brain imaging, the most commonly tested predictions of neurocognitive theories of brain disorders came from assumptions about dysfunctional involvement of particular information processing steps. These problems would lead to exceptionally high or low overall activity in the brain regions to which these processing steps would be localized. Take the example of dyslexia. A neurocognitive theory claiming that children with reading problems have difficulties with the processing of sound and the vision-to-sound mapping of syllables could be tested by investigating whether children with dyslexia have a different level of activity in auditory cortex when listening to speech.

Such predictions can be tested with a traditional univariate analysis of fMRI data. One common problem with such predictions is that it is not always easy to predict the direction of the abnormal activity: Would the dysfunction result in higher or lower overall activity? Furthermore, there might be many ways in which neural processing might be dysfunctional that do not result in a net increase or decrease of overall activity.

Other hypotheses specify in more detail how and why a particular processing step is dysfunctional. A first possibility is that the representations at that stage have different characteristics. In the case of dyslexia, the sound representations in the auditory cortex might contain less information about which speech units or "phonemes" have been heard. We need a method such as MVPA to investigate such a representational hypothesis.

A second possible hypothesis is that the representations at a particular stage are normal, but that other stages of processing have difficulties accessing these representations. In the case of dyslexia, the sound representations in auditory cortex might be fine, but other brain regions might not have access to these sound representations. Data of anatomical and functional connectivity might be useful to study such an access hypothesis.

This wide spectrum of relevant neurocognitive theories applicable to a particular brain disorder calls for a multi-method approach. Boets and colleagues (2013) performed such an MRI study in the context of dyslexia. They differentiated between representational and access theories by applying MVPA and functional/anatomical connectivity analyses. The experimental design included four phoneme conditions: /ba/, /da/, /bu/, and /du/. Within each condition, there was a variety of speakers pronouncing the phonemes. Two groups of subjects were included that were matched on many characteristics except that the individuals in one group were diagnosed with dyslexia and the individuals in the other group were not.

Decoding MVPA was used to investigate the neural representation of these phonemes, more specifically, the degree to which the multi-voxel patterns in a range of ROIs differentiated between the different phonemes. The results of a subset of these ROIs are displayed in Figure 13.5A. The decoding performance was calculated for each phoneme pair. Some phonemes differ only in consonant (black bars), only in vowel (dark gray bars), or in both consonant and vowel (light gray bars). If multi-voxel patterns contain no information about the presented sound, then we would expect a decoding proportion of 0.50. This result was observed for all pairwise comparisons in several ROIs, including the inferior frontal gyrus (IFG, left and right) and primary visual cortex (V1). While we expect V1 to play no role in auditory processing, the left IFG is a well-known language area, frequently referred

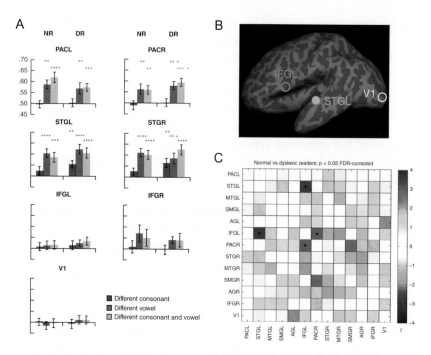

Figure 13.5 Combination of MVPA with functional connectivity analyses to investigate the differences between normal readers (NR) and dyslexic readers (DR). (A) Pair-wise decoding performance of phoneme conditions that differ only in the consonant, only in the vowel, or in both consonant and vowel. Four regions of interest are shown: primary auditory cortex (PAC, left and right), superior temporal gyrus (STG, left and right), inferior frontal gyrus (IFG, left and right), and primary visual cortex (V1). (B) The approximate anatomical location of the four regions of interest. (C) Matrix with the results from null hypothesis testing of the difference in pair-wise functional connectivity between normal and dyslexic readers. Significant differences are highlighted with a black dot.
Panels A and C reproduced with permission from Boets et al., 2013

to as Brocca's area. Nevertheless, no evidence for a neural representation of the sounds was found in this area.

In contrast, areas in the primary auditory cortex (PAC) and nearby temporal regions such as the superior temporal gyrus (STG) showed significant decoding for comparisons of sounds with a different vowel. However, the strength of this decoding was the same in the two subject groups. Thus, as far as can be detected with MVPA fMRI, the phoneme representations were as distinctive in the individuals with dyslexia as they were in the control group. These findings do not seem to support a representational account of dyslexia.

Next, the researchers investigated the functional connectivity between the same ROIs, using the same task-based data. In total there were 13 ROIs, resulting in a 13x13 functional connectivity matrix. Figure 13.5C represents the difference in connectivity between the control group and the group with dyslexia, so that warm colors represent more connectivity in the control group. The IFGL showed a reduced connectivity in the group with dyslexia with several regions, in particular the left STG and the right PAC. Given the aforementioned MVPA result that the IFGL does not contain a neural representation of the sounds while the STG and PAC do, this finding fits with the idea that the regions that contain the sound representations communicate suboptimally with other language regions such as the IFGL. The reduced connectivity in dyslexia was further confirmed by DTI data. Overall, these findings provide a strong support for access theories of dyslexia.

The same combination of MVPA and functional connectivity can be applied to many other disorders. The extent to which the findings support representational or access accounts might vary between disorders. Bulthé and colleagues (2017) performed a very similar study for another neurodevelopmental disorder, dyscalculia, which is characterized by difficulties in arithmetic. The study included MVPA fMRI, functional connectivity, and DTI. One subset of conditions included nonsymbolic magnitudes, more specifically dot patterns. There were four magnitudes: 2, 4, 6, and 8 dots. Decoding MVPA was applied to investigate how strongly these four conditions could be distinguished based on multi-voxel patterns. A relatively large network of regions showed significant decoding for these magnitudes. The decoding was significantly lower in participants with dyscalculia in a subset of these regions in the parietal and prefrontal cortices. Thus, in the case of dyscalculia there was a support for representational theories that assume that dyscalculia is caused by problems with the neural representation of magnitude. The findings from functional and anatomical connectivity were much less clear, and no regions showed reduced connectivity in dyscalculia. Overall, these investigations of neurodevelopmental disorders through a combination of methods reveals the opposite pattern in dyscalculia and dyslexia: representational deficits in dyscalculia, access deficits in dyslexia.

13.5 Clinical Diagnostics with Multi-modal Imaging

For a clinical radiologist or neurologist, diagnosing patients is a daily routine. However, the relevant data used for such a diagnosis change when science makes progress, and become ever more complicated and, very relevant for this chapter, multi-modal. A few examples will suffice. To diagnose a stroke in general and its specific type, the protocol might include computed tomography (CT) imaging with and without a contrast agent and perfusion- and diffusion-weighted MRI (Osborn et al., 2016). The diagnosis of neuropathology in preterm infants might include a combination of T1-, T2-, and diffusion-weighted imaging (Hinojosa-Rodriguez et al., 2017). As a final example, before attributing a patient's headaches to migraine, the neurologist excludes other causes with several imaging methods, including EEG and MRI.

The clinicians will not commit hours of heavy data analysis to each of these imaging modalities to reach their diagnostic conclusion. In the good old days, it often came down to looking at a printout of the data. Today, there are software packages available that typically provide indices that can be computed in a relatively straightforward way based on the raw images, with no intervention necessary from the clinician. Instead, the data processing is automatized and the software provides the relevant measurements in an accelerated fashion. For example, a software package such as Icobrain offers portfolios to compute neural biomarkers relevant in helping in the diagnosis of multiple sclerosis, dementia, and head trauma. While at the moment this approach primarily offers a second opinion and aids the clinician who is in charge, it is not inconceivable that at some point artificial intelligence might surpass the ability of the clinician.

The process of diagnostics can be seen as a complex pattern recognition problem in which the clinician is a highly qualified expert. Box 13.1 brought up artificial algorithms that have recently shown a marked increase in pattern recognition abilities, in some domains already surpassing human capabilities. The more clinicians are faced with input from complex and multi-modal imaging, the bigger share artificial algorithms might have in the diagnostic process. More and more, specialists base their diagnoses on the outcome of specialized processing of clinical images and information from various sources, including artificial intelligence tools (Liu, Cai, Lui, et al., 2015).

We provide a specific example in the context of the diagnosis of Alzheimer's disease. At the moment, routine imaging protocols chiefly serve to exclude other causes of the symptoms and do not yet image the pathological processes underlying Alzheimer's in a sufficiently sensitive manner, in particular not in the early stages of the disease. Nevertheless, images from multiple modalities can already be informative for the diagnosis, including positron emission tomography (PET) and MRI images. Liu and colleagues (Liu, Liu, Cai, et al., 2015) showed that artificial neural networks can be trained to distinguish between different disease types (e.g., Alzheimer's disease [AD], Mild Cognitive Impairment [MCI]) and normal healthy controls (NC) based on a combination of data from PET as well as MRI. To develop and test these algorithms, the authors used the openly available data from hundreds of patients provided by the ADNI consortium (see Box 6.2 in Chapter 6). The sensitivity and specificity of the diagnosis was improved when data from multiple modalities were combined in an intelligent way, resulting in a sensitivity and specificity up to 90% in a relatively easy binary classification (e.g., normal controls versus Alzheimer's). In a multi-class classification that involved four groups, NC, AD, MCI that converted into Alzheimer's, and MCI that did not convert, the overall accuracy based on multiple imaging modalities was 54% (clearly above the chance performance of 25%), with a sensitivity of 52% and a specificity of 87%.

To conclude, advanced methods of data analyses and artificial intelligence applications are important in reaching the full potential of multi-modal neuroimaging in clinical applications as well as fundamental neuroscience.

Summary

- The combination of fMRI and magnetoencephalography/electroencephalography (M/EEG) with multivariate analyses allows researchers to investigate neural representations in high detail in both space and time.
- Both fMRI and EEG can be applied simultaneously, which allows a better integration of the two datasets, but with potential problems with data acquisition and data quality.
- Structural MRI greatly improves the precision of source localization for M/EEG.
- Combining fMRI multi-voxel pattern analysis (MVPA) with connectivity analyses allows researchers to differentiate between representational and access theories of brain disorders.

Review Questions

1. Explain how the rationale behind MVPA can be extended to datasets without voxels such as M/EEG and artificial neural networks.
2. Which type of predictions from neurocognitive theories can be tested with each of the following methods: univariate fMRI analysis, MVPA fMRI, and diffusion tensor imaging (DTI)?
3. Explain how source localization for MEG might be improved by obtaining a structural MRI for each participant.

Further Reading

Cabeza, R., Nyberg, L. & Parck, D. C. (2016). *Cognitive Neuroscience of Aging: Linking Cognitive and Cerebral Aging* (Section I: Methods and Issues). Oxford: Oxford Scholarship Online.

Liu, S., Cai, W., Liu, S., et al. (2015). Multimodal neuroimaging computing: a review of the application in neuropsychiatric disorders. *Brain Informatics*, **2**, 167–180.

(These two reading suggestions give a broad overview of a wide range of imaging methods for two specific domains, aging research and neuropsychiatry.)

CHAPTER FOURTEEN

Causal Methods to Modulate Brain Activity

Learning Objectives

- Understanding the differences and similarities between different methods to modulate brain activity
- Knowing the basics of the physical principles behind methods such as focused ultrasound (FUS), transcranial magnetic stimulation (TMS), and transcranial current stimulation (TCS), and understanding how these principles relate to the strengths and weaknesses of a method
- Learning about the intimate relationship between imaging and stimulation, both in terms of developing hypotheses and predictions and when applying the methods

Imaging methods do not provide causal evidence that a particular brain region or rhythm is necessary for a certain process or behavior. Instead, they provide correlational evidence. In this chapter, we introduce several causal methods that allow researchers to induce changes in brain activity. The effects of stimulation can be measured via changes in behavior, cognitive processing, and neural activity.

None of these causal methods is an "imaging" method, but we cover them nevertheless because they are highly relevant to test predictions resulting from the correlational evidence obtained through imaging. In addition, the application of these causal methods often involves imaging, such as magnetic resonance imaging (MRI), to determine the anatomical location where the causal method will be applied.

Here we only cover direct methods for modulating neural activity by influencing the physical properties of the neural tissue. There is a much wider range of approaches to *change neural activity indirectly*. Medication is an obvious example. It results in very nonspecific neuromodulation given that potential effects on neural activity will be distributed across the whole nervous system or at least complete neurotransmitter systems. More specific indirect neuromodulation is not difficult; in fact, we all do it every day. By having you read this sentence, we alter your brain activity. BY PUTTING IT IN CAPITAL LETTERS, WE MIGHT EVEN STRENGTHEN THAT EFFECT. Telling your friends how much they mean to you will change their brain activity, and their reaction will change yours. A more specific set of methods falls somewhat in between indirect and direct methods of neuromodulation and involves **neurofeedback**. Here neural activity is measured and is fed back in real time to the participant through a sensory channel (e.g., a visual display or earplugs). The participant uses this feedback to learn how to alter their brain activity and to use that knowledge when they are no longer connected to the measurement device. The feedback loop is effective, in the sense that participants can learn how to control particular aspects of brain activity (Sitaram et al., 2017). Nevertheless, there is not sufficient evidence (and hence no US Food and Drug Administration [FDA] approval) to consider it as an effective treatment for disorders such as depression and ADHD, even though it is sometimes applied in that context. Overall, among the indirect methods for neuromodulation and treatment, the most specific and most effective approach is probably still old-school communication and psychology.

Turning back to the direct causal methods, it is relevant to start with two general points. First, the causal methods include methods that directly alter brain activity by the local application of magnetic fields or electrical currents. As a result, we change neural activity and look for changes at the behavioral level, hence the denotation "causal." Even though we hereby use the traditional distinction between "correlation" and "causality," we should not take it too far. Correlational data can be very relevant to infer causality, albeit not with absolute certainty (see, e.g., Weber and Thompson-Schill, 2010). At the same time, it is dangerous to naively infer causality from results obtained with a causal method. Inference is tricky, as we learned in the context of forward and reverse inference. There are many ways in which altered brain activity can influence behavior directly or indirectly. For example, stimulating region A might change behavior, not because activity in region A is directly causing the behavioral change but because the stimulation in region A indirectly affects neural activity in a distant region B, which is then causing the behavioral change. Thus, a causal method also does not provide absolute certainty about the presence or absence of causality.

Second, although all causal methods have "stimulation" in their name, it is important to note that this term refers to what is being applied at the physical level and not to its effect on neural processing. Indeed, while the "stimulation" at the physical level can sometimes result in stimulation, or excitation, at the neural level it can also interfere, hamper, or inhibit neural processing.

The causal methods are ordered in terms of their assumed spatial specificity. We therefore look first at the methods that offer the highest spatial resolution: microstimulation and deep brain stimulation, followed by focused ultrasound (FUS), transcranial magnetic stimulation (TMS), and transcranial current stimulation (TCS). We also briefly touch upon the ethical concerns related to neural stimulation methods (see Box 14.1).

14.1 Microstimulation and Deep Brain Stimulation

Microstimulation and deep brain stimulation (DBS) require the insertion of an electrode into the neural tissue. A small electrical current is applied through the electrode that influences the electrical activity of neurons near the tip of the

Box 14.1 Ethical Concerns Related to Noninvasive Neuromodulation

Methods for neuromodulation raise ethical concerns. For example, is it even appropriate to influence someone's brain activity in such a way? Given that neuroscientists believe that our mind is a consequence of brain activity, it naturally follows that we manipulate the mind when we electrically, magnetically, or sonically alter neural activity.

These ethical considerations are important to keep in mind when engaging in this research. However, now and in the future, we should also consider the limitations of the available techniques when talking about ethical consequences. Given the spatial resolution of these methods, noninvasive neuromodulation can improve or decrease performance in particular tasks, it might bias us to rely on one strategy more than another, but it does not fundamentally alter the content of our mental life.

Let us envision the future and assume that at some point we would have a noninvasive technology that affords us the precision that microstimulation offers us today (very unlikely, because physically this would be almost impossible), or that the invasive technology would become so harmless that we would be able apply it on a much wider scale (also very unlikely, because of biomedical hazards). Even in this very unlikely vision of the future, we would only be able to do what we can do now with microstimulation – namely, stimulating or inhibiting large populations of neurons at one or a small number of foci. Again, we would be able to induce more or less of what is already there: more or less emotional engagement (perhaps through stimulating amygdala), inducing emotional indifference (amygdala silencing), helping with overall memory encoding and recall, and so on. This is all very impressive, and there are important clinical applications, as we mentioned in drug-resistant forms of obsessive-compulsive disorder or depression.

Ethical discussions do not typically target these clinical applications with their obvious benefits. When people become afraid of neuromodulation, it seems to be that their fears are induced by other potential applications that require a technology of a very different level. For example, neuromodulation might allow us to manipulate the finer content of our mental life, such as the exact memories that we have. The premise of the movie *Eternal Sunshine of the Spotless Mind* is an interesting illustration. The character played by Kate Winslet has all her memories of her ex erased. Hollywood loves such scenarios, but in reality this would require modulating the activity of thousands of neurons at the single neuron level in human beings, as well as a perfect understanding of how the activity of each of these neurons is related to the memory of a particular person. This is not in our power – not now, and not in the foreseeable future.

Consider face perception. Transcranial magnetic stimulation studies have shown influences of the stimulation of face areas on the proficiency of face perception. There are small effects of such stimulation on how well we recognize faces and their expressed emotions (e.g., Pitcher et al., 2008). Microstimulation of a face patch has revealed more specific and larger effects, so that the geometry of a face can change in appearance (Parvizi et al., 2012). However, individual faces are coded by the pattern of activity across thousands of face-selective neurons. If we want to evoke the pattern of activity associated with a particular face, we would need to individually modulate the activity of thousands of neurons with single-neuron resolution, and it would have to be the correct neurons. That is science fiction and will remain fictional in the foreseeable future. Of course, the history of science is replete with amazing and unexpected paradigm shifts, so who knows what the far future will bring?

electrode. The larger the current, the wider the area in which neurons will be influenced by the current and the stronger the influence on the neurons that are closest. Nearby neurons could be damaged by the current if it is too strong (in addition to the neurons that are inevitably destroyed by inserting the electrode). A relatively strong current that does not exceed the threshold for neuronal damage will induce action potentials. A weaker current might not induce any action potentials but might still result in a change in the membrane potential of the nearby neurons and as such influence neural processing.

The choice of the best current strength can sometimes seem more a matter of intuition than of exact science, except when the electrode is inserted in a region where stimulation results in obvious behavioral effects. We will focus on one example, the frontal eye fields (FEF). This premotor area in the frontal cortex has been investigated in numerous studies with monkeys and has also been found in humans. The responses of neurons in the FEF are related to eye movements, and neurons that respond to eye movements in the same direction tend to be clustered in the same part of the FEF (topographic organization). Microstimulation in this area with currents of less than 50 μA elicits a saccade (eye movement), the direction of which depends on the exact location of the electrode within the FEF topographic map. The saccadic threshold, defined as the current that is sufficient to elicit an eye movement, provides a straightforward reference to define current in terms of its physiological effect. Many studies are more interested in microstimulation effects at subthreshold levels, which are then expressed in percentages of the saccadic threshold (e.g., Armstrong and Moore, 2007).

Microstimulation and deep brain stimulation refer to two different applications of this invasive electrical stimulation. Microstimulation in humans is primarily restricted to patients who suffer from severe, untreatable epileptic seizures. In some of those patients, neurologists implant recording and stimulation electrodes to better determine the source of the seizures. The implanted electrodes are removed prior to surgery. In some cases, it is possible to take some time to use the implanted electrodes to also characterize the neural responses for research purposes.

We will restrict ourselves to one intriguing example of microstimulation in this context, the results of which were published in a paper by Parvizi and colleagues (2012). They implanted electrodes in the visual cortex of one patient. The recorded electrical activity indicated that a few of the electrodes were located in a fusiform

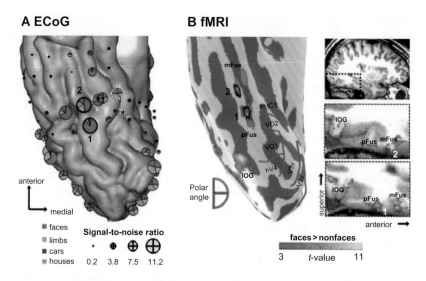

Figure 14.1 Invasive microstimulation of face-selective patches in the human brain. The location of the two channels used for brain stimulation is indicated with 1 and 2 in each panel. (A) Location of the intracranial electrodes used for electrophysiological recordings, so-called electrocorticography (ECoG). For each electrode, the neural responses in four conditions (faces, limbs, cars, houses) are shown with a pie chart. The diameter of each pie chart reflects the signal-to-noise ratio of the channel. The anatomical image shows a ventral view (view from below) of the occipital and posterior temporal cortex. (B) Face selectivity as measured with functional MRI (fMRI). Blue, green, and red lines represent the meridian representations in part of the retinotopic cortex. The left image shows a ventral view of the inflated surface, the right images a few sagittal slices.
Reproduced with permission from Parvizi et al., 2012

face-selective area as defined by functional MRI (fMRI) in the same patient (Fig. 14.1). A short stimulation through these electrodes influenced the perception of faces by the patient. One of his verbal descriptions of this effect is as follows: "You almost look like somebody I've seen before, but somebody different. That was a trip. … It's almost like the shape of your face, your features drooped" (Parvizi et al., 2012, p. 14198). The data quality and the number of subjects in such a study are necessarily very limited, given the clinical context to which such data collection is restricted, but it is obviously a very intriguing finding.

The term "deep brain stimulation" or DBS refers to the same method of micro-stimulation but as applied in the deep structures of the brain such as the thalamus and basal ganglia. The original application of DBS was used as a treatment for Parkinson's disease, for which it is an FDA-approved treatment (Deuschl et al., 2006). It is also being tested in the context of other syndromes, including severe forms of obsessive-compulsive disorder (Greenberg et al., 2006) and depression (Mayberg et al., 2005) that do not respond to other treatments. The symptoms are alleviated during the stimulation, but they return afterward. Thus, the implanted electrodes are meant to stay in place for as long as possible.

Deep brain stimulation typically involves a repetitive and chronic stimulation across a long period of time – a kind of neural pacemaker. This chronic stimulation can function as a treatment through various mechanisms: enhancing activity, inhibiting activity, or synchronizing activity. For example, in the case of depression, the stimulation is applied to the subgenual cingulate region, a structure in which the activity is elevated in some depressive patients. Stimulation in white matter near this region is thought to reduce this elevated activity, resulting in less depression.

14.2 Focused Ultrasound Stimulation (FUS)

Physically, sound is characterized as a wave of air displacement. This mechanical movement is also why we can hear sounds, because airwaves make the eardrum move back and forth, and the resulting movements in the inner ear activate the auditory receptor cells. However, the frequency range that we can hear is only a very small fraction of the possible spectrum of frequencies. A frequency of 20 kHz is too high to be detectable by human ears. Waves with a frequency beyond the hearing range are referred to as "ultrasound". Focused ultrasound stimulation typically includes frequencies of a few hundred kHz. While we are used to thinking of sound as a wave that propagates through a large volume of space, these high-frequency waves are much more restricted in space. The transducers used for FUS are designed to limit these waves even further in space, resulting in a relatively focused volume of space in which the waves propagate.

Given that FUS is applied transcranially, the bone reduces the amplitude dramatically, with a factor of 4. In contrast, however, to the light waves used with functional near-infrared spectroscopy (fNIRS), the sound waves are not scattered when going through the bone (Legon et al., 2014). The region stimulated by FUS looks a bit like a rugby ball, with the long axis being orthogonal to the scalp surface. In lateral directions, the spatial resolution is better than other noninvasive stimulation methods (see the following sections), reaching a resolution of only a few millimeters. The main focus of stimulation can be deeper than with these other methods, although this potential has not yet been tested in human studies. Given the relatively high spatial precision of FUS, it is typically guided by a structural MRI.

It is important to consider the intensity of the ultrasound waves. With high intensities, the waves contain so much energy that the tissue heats up and damage occurs. Such high-intensity FUS can be used and is being used to lesion brain structures. When used for neural stimulation, the waves have a relatively low intensity, referred to as low-intensity FUS (Rezayat and Toostani, 2016). In this low-intensity regime, the induced thermal energy is very low and does not lead to any harm.

Focused ultrasound stimulation is a relatively new method. It has not been fully determined yet how FUS influences neural processing. Given the low intensity of the waves, most of the effect on neural processing is not due to the tissue heating up. A non-thermal form of energy, which is very likely behind most of the effects, is

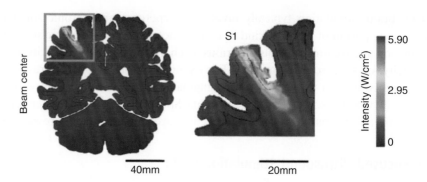

Figure 14.2 Simulation of the area of stimulated tissue during the application of FUS to somatosensory cortex S1. The coronal slices show a projection of FUS fields as measured in a realistic brain model. The coronal slice is taken at the anterior-posterior center of the beam.
Figure adapted with permission from Legon et al., 2014

mechanical energy. The high-frequency airwaves cause very small displacements of cells, and these displacements influence the properties of receptors such as voltage-gated sodium and calcium channels (Rezayat and Toostani, 2016).

Focused ultrasound stimulation was first validated in animal studies, but recently there have been several convincing demonstrations in humans. For example, Legon and colleagues (2014) showed that FUS applied to the somatosensory cortex modulates somatosensory evoked potentials measured through electroencephalography (EEG) and enhances performance in discrimination tasks. They calculated the area of stimulated tissue as shown in Figure 14.2. There are no neural measurements to confirm that this calculation corresponds to the area of tissue with affected neural responses, except the observation that FUS displaced 1 cm anterior or posterior did no longer have an effect on somatosensory potentials. In another study, Lee and colleagues (2016) stimulated the primary visual cortex with FUS and observed changes in blood-oxygenation-level dependent (BOLD) fMRI signals, electro-physiological responses, and accompanying phosphene perception. Despite these exciting results, many questions remain, such as why there is a large minority of participants who are unresponsive to the stimulation (Lee et al., 2016), and whether systematic comparisons will allow us to more closely compare the effective spatial precision of FUS and TMS.

14.3 Transcranial Magnetic Stimulation (TMS)

The physical principle behind TMS will sound familiar to someone who has been studying the physics of MRI because of the central role of electromagnetic induction. In TMS, a coil is placed over the skull and an electrical current is applied. This electrical current induces a magnetic field, which, in turn, causes another electrical current in the brain (Fig. 14.3A). The shape of the magnetic field and of the induced

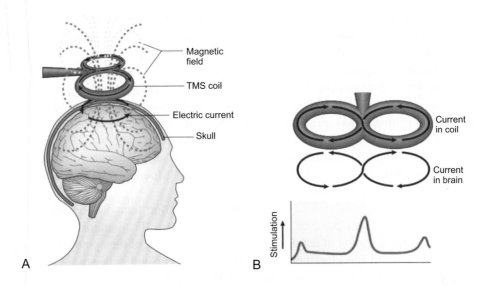

Figure 14.3 Illustration of transcranial magnetic stimulation (TMS) and coil design. (A) An electrical current in the coil (thin black arrows drawn in the coil) induces a magnetic field orthogonal to the coil (red lines). This magnetic field passes through the skull and induces electrical currents in an electrical field that runs parallel to the coil (thick black line). (B) Illustration of the spatial distribution of stimulation induced by a figure eight–shaped coil.
Figure reproduced with permission from Ridding and Rothwell, 2007

current depend on the shape of the coil, which is a circle in the simplest design but can also take other forms, such as a figure eight–shaped coil. The latter provides a more focused magnetic field at the center where the two coils meet (Fig. 14.3B) and so offers greater precision in terms of the location of altered neural activity.

The exact properties of this second electrical current and the effect that this current has on neural activity depends on several parameters, which make it difficult to predict the exact effect of TMS on neural activity. Some parameters can still be modeled, such as the distance from the coil: The strongest effect will be induced underneath the coil, and the effect will gradually dissipate with longer distance. Other parameters involve biological factors, such as the conductivity of tissue and the orientation of axons. These biological factors are more difficult to fully characterize.

The effect of distance tends to restrict the application of TMS to superficial structures. Nevertheless, some coil designs allow for the stimulation of less superficial structures, at the expense of spatial precision (Zangen et al., 2005).

As with all forms of brain stimulation, the induced electrical current can have a variety of effects on neural information processing. On the one hand, the stimulation can result in interference or noise induction and as such hamper normal processing and performance. On the other hand, the electrical stimulation can result in actual neural stimulation and mimic the effect of excitatory input to a region.

Examples of the latter are the induction of movements when TMS is applied to primary motor cortex and the occurrence of phosphenes after application of TMS to the visual cortex (e.g., Meyer et al., 1990).

Transcranial magnetic stimulation probably has a spatial resolution of close to 1 centimeter, and cannot compete with the resolution of invasive techniques such as microstimulation and DBS. Regions that are more than a centimeter apart can be dissociated through TMS. For example, Pitcher and colleagues (2012) showed that (late) TMS of the occipital face area only affects face processing, while TMS at the same timing (105 ms after stimulus onset) only affects body processing when applied to the extrastriate body area. This double dissociation is found even though the two regions are less than 2 cm apart.

Transcranial magnetic stimulation also has a very good temporal resolution, at least when only a single pulse or a double pulse is applied. The temporal resolution is limited by the duration of the pulse(s) and by the number of time points tested by the researchers. In the aforementioned study of Pitcher and colleagues (2012), a difference was found between stimulation at 45 and 105 ms post-stimulus, while no effects were found at intermediate times tested at intervals of 20 ms. The design of this study would therefore provide a temporal resolution of 20 ms. The possibility of investigating when regions are involved causally in a particular behavior has been referred to as causal chronometry (Pascual-Leone et al., 2000).

There is also a more sustained version of TMS, referred to as repetitive TMS (rTMS). Here multiple pulses are applied for a particular period of time and frequency. Repetitive TMS does not have a good temporal resolution but might induce a stronger effect. For this reason, repetitive TMS also involves a higher risk, although it is widely considered to be a safe technique when applied appropriately (Rossi et al., 2009). It has been shown that rTMS can induce seizures in a very small minority of participants, and primarily in patients who were already susceptible (e.g., due to medication).

One possible approach to combine the two variants of TMS is to first apply rTMS to establish the existence of a causal link and then apply single/double-pulse TMS to investigate this link with a higher temporal resolution. As an example, consider the study by Pitcher and colleagues (2008). The authors were interested in the potential role of the occipital face area (OFA) in emotion recognition. The OFA is located near the surface of the skull and can therefore be stimulated with TMS, in contrast to the fusiform face area (FFA). Pitcher and colleagues used a combination of structural and functional MRI to determine the location of the OFA in each individual participant (Fig. 14.4). In a first set of experiments, they applied repetitive TMS with a frequency of 10 Hz for 500 ms (Fig. 14.5A). Transcranial magnetic stimulation of the right OFA resulted in lower performance in recognizing emotions from face images, while identity recognition was not affected. In a later experiment, the authors applied double-pulse TMS with an interval of 40 ms between the pulses (Fig. 14.5B). The experiment included multiple timing conditions with a 40 ms difference between conditions, with the earliest condition including two pulses

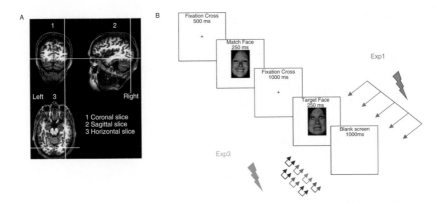

Figure 14.4 Determination of the anatomical coordinates of the region of interest and overview of the experimental methods of Pitcher et al. (2008). (A) The Talairach coordinates of the occipital face area in a group study were used to determine the anatomical location of the occipital face area (OFA). These coordinates were then transformed to the subject's native space in order to obtain subject-specific coordinates for the stimulation. (B) Illustration of the trial procedure and the TMS protocol. Experiment 1 included a repetitive stimulation of 10 Hz for 500 ms starting at stimulus onset (illustrated in blue). Experiment 3 included a double-pulse TMS in 7 conditions with different timings (each illustrated in a different color).
Figure adapted with permission from Pitcher et al., 2008

applied 20–60 ms after stimulus onset, and the latest condition at 250–290 ms. Transcranial magnetic stimulation of the right OFA only affected emotion recognition in the condition with timing 60–100 ms after stimulus onset, suggesting that the causal influence of OFA on emotion recognition occurs relatively early after stimulus onset.

For TMS, it is important to have proper control conditions. Even when researchers are only interested in one particular brain region and timing condition, the experimental paradigm should include at least one condition that controls for potential placebo effects. One possibility is the use of a sham condition, which often involves turning the coil by 90 degrees so that the magnetic field does not influence neural activity. Such a sham condition is easily detected by participants, because the common side effects of real stimulation, such as scalp sensations or muscle twitching, are not present in the sham condition. An alternative control condition that is frequently used is stimulation of the vertex, which is the highest point of the skull and close to the postcentral gyri and electrode position Cz in the EEG.

In a clinical context, TMS has a major diagnostic value in testing the connectivity between the motor cortex and peripheral muscles in motor-related disorders and after stroke (for review, see Groppa et al., 2012). The efficacy of TMS as part of a clinical treatment of disorders related to the central nervous system has been tested in many domains, but its efficacy is not always as strong as hoped for. In major depression, some positive evidence has been reported. In this case, repetitive TMS

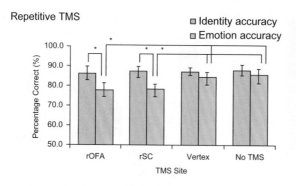

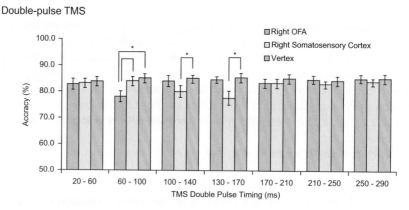

Figure 14.5 The influence of repetitive TMS and double-pulse TMS on face identity and face emotion recognition. The asterisks (*) denote a comparison that yields a statistically significant difference. Panels adapted with permission from Pitcher et al., 2008

is used as an alternative to the classical and very impactful electroconvulsive therapy ("electroshocks") for treating patients. According to the review by Brunelin and colleagues (2007), repetitive TMS is primarily applied to the dorsolateral prefrontal cortex, with an interaction between the side of stimulation (left or right) and the frequency of stimulation (high and low frequency stimulation). Low-frequency stimulation is intended to inhibit cortical excitability, while high-frequency stimulation is used to stimulate neural activity. The strength of the effect is illustrated by numbers such as 37% responders (= meaningful reduction in symptom severity) in the TMS group versus 20% responders in a placebo group. Ten years later, it is still recommended as a possible therapy for patients who are treatment resistant or intolerant (Perera et al., 2016).

Transcranial magnetic stimulation is also applied and is FDA approved in the context of migraine. Here treatment might involve a TMS device that can be taken home and self-applied by the patient. Lipton and colleagues (2010) showed that single-pulse TMS over the visual cortex (occipital bone) reduces the probability of a headache pain in migraine attacks with a visual aura two hours after pain onset from 78% in the sham TMS group to 61% in the TMS group. This is a positive effect that can make a meaningful difference for some patients.

14.4 Transcranial Current Stimulation (TCS)

With transcranial current stimulation (TCS), a small current is applied to the skull. The basic equipment for the simplest version of TCS is straightforward: a battery and two electrodes (see Fig. 14.6). One electrode is positively charged, referred to as an anode, the other electrode is the negative, referred to as a cathode. The current flows from the anode to the cathode. Warning: Please do not try this at home, in case this simple description would persuade a do-it-yourself reader! A battery and electrodes are cheap and easy to work with, but not necessarily safe. Those TCS devices that are certified for human use come with many additional features to ascertain safety and proper control of various parameters. As a consequence, these devices are disappointingly expensive, easily running into several thousand dollars.

The electrical current will influence cortical excitability. At the site of the anode, the current will depolarize neurons and as such increase cortical excitability. The opposite effect is seen at the cathode.

Several parameters are important to consider (Nitsche et al., 2008). First, current strength will determine not only the effect size at the neural level but also side effects. Studies typically use current strengths of 1–2 mA, which is enough to generate at least some effect but still keep the side effects under control. At this strength, skin sensations at the start and end of stimulation are frequently noticed,

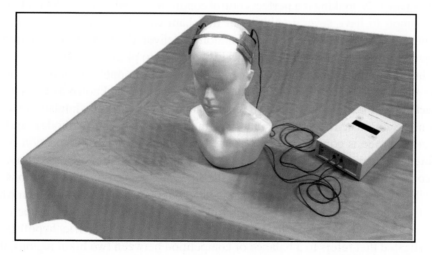

Figure 14.6 The equipment used for transcranial current stimulation. The anode is shown in red, the cathode in blue.

skin irritation (e.g., redness) is regularly present but does not indicate skin damage, and major side effects such as headaches are rare.

Second, the contact area of the electrodes is relatively large, often 25 cm^2 or more. Given that current density should be controlled, smaller electrodes might require the use of smaller current strengths to avoid aversive side effects. Because of the use of large electrodes, the relatively uniform delivery of the current across the electrode area, and the way in which the current flows in the skull, TCS has a very poor spatial resolution, even relative to TMS. It would be unrealistic to expect that TCS would be able to dissociate regions that are only 2 cm apart, as was shown for TMS.

Third, the duration of stimulation is important to consider. The cumulated effect of a longer stimulation will be larger than of a shorter stimulation, and a longer stimulation might also induce a longer aftereffect. In motor cortex, these after-effects can even be longer than the stimulation, with aftereffects up to 1 hour after stimulation for less than 15 minutes (for review, see Nitsche et al., 2008). As a consequence, TCS has a very poor temporal resolution. This property of TCS also affects experimental design: Different stimulation conditions are often not com-bined in a single subject by a repeated-measures approach but rather through a between-subject design unless the experiment includes multiple sessions.

Transcranial current stimulation studies typically include multiple conditions involving different subjects. The minimum number is one stimulation condition and one no-stimulation or sham condition. Often the sham condition includes the same electrode positioning and two very short current deliveries at the start and at the end of the period in which stimulation is continuously applied in the experi-mental condition. As such, the sham condition mimics the minor skin sensations in the experimental condition, because these sensations are limited to the start and the end of current delivery. Through this approach, subjects cannot distinguish real TCS from sham TCS, making it a perfect control condition (Gandiga et al., 2006). It is not uncommon to have several subjects in the sham condition reporting side effects during the interval in which no stimulation is delivered, as much as reported by subjects during actual stimulation. This is likely due to placebo effects.

Thus far we have assumed that current always goes in one direction. This is the case when a direct current is applied, and this technique is known as **transcranial direct current stimulation (TDCS)**. Transcranial direct current stimulation studies often use one electrode for stimulation (anode) or inhibition (cathode), and the other electrode is considered a reference electrode. Although the location of the reference electrode would in such a case not be the focus of attention, it is important to consider, because it will determine the flow of the current. Many options are possible: a location at the same side of the head but on top of a cortical region which is not considered relevant for the experimental questions, a location on the other side of the head, or even on the shoulder on the other side. If a hypothesis is investigated that refers to a balance or competition between two brain regions, then it might also be relevant to place the anode on top of one of these regions and the cathode on top of the other one.

Other variants of TCS involve an alternating current. In such cases, both electrodes have the same function and labels such as "anodal," "cathodal," and "reference electrode" are no longer used to differentiate the two electrodes. When this current is alternating at a fixed frequency, the method is referred to as **transcranial alternating current stimulation (TACS)**. This method is particularly useful for testing hypotheses that particular frequency ranges might be involved (see the chapters on EEG for a few examples). When the current is not simply alternating but is modulated according to a random frequency spectrum, the method is known as **transcranial random noise stimulation (TRNS)**. Enhancement of cortical excitability through TRNS might be related to relatively high frequencies, 100 Hz and more (Terney et al., 2008).

All these methods have relatively small effects on neural activity because of the weak currents that can be used. It is thus unrealistic to expect large and immediate effects on behavior. Nevertheless, TCS seems to show robust effects in some specific contexts. First, a small change in cortical excitability might have a particularly large effect on neural activity and related behavior when a task is performed at threshold. Second, whereas no immediate effects might exist on behavior, effects might become larger in paradigms in which small effects can accumulate over time. This would be the case in long-term training paradigms in which training effects are built up across time.

Many studies have been performed that have both characteristics. One example is a recent study by Van Meel and colleagues (2016). They studied the effect of anodal TDCS in a perceptual learning paradigm in which participants had to recognize images of objects that were shown only very briefly (Fig. 14.7). There were two subject groups, with 12 participants in each: anodal stimulation of the right lateral occipital complex (LOC), a region thought to be involved in object recognition, and sham stimulation. The reference electrode was positioned on the left shoulder. All subjects were tested for four successive days. The first training day showed no difference in behavioral performance, illustrating the fact that the short-term effect of TDCS on behavior is negligible in the short term, even when stimuli are presented near the threshold level. Nevertheless, the improvement in performance from the first to the last day was larger in the anodal TDCS group compared with the sham condition. Thus, anodal TDCS stimulation can increase the training effect accumulated across multiple days.

Another illustration of the accumulating effects of multiple TDCS sessions is given in a study by Cohen Kadosh and colleagues (2010). Subjects learned to associate a new set of artificial symbols with numerical magnitudes during six sessions. Transcranial direct current stimulation was applied for 20 minutes at the beginning of each session. The two electrodes were positioned on top of the left and right parietal lobes. Fifteen subjects were divided across three groups: anodal stimulation in the left lobe (and cathodal in the right), anodal stimulation in the right lobe, and sham. The results suggested that the numerical magnitudes were learned more readily by the group receiving anodal stimulation in the right parietal

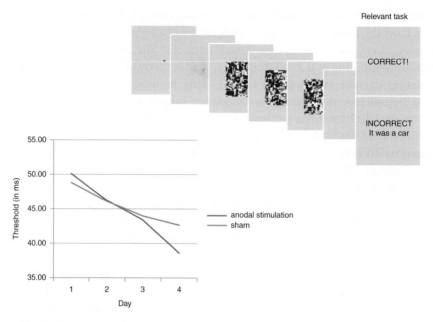

Figure 14.7 The application of TDCS in the context of perceptual learning. The top shows the trial sequence, with an image of a car followed by several masking images. Results are expressed in terms of the threshold, which is the stimulus duration needed for the identification of images. The threshold improves due to training, and this improvement is larger for the condition with anodal TMS.
Adapted from Van Meel et al., 2016

lobe, in agreement with a specific role of this cortical region for numerical processing (Fig. 14.8). As shown in Figure 14.8, for familiar everyday digits the participants of both groups show a linear relationship between the objective magnitude of digits and their subjective magnitude according to the participants. For the new artificial digits, participants showed a similar linear relationship in the anodal stimulation group, while the other groups did not. Although the small number of subjects ($N = 5$) per group is a disadvantage of this particular study for drawing strong conclusions, it illustrates the potential that TDCS might provide for enhancing training effects that accumulate across days. Recent studies from the same group used TRNS to confirm beneficial effects of behavioral training combined with cortical stimulation (Cappelletti et al., 2013; Snowball et al., 2013).

Overall, the field of TCS is still in transition, and further studies with larger sample sizes are needed for a more accurate estimate of the actual effect size of current TCS protocols. Some have voiced doubts about this effect size. A recent study even went through the trouble of measuring currents elicited by TCS applied to human cadaver heads (Voroslakos et al., 2018). Their findings suggested that common TCS protocols do not induce effective currents in the brain. This is a wake-up call to the need for further experiments to improve the existing protocols and experimental designs. It is also a perfect illustration of the multidisciplinary nature

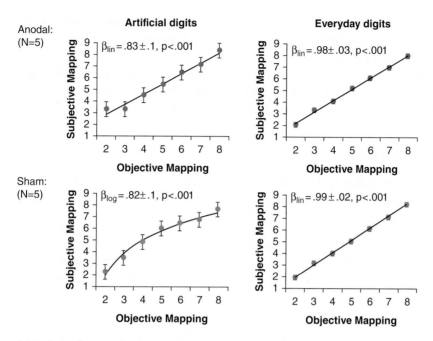

Figure 14.8 The application of TDCS in the context of numerical cognition for two subject groups, anodal stimulation and sham. Results show the relationship between subjective and objective magnitude for artificial digits (*left*) and for everyday digits (*right*).
Figure reproduced with permission from Cohen Kadosh et al., 2010

of human brain imaging that we end this book with a study on dead human brains, just in case the reader may already have forgotten the dead salmon!

Summary

- There is a wide variety of methods for neuromodulation that allow researchers to test the causal link between neural activity and behavior.
- In order of decreasing spatial resolution, the noninvasive methods include focused ultrasound stimulation (FUS), transcranial magnetic stimulation (TMS), and transcranial current stimulation (TCS).
- In order of decreasing temporal specificity, the list includes single-/double-pulse TMS, FUS, repetitive TMS, and TCS.

Review Questions

1. Explain the extent to which the availability of anatomical images of individual participants is relevant for the different methods of noninvasive neuromodulation.

2. Describe and explain the differences in spatial and temporal resolution between transcranial magnetic stimulation (TMS) and transcranial current stimulation (TCS).
3. Explain the difference in the elicited neural modulation when an electrical current is applied through an invasive electrode, as in microstimulation, or through a noninvasive scalp electrode, as in TCS.

Further Reading

Knotkova, H. & Rasche, D. (2016). *Textbook of Neuromodulation*. New York: Springer-Verlag. (This book provides a much more in-depth overview of techniques for neuromodulation and stimulation.)

Woods, A. J., Antal, A., Bikson, M., et al. (2016). A technical guide to tDCS, and related non-invasive brain stimulation tools. *Clinical Neurophysiology*, **127**(2), 1031–1048. (This paper provides a useful overview of TCS, covering topics such as how it works, which parameters to consider, and how to set up the experimental design.)

Glossary

Action potential.   A rapid rise and fall of the membrane potential of a neuron. It has a characteristic temporal envelope that is caused by the involved molecular mechanisms. It propagates through the axon of the neuron and is the major format for communication in the brain.

Additivity.   Property of a linear system, so that the response to a complex stimulus, AB, that is composed of two simple stimuli, A and B, is equal to the sum of the response to A and the response to B. Additivity is often an assumption in the modeling of hemodynamic responses. The same assumption also underlies the (Donders) subtraction method.

Adjacency matrix.   A square matrix that represents a finite graph. Each entry of the matrix indicates a link between two nodes of the graph.

Alpha (α) band.   A frequency band of M/EEG activity, approximately including the frequency range 8–13 Hz. It is sometimes also referred to as the alpha wave.

Alternating current (AC) amplifier.   An electric device that amplifies the alternating current signal. See also direct current (DC) amplifier.

Alternating current (AC) noise.   Electromagnetic noise due to alternating current noise sources, mainly the power supply. Also referred to as powerline noise or mains noise.

Amplitude spectral density (ASD).   Standardized amplitude spectrum.

Amplitude spectrum.   Spectrum of the amplitude of frequency components at the different frequencies in a signal.

Analog-to-digital (AD) converter.   An electric device that converts an analog signal to a digital signal.

Analog-to-digital (AD) level.   Amount of information per digital sample. The unit is the bit.

Arterial spin labeling (ASL).   An fMRI method that measures blood flow by labeling water molecules that move because of perfusion.

Artifacts.   Distortions seen in images or electrophysiological time series. The distortions are unwanted but sometimes impossible to avoid. Image and signal-processing steps are needed to minimize the impact of the distortions in statistical data processing.

Auditory brainstem response (ABR).   A series of seven evoked potentials that appear within 10 ms from an auditory click stimulus. Each peak corresponds to activity of auditory nerves and nuclei in the brain stem.

Auditory evoked potential (AEP).   An evoked potential in response to an auditory stimulus.

Autocorrelation.   A correlation of a signal with itself when translated. If time is the dimension over which the translation happens, we refer to a temporal autocorrelation. An autocorrelation reflects a dependence between successive data points.

Average reference.   A montage method in which the reference signal is an average signal, such as the average of all EEG electrodes.

Axial diffusivity (AD) .   The amount of diffusion along the direction of maximal diffusion.

Axial gradiometer.   MEG sensor with two pick-up coils. The coils turn around the common axis in different planes/heights.

Band-cut filter.   A filter to remove a band of frequency components. Also known as a notch filter.

Beta band.   A frequency band of M/EEG activity. The range is approximately 13–30 Hz.

Beta-series correlations.   Method for functional connectivity analysis that includes fitting the effect of individual events through a general linear model and analyzing the variation across time in the resulting beta estimates.

Beta value.   Value obtained through model fitting that provides an estimate of how much and in which direction an independent variable (e.g., regressor of interest) predicts changes in a dependent variable (e.g., fMRI signal in a voxel).

Bipolar derivation.   A montage method in which an EEG signal is derived relative to another scalp electrode signal.

Block design.   Experimental design in which trials of a particular condition are grouped in time to form a block of trials. Within blocks, the hemodynamic responses associated with individual trials add together to generate a strong cumulative signal.

Blood oxygenation.   The ratio of oxygenated to deoxygenated hemoglobin.

Blood-oxygenation-level dependent (BOLD) functional magnetic resonance imaging (fMRI).   fMRI in which the measured signal is intended to be sensitive to the level of blood oxygenation.

Brain extraction.   The delineation of the parts of images that contain brain tissue, in order to restrict further analyses to only these parts.

Cerebrospinal fluid (CSF).   Body fluid that is found in and around the brain, in particular in the ventricles and surrounding the cerebral cortex.

Circular analyses.   Statistical analyses in which analysis steps are mutually dependent while they should be independent. This might happen because one or more earlier steps in the analysis stream are informed by the outcome of later steps, or because data are selected in ways that are not statistically independent from tests that are performed in later steps.

Circular mean.   Mean in circular statistics. Also known as vector mean or directional mean.

Circular statistics.   Statistics for circular-valued data, such as phase. Also known as directional statistics or spherical statistics.

Coil.   A loop of wire that is used to transmit or receive an electrical current. This current can induce or be induced by a magnetic field.

Condition-rich design.   Experimental design in which many individual conditions are identified. This contrasts with the typical design in a human neuroimaging experiment that typically only includes a low number of conditions. Condition-rich designs have been developed for the purpose of multi-voxel pattern analysis.

Contact impedance.   Electrical impedance between an EEG electrode and the scalp. Less than 5 kΩ is recommended for a good signal-to-noise ratio.

Convolution.   Mathematical operation in which the integral is taken of the point-wise multiplication of a time series with a function that is translated in time.

Coregistration.   Step in the preprocessing of fMRI images. Coregistration brings different image modalities, such as a functional scan and an anatomical volume, in one and the same spatial coordinate frame.

Correlational multi-voxel pattern analysis (MVPA).   MVPA approach that involves the computation of correlations between multi-voxel patterns.

Cluster-wise correction.   Correction for multiple comparisons that combines an uncorrected threshold at the voxel level with a further threshold incorporating cluster size: the number of adjacent voxels that cross the uncorrected threshold.

Computerized tomography (CT) scanning.   Three-dimensional imaging with X-ray images. CT scanning is rarely used in studies looking for brain/behavior relationships, but it is very useful for the diagnosis of a wide range of diseases that affect the nervous system.

Cyclotron.   Machine to create radionuclides, such as used in the radioactive tracers for PET imaging.

Decoding multi-voxel pattern analysis (MVPA).   MVPA approach that involves the training and cross-validation of pattern classifiers.

Deep brain stimulation (DBS).   Method to influence neural activity locally by applying a small electrical current through an electrode that is inserted deep in the brain.

Default mode network.   Network of regions with strong functional connectivity that are most strongly activated when participants are not engaged in a particular task.

Delta band.   A frequency band of M/EEG activity. The band includes approximately 1 to 4 Hz. For healthy adults, the slow activity appears during deep sleep.

Dephasing.   The gradual decrease in correspondence between elements (protons, neuronal responses, electrophysiological signals) in the phase of oscillatory changes.

Depolarization.   Change in the membrane potentials to less negative values. This is what happens when a neuron receives excitatory synaptic input.

Design matrix.   The matrix that contains all independent variables included in the general linear model, typically involving regressors of interest (e.g., the time onsets of experimental conditions) as well as covariates or potential confounds (e.g., motion-correction parameters).

DICOM.   DICOM is a standard format for medical images. DICOM stands for Digital Imaging and Communications in Medicine. The format was traditionally used by many MRI scanners, but it is converted into other formats for data analysis.

Diffusion.   Phenomenon that molecules tend to move around in a medium in such a way that they spread out as evenly as possible.

Diffusion tensor imaging (DTI).   Imaging approach based on diffusion-weighted imaging that is used to investigate structural connectivity in the brain.

Diffusion-weighted imaging (DWI).   Imaging with MRI pulse sequences that are sensitive to molecular diffusion.

Direct current (DC) amplifier.   An electric device which amplifies the direct and alternating current signals. See also alternating current (AC) amplifier.

Direct influence.   An influence from one brain region to another without intermediate regions; this influence explains the correlation in activity between the two regions.

Discrete Fourier transform (DFT).   A mathematical operation that transforms a discrete time domain signal into a discrete frequency domain signal.

Donders subtraction method.   See subtraction method.

Double dipping. Colloquial term for a statistical approach in which the same data are used for selecting relevant data and for performing analyses that are restricted to these relevant data.

Down-sampling. A signal resampling method to decrease the number of samples. Original samples are interpolated and resampled with a lower sampling frequency. Alternatively, the original sample points are subsampled, e.g., one in every five samples.

Echo time (TE). The time interval between excitation (or refocusing by a gradient switch) and data acquisition.

Edited spectrum. Method applied in the context of magnetic resonance spectroscopy. It computes the contribution of a metabolite in peaks that reflect multiple metabolites from the effect that the suppression of one peak has on other peaks.

Effective connectivity. Functional connectivity between brain regions that implies a direction in the connectivity (which region drives the other).

Efficiency. Index to measure the amount of resources (e.g., time) that are needed to implement a method or design. Efficiency is an important consideration when comparing experimental designs for hemodynamic imaging. It is affected negatively by correlations between independent variables.

Electrically shielded room. A room that is covered by conductive materials. The materials prevent the electric activity outside of the room to enter. Also referred to as a Faraday cage.

Electrocardiography (ECG). Method to measure electrophysiological activity of the cardiovascular system.

Electrocorticography (ECoG). Method to measure EEG from the cortical surface. The electrodes are placed on the pia mater of the brain.

Electrode. A piece of conductive material which makes electric contact with an object of measurement, such as a neuron, brain tissue, skull, or scalp.

Electroencephalography (EEG). Method to record electric signal due to brain activity. The signal is recorded from the electrodes on scalp, skull, cortical surface, or in brain tissue.

Electromyography (EMG). Method to measure electric signal due to muscular activity.

Electrooculography (EOG). Method to measure electric activity due to eye movements.

Event-related design. Experimental design in which trials of different conditions are ordered in a pseudo-random sequence so that successive trials are often from a different condition. Depending on the length of the inter-trial interval, the event-related design can be rapid (short interval; typically only a few seconds) or slow (long interval; often more than 10 seconds).

Event-related potential (ERP). An M/EEG component that appears in response to an external stimulus or an internal event.

Event-related synchrony. An increase in signal amplitude relative to the pre-event baseline level. The amplitude is computed from a time-frequency signal.

Evoked potential (EP). An M/EEG response to an external stimulus. Also see event-related potential.

Excitatory postsynaptic potential (EPSP). See postsynaptic potential (PSP).

Extracellular recordings. The measurement of the electrical signals from single neurons or populations of neurons by means of an electrode that is brought near (but not in) these neurons or populations.

False discovery rate (FDR). An approach to correct for multiple comparisons that controls the proportion of incorrectly rejected null hypotheses based on the observed distribution of uncorrected p-values. If we apply the FDR correction with a corrected $p = 0.05$, then 1 out of 20 of activated voxels/regions is a false positive.

Family-wise error (FWE) correction. Method to control for the probability of a type-I error (claiming that there is an effect while there is none) at the "family" level of all relevant voxels, so that the probability to find one or more voxels with a lower p-value is 0.05 if the null hypothesis of no effect is true. This approach is related to Bonferroni correction, but takes into account the covariance between voxels which reduces the number of independent tests.

Fast Fourier transform (FFT). A computer algorithm to perform a discrete Fourier transform (DFT).

Field inhomogeneity. Small spatial variations in the local magnetic field. It contributes to T2* decay.

Field of view (FOV). The size of the imaged volume or slice.

Filtering. The attenuation of parts of the measured frequency spectrum. We distinguish between low-pass filtering (higher frequencies are attenuated), band-pass filtering (lowest and highest frequencies are attenuated, middle frequencies remain), and high-pass filtering (lower frequencies are attenuated).

Flatmap. Visualization of the cortical surface as a two-dimensional sheet. The creation of a flatmap requires that cuts are made in the surface so that the original three-dimensional layout of the surface can be represented in two dimensions.

Flip angle. The angle in which spins are flipped by the radio frequency (RF) pulse.

Focused ultrasound stimulation (FUS). Noninvasive method for modulating brain activity by applying focused sound waves in the ultrasound frequency range. The waves probably affect neural activity by causing very small displacements of cells, as such influencing the properties of receptors such as voltage-gated sodium and calcium channels.

Forward inference. Statistical inference that activation in a brain region is related to a particular cognitive process because it was observed that if the cognitive process is manipulated, then this specific brain region is activated.

Fourier analysis. Method to decompose a signal into a sum of frequency components, each with a particular amplitude and phase.

Fractional anisotropy (FA). The difference in diffusion depending on the direction in which it is computed. It is computed by taking the difference between the length of each diffusion axis and the mean diffusion, followed by a further normalization for the total diffusion.

Frequency. The speed with which a signal is changing. It is expressed in hertz (Hz), for which the unit of time is a second. A signal with frequency 1 Hz is a signal that goes up and down one time per second.

Frequency components.   Elementary functions that together make up a signal. Each component has a different frequency, ranging from slow to fast. Each component is determined by three parameters: frequency, amplitude (how much it is going up and down), and phase (when it is going up and down). Apart from the changes that can be induced by altering these parameters, the components are the same. In most methods of signal processing, sinusoidal functions are used.

Frequency-encoding (FE) gradient.   A gradient that is applied during data acquisition, so that nuclei at different positions along the gradient have a different resonance frequency.

Frequency spectrum.   The range of frequencies in a signal. Its limits depend on sampling duration and sampling frequency.

Full width at half maximum (FWHM).   Index that captures the width of a function, typically the function that is applied during spatial smoothing. The index captures how wide the function is when the function is at half of its maximal height.

Functional connectivity.   Relationship between brain regions in how their neural activity varies across time.

Functional localization.   The enterprise of trying to pinpoint where mental functions are localized in the brain.

Functional localizer.   Experiment that is intended to localize regions of interest (ROIs) through functional activity. It is typically only a small part of a larger study that includes other manipulations, the effect of which is tested in the localized ROIs.

Functional magnetic resonance imaging (fMRI).   The use of nuclear magnetic resonance in order to measure the hemodynamic changes related to neural activity.

Functional magnetic resonance imaging (fMRI) adaptation.   Experimental design and method that is developed to measure how neural responses depend on whether successive stimuli are the same or different. This stimulus-specific adaptation is often used as a measure of how sensitive the neuronal population in a voxel or region is to the stimulus change.

Functional near-infrared spectroscopy (fNIRS).   An imaging technique that measures the hemodynamic response through its effect on the light reflectance of neural tissue in the near-infrared part of the spectrum.

Fusiform face area (FFA).   Region in the human cortex principally in the lateral fusiform gyrus. It is defined by a higher hemodynamic response to pictures containing faces than to pictures containing other objects.

Galvanic skin response (GSR).   A measure of skin conductance which changes due to activity of sweat glands.

Gamma band.   A frequency band of M/EEG activity, going from 30 Hz and higher. The lower gamma band is approximately 30–60 Hz, and the higher gamma band is approximately 60–200 Hz.

Gastric evoked potential (GEP).   An evoked potential due to a gastric stimulus, such as oral gustatory application of 10% sucrose.

General linear model (GLM).   Statistical approach to capture the linear relationship between multiple dependent variables and a set of independent variables. With only one dependent variable, the GLM is a multiple linear regression. In the case of neuroimaging, the dependent variables can refer to the signal of voxels (fMRI) or electrodes (EEG/MEG).

Gradient. A gradual, primarily linear, change in field strength over space. Gradients constitute an important part of pulse sequences for MRI.

Gradient-echo echo-planar imaging (GE-EPI) sequence. An MRI pulse sequence that involves the successive acquisition of different planes/slices and by which echoes are created through gradient reversals. This sequence is used very often for BOLD fMRI.

Gradiometer. A multi-coil magnetometer used for bio-magnetic sensing, such as MEG.

Granger causality. Method to model the statistical dependence between time series by analyzing whether one time series can be predicted (in time) by the other.

Graph theory. Framework for the study of graphs that are composed of nodes with pair-wise connections. The analysis results in the characterization of complex systems through a small set of network parameters.

Ground electrode. An electrode that is connected to the earth. The path carries the short-circuited or faulty current away from the test participant. It could also provide recording reference level for EEG recording.

Half-life. The time it takes before a quantity reduces to half its value. In the current context, it primarily refers to the half-life of injected contrast agents or radioactive tracers.

Head position indicator (HPI) coil. Metal coil that is attached to the head of test participants to monitor head position in a MEG helmet. At least three HPIs are attached to detect head position change during MEG measurement.

Hemodynamic response function (HRF). The change in blood circulation over time in response to a change in neuronal activity.

Hemodynamics. Changes over time in blood circulation.

Hemoglobin. Protein that is present in blood and is responsible for the transport of oxygen and carbon dioxide. It is referred to as deoxygenated hemoglobin or deoxyhemoglobin when the oxygen is removed.

High-cut filter. A filter to remove frequency components higher than a threshold. Also known as a low-pass filter.

Hilbert transform. A mathematical operation that gives the orthogonal component of a real-valued signal. The original and orthogonal signals are combined as a complex-valued signal, the analytic signal.

Histology. An invasive methodology for studying brain anatomy at high spatial resolution. It typically involves cutting the brain in pieces, such as slices.

Hyperacuity. Property of a measurement system that is able to pick up a signal that has a higher frequency than the intuitive or theoretical limit of the system given its sample rate. In the context of human fMRI, it refers to the ability to measure a functional property that is organized at a finer scale than the voxel size.

Independent component analysis (ICA). Statistical method that tries to identify the sources that compose a signal by searching for components that are statistically independent.

Inflated brain. Visualization of the cortex in which the massive indentation of the cortical surface is neutralized through a process akin to inflating a balloon.

Inhibitory postsynaptic potential (IPSP). See postsynaptic potential (PSP).

Inion.   An anatomical landmark where the external occipital protuberance crosses with the midsagittal line.

Initial dip.   Transient decrease in local MRI signal due to a decrease in blood oxygenation. This is the first part of the hemodynamic response, but it is not typically observed in human imaging because it is local, transient, and small.

In-plane voxel size.   The size of voxels within brain slices, which is equal to the field of view divided by the number of voxels.

International 10–20 system.   A standardized EEG electrode placement that specifies 19 electrode locations on the scalp. The locations are determined based on anatomical landmarks of the head, namely, nasion, inion, left and right preauricular points.

Inter-trial phase coherence (ITPC).   An index of phase consistency across trials of an event-related paradigm study. It corresponds to the length of the mean phase vector. Zero corresponds to random (no phase coherence), and one corresponds to perfectly consistent phase. Also known as phase-locking factor (PLF).

Intracranial recordings.   Another name for electrocorticography.

Jennifer Aniston neuron.   One of the most famous neurons in the human brain. Very similar to, but not to be confused with, the Halle Berry neuron and the grandmother neuron.

Jitter.   Variation in inter-stimulus or inter-trial intervals.

***k*-space.**   The characterization of the MR signal as an amplitude and phase spectrum in a polar coordinate system with the frequency and the orientation of the components as dimensions.

k-Complex.   An EEG waveform which appears during Stage 2 non-REM sleep. The waveform is sharply bi-phasic.

Larmor frequency.   The frequency of the spin of a nucleus. It differs between different elements and depends linearly on magnetic field strength.

Lateral occipital complex (LOC).   Region in the human cortex, primarily in the lateral occipital cortex but extending into the temporal and parietal lobes. It is defined by a higher hemodynamic response to pictures containing objects than to pictures without objects (e.g., random patterns). It can be further divided into sub-regions, such as lateral occipital (LO) and posterior fusiform (PF or pFs).

Linear regression.   Statistical approach to capture the linear relationship between a dependent variable and one or more independent variables. We refer to simple linear regression if there is only one independent variable; otherwise, it is a multiple linear regression.

Linear system.   An input-output system of which the response (output) to a complex stimulus (input) can be estimated from the responses to the simple stimuli that make up the complex stimulus. This property is referred to as additivity.

Local field potentials (LFPs).   Slow-frequency (below 200 Hz) potential changes measured by an invasive electrode.

Low-cut filter.   A filter to remove frequency components lower than a threshold. Also known as a high-pass filter.

Magnetically shielded room.   A room that shields an environmental electromagnetic field for MEG and MCG. The room is covered by highly permeable materials and conductive materials that channel electromagnetic fields away from the inside of the room. An active noise cancellation system may also be added.

Magnetic resonance imaging (MRI). The use of nuclear magnetic resonance to obtain two- or three-dimensional images.

Magnetic resonance spectroscopy (MRS). The use of nuclear magnetic resonance in order to quantify the concentration of metabolites by measuring the spectrum of spin frequencies.

Magnetic resonance spectroscopy imaging (MRSI). MRS application that results in a three-dimensional image.

Magnetocardiogram (MCG). The magnetic signal due to cardiac activity.

Magnetocardiography (MCG). Method to record magnetic signal due to cardiovascular activity.

Magnetoencephalography (MEG). Method to record magnetic signal due to brain activity. A high sensitivity magnetometer, referred to as a Superconducting QUantum Interference Device (SQUID), is used to measure the weak signal.

Magnetometer. Sensor for magnetic field signals. In MEG literature, it often refers to a single coil magnetometer.

Matched Filter Theorem. Theorem in signal processing that states that it is best to filter the data with a filter kernel that has the same amplitude spectrum as the signal that one wants to measure among noise with a different amplitude spectrum.

Mean diffusion (MD). A measure of the amount of diffusion in a voxel, independent of the direction.

Mediated influence. An influence from one region to another that is caused by an indirect route through a third region.

Membrane potential. Electrical potential difference between the inside of a neuron and its outside medium.

Microstimulation. Method to influence neural activity locally by applying a small electrical current through an invasive electrode.

MNI templates. Anatomical templates created by the Montreal Neurological Institute.

Monopolar derivation. Method to derive voltage signal relative to a single reference level, e.g., EEG signal referenced to linked earlobes.

Montage. Method to rereference EEG signal to a biological baseline. Also see reference.

Morlet wavelet. A basis function of wavelet analysis. It is the product of a sinusoid and the Gaussian function.

Morphometry. A quantitative analysis of the form/shape of an entity, in the present context of the brain anatomy (brain morphometry).

Motion correction. Step in the preprocessing of fMRI images. It compensates for changes in the position of the head in images that were acquired at different points in time.

Motion-correction parameters. The transformation parameters that describe how each image in an fMRI dataset has to be transformed in order to correct for motion.

Multiband imaging. See multi-echo imaging.

Multi-channel phased-array coils. Multiple surface coils that form an array, ideally surrounding a volume in such a way that they provide high sensitivity that is relatively homogeneous in the volume.

Multi-echo imaging. Imaging methods that allow the acquisition of multiple slices after one radio frequency (RF) pulse, resulting in a marked acceleration of imaging. This allows for shorter repetition times and higher temporal sampling rates.

Multi-modal imaging. The combination of information from different imaging modalities in one study or analysis.

Multiple comparisons problem. The analysis of neuroimaging data typically includes a high number of statistical comparisons. In such a case it is required to correct for the number of independent comparisons that are done.

Multi-voxel pattern analysis (MVPA). Statistical analysis of fMRI data that takes as input the variation of signal/response across voxels, so-called multi-voxel patterns. Given that each voxel is a variable, it is a special case of more general multivariate pattern analysis.

Nasion. An anatomical landmark where the frontal nasal bone suture crosses the midsagittal line. It corresponds to the lowest point of the ridge of the nose.

Neurovascular coupling. Effect of neural activity on blood circulation.

NIfTI. Standard format for MRI images developed by the Neuroimaging Informatics Technology Initiative. Its conception was motivated by the desire to increase the ease of exchanging files between different software packages. The major software packages for MRI data analysis can handle NIfTI images for input and output.

Node degree. A graph theoretical parameter that reflects the number of nodes to which a node is connected.

Normalization. This concept can refer to two procedures. First, the alignment of data of individual participants with a common spatial reference space. Second, the normalization of signal values by a reference value, such as the signal value measured in a baseline condition.

Notch filter. See band-cut filter.

Nuclear magnetic resonance. The phenomenon that nuclei with a magnetic moment absorb energy if the oscillation frequency of a magnetic field matches the Larmor frequency of the nuclei.

Nuisance regressors. Independent variables that we might expect to predict part of the variation in the fMRI signal, but that are not of primary interest to the researcher.

Object-selective cortex. Region in the human cortex, primarily in the occipital but extending into the temporal and parietal lobes. It is defined by a higher hemodynamic response to pictures containing objects than to pictures with objects (e.g., random patterns).

Olfactory evoked potential (OEP). An evoked potential in response to an olfactory stimulus, such as a puff of vanillin solvent in the nasal cavity.

One-back counterbalancing. Ordering of trials so that each condition is equally likely to follow each other condition. A purely random ordering of trials is not guaranteed to satisfy one-back counterbalancing, which is why this constraint is often introduced. One-back counterbalancing is a special case of more general N-back counterbalancing.

One-back task. Behavioral task in which participants have to compare a current trial with the preceding trial. This task is often used in cognitive neuroimaging. The one-back task is a specific case of N-back tasks, in which participants have to compare a current trial T with trial $T - N$.

Optical imaging.   Imaging approach in which measurements are made by light sensors, ranging from arrays of individual detectors to microscopes. Functional near-infrared spectroscopy is an example of an optical imaging method that is noninvasive and often used in human research. There are also invasive optical imaging methods that are used only in animals and that provide columnar resolution or even single-neuron resolution.

Parametric design.   Experimental design in which a particular parameter or dimension is manipulated quantitatively in more than two steps.

Partial correlation.   The correlation that remains between two variables after taking into account the correlations with other variables.

Partial phase locking (PPL).   A transient phase locking among oscillatory components.

Path length.   A graph theoretical parameter that reflects the number of nodes that have to be passed to move from one node to another.

Percent signal change (PSC).   Signal change in comparison with a baseline condition, expressed as a percentage.

Phase.   A point in a cycle of oscillation, expressed as an angle.

Phase coherence.   Coherence of phase between two signals.

Phase-encoding (PE) gradient.   A gradient that is applied after an RF pulse and before the signal is acquired, and that allows the decoding of spatial position through the differences in phase induced in nuclei at different positions along the gradient.

Phase locking.   Oscillations with a constant phase lag. The phase locking with lag = 0 is synchrony.

Phase-locking factor (PLF).   See Inter-trial phase coherence (ITPC).

Phase-locking index (PLI).   An index of phase coherence. Zero corresponds to random and one corresponds to perfect phase locking. Also known as the synchrony index (SI) and the single trial phase-locking value (S-PLV).

Phrenology.   An outdated pseudo-science that claimed that outer features of the skull would be related to mental functions.

Planar gradiometer.   MEG sensor with two pick-up coils. The coils turn in a figure-eight shape in the same plane.

Point-spread function (PSF).   A function that characterizes the broader spread of signal when a very small point in the brain is activated. The width of this function is a useful index for spatial resolution. The lower this width, the higher the resolution.

Positron emission tomography (PET).   Method to measure local blood volume that is based on sensitivity for the emission of positrons from an injected radioactive tracer.

Postsynaptic potential (PSP).   A membrane potential that is generated at the postsynaptic terminal of a chemical synapse. The potential increases when positive ions (e.g., Na+) flow into the cell via an excitatory synapse, i.e., excitatory postsynaptic potential (EPSP). Conversely, the potential decreases as negative ions (e.g., Cl-) flow into the cell via an inhibitory synapse, i.e., inhibitory postsynaptic potential (IPSP).

Power spectral density (PSD).   A standardized power spectrum.

Power spectrum.   Frequency spectrum in power of amplitude.

Preauricular point.   An anatomical landmark where the posterior root of the zygomatic arch (cheek bone) lies immediately in front of the upper end of the tragus.

Principal component analysis (PCA).   Statistical method that tries to identify a small number of components that explain most of the variance in the data. The resulting data reduction is most successful if the variables in the data show a high degree of covariance.

Psychophysiological interaction (PPI).   Dependence of functional connectivity on an experimental manipulation such as task or presented stimuli.

Pulse sequence.   The temporal sequence of radio frequency (RF) pulses and timing and duration of gradients.

Radial diffusivity (RD).   The amount of diffusion along the two directions orthogonal to the direction of maximal diffusion.

Radio frequency (RF) pulse.   A magnetic field that is applied for a very short time (pulse) and that oscillates in a frequency that is in the same part of the frequency spectrum as radio waves.

Random-effects analysis.   A statistical analysis that takes into account that data are structured according to a hierarchy of factors. In the present context, it mainly refers to analyses that isolate the hierarchical level of subjects, which is needed to test the variance of effects across subjects and hence for any conclusions that generalize from the measured subject sample to the population. Random-effects analyses stand in contrast with fixed-effect analyses that typically do not allow generalizations toward the population.

Rapid counterbalanced event-related design.   An event-related experimental design with a relatively short interval between successive trials and a counterbalancing of condition order.

Rapid eye movement sleep (REM sleep).   A sleep stage characterized by rapid eye movements and the EEG pattern similar to the awake stage. Also known as paradoxical sleep.

Reference.   See montage.

Reference electrode.   An electrode that provides a reference voltage signal.

Reference image.   The image that is used as the reference image that would remain unchanged. Other images are transformed to align them with the reference image.

Region of interest (ROI).   A brain region that is of particular interest. It is delineated through anatomical and/or functional criteria.

Region-of-interest (ROI) analysis.   Analysis that is performed only on a subset of the data, such as a local cluster of voxels or electrodes.

Regressors of interest.   The independent variables that specify the occurrence of experimental conditions in which a researcher is interested.

Repetition time (TR).   The time interval between successive excitations of the same spatial position.

Repetitive transcranial magnetic stimulation (rTMS).   A form of transcranial magnetic stimulation in which the induced magnetic field is applied repeatedly at a particular frequency, as such forming a train of pulses.

Representational similarity analysis (RSA).   Comparison of datasets from different sources by studying the similarity structure in the datasets.

Reslicing.   The creation of a new, discrete image after a continuous transformation was applied to an original (also discrete) image. A discrete image is sampled at discrete points (pixels or voxels).

Resting potential. The membrane potential when an neuron is at rest and receives no synaptic input.

Resting-state fMRI (RS fMRI). Functional MRI scan during which participants are asked to rest and no stimuli or task manipulations are presented. RS fMRI scans are used for studying functional connectivity.

Retinotopy. The systematic mapping of the input of the receptors in the retina onto an array of neurons, so that nearby neurons receive input from nearby receptors in the retina.

Reverse inference. Statistical inference that activation in a brain region in a new study is related to a particular cognitive process because the region is activated in the new study and other studies in the literature found that the region is activated when this cognitive process is involved.

Rigid transformation. A transformation of an image that is a combination of rotations and translations.

Sampling frequency. The number of samples per second by which a signal is measured.

Scalogram. A time-frequency representation of a wavelet-transformed signal.

Scrubbing. Data-processing method that involves the demarcation and exclusion from further analysis of data points with unwanted characteristics, such as subject motion.

Second-level (random-effects) (group) analysis. A statistical approach that tests the size of an effect against the variability across participants. The input to this analysis is the contrast maps that have been computed per participant; this is the first-level analysis.

Seed region. A region of interest, the data of which are taken as the reference to compare with the other voxels/regions in a dataset.

Sensitivity. In general, "sensitivity" refers to the ability to detect a signal when it is present. For example, it could be specified as the proportion of datasets in which a significant effect is found when the effect was indeed present. Sensitivity also has a specific meaning in signal detection theory where it refers to the overall ability to differentiate between situations in which a signal is present versus situations in which it is not present.

Shared influence. This concept refers to a scenario in which two brain regions receive (share) input from a third region.

Short time Fourier transform (STFT). A method to obtain a time-frequency representation from a time-domain signal. The discrete Fourier transform is applied to a short segment of the time signal.

Signal contrast. The difference in signal between different tissues.

Signal-to-noise ratio (SNR). Index to express the proportion of a measurement that is related to factors of interest ("signal") relative to factors of no interest ("noise").

Single trial phase-locking value (S-PLV). See phase-locking index (PLI).

Single-voxel spectroscopy (SVS). A magnetic resonance spectroscopy method that measures one volume or voxel of interest.

Sleep spindle. An EEG waveform which is characteristic in EEG signal during Stage 2 non-REM sleep. The waveform is a burst of activity ("spindle") in 11–15 Hz.

Slice-selection gradient. The gradient that determines which brain slice is being excited by the radio frequency (RF) pulse that is being applied at the same time as the gradient.

Slice timing. Step in the preprocessing of functional MRI images. It compensates for the difference in acquisition time between slices.

Slow-wave sleep (SWS). A sleep stage characterized by slow EEG activity, e.g., delta band activity. Also referred to as deep sleep.

Smoothing. Procedure that increases the similarity between nearby data points, either in time (temporal smoothing) or in space (spatial smoothing).

Somatosensory evoked potential (SEP). An evoked potential in response to a somatosensory stimulus, such as a vibration to a fingertip.

Source localization. The estimation of the spatial location from which individual components of a signal originate.

Spatial resolution. The smallest unit of space that can be resolved. It will determine which scale of organization can be picked up.

Specific absorption rate (SAR). A safety index that indicates how much energy a tissue can absorb without undergoing a threshold increase in temperature.

Spectrogram. A matrix that shows a variable, often the amplitude or phase of a signal, as a function of frequency and of time.

Spin-echo echo-planar imaging (SE-EPI) sequence. An MRI pulse sequence that involves the successive acquisition of different planes/slices and that includes the creation of a spin echo by using a refocusing radio frequency (RF) pulse.

Stage 2 sleep. A sleep stage that is characterized by transient EEG activities, such as sleep spindles and K-complex. It is a shallow sleep stage (in contrast to deep sleep).

Statistical parametric mapping (SPM). Statistical approach to the analysis of imaging data. The acronym is also used to refer to the software package developed by the groups that proposed this statistical approach.

Steady-state evoked potential (ssEP). M/EEG response not to a single but to oscillatory stimulation. Modality of the stimulation is added to the abbreviation, e.g., ssVEP for visual oscillatory stimulation.

Stereo EEG (sEEG). EEG recorded from electrodes inserted into the brain tissue in vivo.

Structural equation modeling (SEM) . General statistical method to model correlational data that can be modeled as a complex graph model, potentially also including latent variables.

Structural magnetic resonance imaging. The use of magnetic resonance imaging to image the anatomy or structure of the brain.

Subtraction method. Comparison of two experimental conditions by subtracting the results of one condition from the other. These results can take various forms, such as reaction time measurements or fMRI signal.

Superconducting QUantum Interference Device (SQUID). A high-sensitivity magnetometer for very weak magnetic field signals, such as MEG. It consists of super conductive coils and Josephson junctions.

Surface-based morphometry. Morphometric analysis in which quantitative indices are computed in surface space.

Surface-based normalization. Normalization of an individual cortical surface to a surface template.

Surface extraction. Extraction of the cortical surface. Each brain has two surfaces, one per hemisphere. A surface is made out of vertices.

Surface flattening.   Creating a two-dimensional sheet from the original three-dimensional warping of the cortical surface.

Surface rendering.   Visualization of the extracted cortical surface.

Synchrony index (SI).   See phase-locking index (PLI).

T1 recovery.   The recovery of the magnetization along the longitudinal orientation, which reflects the realignment of the spins with the direction of the static magnetic field.

T2 decay.   The loss of transverse magnetization in the direction of the oscillating field applied by the radio frequency (RF) pulse due to the loss in phase coherence related to spin-spin interactions.

T2* decay.   The total dephasing as a consequence of spin-spin interactions, field inhomogeneity, and tissue susceptibility. T2* decay is always faster (more dephasing) than T2 decay.

Talairach atlas.   A historical and famous anatomical atlas of the human brain based on one individual.

Temporal resolution.   The smallest unit of time that can be differentiated by a method.

tesla (T) .   The standard unit of magnetic field strength.

Theta band.   A frequency band of M/EEG activity; 4–8 Hz.

Tissue segmentation.   Segmentation of the brain into its different tissue types, often including white matter, gray matter, and cerebrospinal fluid.

Tissue susceptibility.   The effect of tissue on the Larmor frequency of a nucleus. It contributes to T2* decay.

Tractography.   The delineation of white matter tracts, typically based on diffusion tensor imaging (DTI) scans.

Transcranial current stimulation (TCS).   An uninvasive technique for modulating neural activity that involves two electrodes and a battery. Current flows from one electrode (anode) to the other (cathode). This current influences cortical excitability. It can involve a direct current (transcranial direct current stimulation, or TDCS), an alternating current (transcranial alternating current stimulation, or TACS), or a current that changes over time in a more random manner (transcranial random noise stimulation, or TRNS).

Transcranial direct current stimulation (TDCS).   A form of transcranial current stimulation that involves an uninvasive technique for modulating neural activity that involves two electrodes and a battery. Current flows from one electrode (anode) to the other (cathode). This current influences cortical excitability.

Transcranial magnetic stimulation (TMS).   Modulation of neural activity by inducing current in neural tissue through electromagnetic induction. Depending on where TMS is applied, it can degrade the normal function (interference) or enhance it (stimulation).

Transformation matrix.   Matrix with numbers that describe how an image has to be transformed (translated, rotated, resized).

Univariate analysis.   An analysis that is focused on single variables. The standard approach to fMRI data analysis is sometimes referred to as a univariate or voxel-wise analysis because its computations (e.g., estimation of a multiple regression model) are initially performed for each individual voxel separately.

Up-sampling.   A signal resampling method to increase the number of samples. Original samples are interpolated and resampled in a higher sampling frequency.

Vertex.   A vertex (plural: vertices) is the element from which a cortical surface is built, similar to how a brain slice is composed of voxels. A technical difference is that a vertex is a point (vertices are connected with lines), while a voxel is a volumetric unit.

Visual area 1 (V1).   The area where the visual signals coming from the retina first enter cortex, also referred to as primary visual cortex. V1 is regularly featured in examples in the book because the properties of this area are well known, and as such this area is a useful target in studies that validate new methods.

Visual evoked potential (VEP).   An evoked potential in response to a visual stimulus.

Volume-based normalization.   Normalization using the three-dimensional space in which brains exist, with the dimensions left/right, anterior/posterior, and superior/inferior.

Volume conduction.   Electric conduction between an electrode and a generator.

Voxel.   The volume element from which three-dimensional MRI images are composed, in the same way as pixel means "picture elements."

Voxel-based lesion-symptom mapping.   A statistical analysis that investigates the relationship between the presence of a lesion in voxels and the severity of behavioral symptoms.

Voxel-based morphometry (VBM).   Morphometric analysis in which quantitative indices are computed in voxel space.

Water suppression.   Suppression of the signal of water in magnetic resonance spectroscopy to avoid that it would dominate the obtained frequency spectrum.

Wavelet transform.   A mathematical operation to transform a signal to a linear combination of wavelet functions.

References

Aguirre, G. K., Zarahn, E., & D'Esposito, M. (1998). The variability of human, BOLD hemodynamic responses. *Neuroimage*, **8**, 360–369.

Albert, M. S., Dekosky, S. T., Dickson, D., et al. (2011). The diagnosis of mild cognitive impairment due to Alzheimer's disease: recommendations from the National Institute on Aging-Alzheimer's Association workgroups on diagnostic guidelines for Alzheimer's disease. *Alzheimers & Dementia*, **7**, 270–279.

Alexander, A. L., Lee, J. E., Lazar, M. & Field, A. S. (2007). Diffusion tensor imaging of the brain. *Neurotherapeutics*, **4**, 316–329.

American Electroencephalographic Society. (1994). Guideline thirteen: guidelines for standard electrode position nomenclature. *Journal of Clinical Neurophysiology*, **11**, 111–113.

Armstrong, K. M. & Moore, T. (2007). Rapid enhancement of visual cortical response discriminability by microstimulation of the frontal eye field. *Proceedings of the National Academy of Sciences of the United States of America*, **104**, 9499–9504.

Aserinsky, E. & Kleitman, N. (1953). Regularly occurring periods of eye motility, and concomitant phenomena, during sleep. *Science*, **118**, 273–274.

Attwell, D. & Iadecola, C. (2002). The neural basis of functional brain imaging signals. *Trends in Neurosciences*, **25**, 621–625.

Attwell, D. & Laughlin, S. B. (2001). An energy budget for signaling in the grey matter of the brain. *Journal of Cerebral Blood Flow and Metabolism*, **21**, 1133–1145.

Bagozzi, R. P., Verbeke, W. J. M. I., Dietvorst, R. C., Belschak, F. D., Van Den Berg, W. E. & Rietdijk, W. J. R. (2013). Theory of mind and empathic explanations of Machiavellianism: a neuroscience perspective. *Journal of Management*, **39**, 1760–1798.

Bandettini, P. A. & Cox, R. W. (2000). Event-related fMRI contrast when using constant interstimulus interval: theory and experiment. *Magnetic Resonance in Medicine*, **43**, 540–548.

Barnea-Goraly, N., Kwon, H., Menon, V., Eliez, S., Lotspeich, L. & Reiss, A. L. (2004). White matter structure in autism: preliminary evidence from diffusion tensor imaging. *Biological Psychiatry*, **55**, 323–326.

Bartels, A. & Zeki, S. (2000). The neural basis of romantic love. *Neuroreport*, **11**, 3829–3834.

Başar, E. (2012). A review of alpha activity in integrative brain function: fundamental physiology, sensory coding, cognition and pathology. *International Journal of Psychophysiology*, **86**, 1–24.

Bates, E., Wilson, S. M., Saygin, A. P., et al. (2003). Voxel-based lesion-symptom mapping. *Nature Neuroscience*, **6**, 448–450.

Beckmann, C. F., Deluca, M., Devlin, J. T. & Smith, S. M. (2005). Investigations into resting-state connectivity using independent component analysis. *Philosophical Transactions of the Royal Society of London. Series B Biological Sciences*, **360**, 1001–1013.

Bennett, C. M., Miller, M. B. & Wolford, G. L. (2009). Neural correlates of interspecies perspective taking in the post-mortem Atlantic Salmon: an argument for multiple comparisons correction. *Neuroimage*, **47**, S125.

Bennett, C. M., Wolford, G. L. & Miller, M. B. (2009). The principled control of false positives in neuroimaging. *Social Cognitive and Affective Neuroscience*, **4**, 417–422.

Berger, H. (1929). Über das Elektrenkephalogramm des Menschen [On the human electroencephalogram]. *Archiv für Psychiatrie und Nervenkrankheiten*, **87**, 527–570.

Bernstein, M. A., King, K. F. & Zhou, X. J. (2004). *Handbook of MRI Pulse Sequences*. New York: Elsevier Academic Press.

Bertholdo, D., Watcharakorn, A. & Castillo, M. (2013). Brain proton magnetic resonance spectroscopy: introduction and overview. *Neuroimaging Clinics of North America*, **23**, 359–380.

Bickart, K. C., Wright, C. I., Dautoff, R. J., Dickerson, B. C. & Barrett, L. F. (2011). Amygdala volume and social network size in humans. *Nature Neuroscience*, **14**, 1217.

Bloch, F., Hansen, W. W. & Packard, M. (1946). Nuclear induction. *Physical Review*, **69**, 127.

Boets, B., Op de Beeck, H. P., Vandermosten, M., et al. (2013). Intact but less accessible phonetic representations in adults with dyslexia. *Science*, **342**, 1251–1254.

Borogovac, A. & Asllani, I. (2012). Arterial spin labeling (ASL) fMRI: advantages, theoretical constrains, and experimental challenges in neurosciences. *International Journal of Biomedical Imaging*, **2012**, Article ID 818456.

Box, G. E., Jenkins, G. M., Reinsel, G. C. & Ljung, G. M. (2015). *Time Series Analysis: Forecasting and Control*. New York: John Wiley & Sons.

Boynton, G. M., Engel, S. A., Glover, G. H. & Heeger, D. J. (1996). Linear systems analysis of functional magnetic resonance imaging in human V1. *Journal of Neuroscience*, **16**, 4207–4221.

Bracci, S. & Op de Beeck, H. (2016). Dissociations and associations between shape and category representations in the two visual pathways. *Journal of Neuroscience*, **36**, 432–444.

Bracci, S., Ritchie, J. B. & Op de Beeck, H. (2017). On the partnership between neural representations of object categories and visual features in the ventral visual pathway. *Neuropsychologia*, **105**, 153–164.

Brillinger, D. R. (2001). *Time Series: Data Analysis and Theory*. Philadelphia, PA: SIAM.

Brunelin, J., Poulet, E., Boeuve, C., Zeroug-Vial, H., D'Amato, T. & Saoud, M. (2007). Efficacy of repetitive transcranial magnetic stimulation (rTMS) in major depression: a review. [In French.] *L'Encéphale*, **33**, 126–134.

Buckner, R. L. (1998). Event-related fMRI and the hemodynamic response. *Human Brain Mapping*, **6**, 373–377.

Buckner, R. L., Krienen, F. M. & Yeo, B. T. (2013). Opportunities and limitations of intrinsic functional connectivity MRI. *Nature Neuroscience*, **16**, 832–837.

Bullmore, E. & Sporns, O. (2009). Complex brain networks: graph theoretical analysis of structural and functional systems. *Nature Reviews Neuroscience*, **10**, 186–198.

Bulthe, J., De Smedt, B. & Op de Beeck, H. P. (2014). Format-dependent representations of symbolic and non-symbolic numbers in the human cortex as revealed by multi-voxel pattern analyses. *Neuroimage*, **87**, 311–322.

Bulthe, J., Van den Hurk, J., Daniels, N., De Smedt, B. & Op de Beeck, H. P. (2014). A validation of a multi-spatial scale method for multivariate pattern analysis. In *Pattern Recognition in Neuroimaging. International Workshop on Pattern Recognition in Neuroimaging*. Tubingen, Germany: IEEE.

Cacioppo, J. T., Tassinary, L. G. & Bertson, G. (2007). Psychophysiological science: interdisciplinary approaches to classic questions about the mind. In J. T. Cacioppo, L. G. Tassinary & G. Bertson (Eds.), *Handbook of Psychophysiology*. Cambridge: Cambridge University Press.

Cappelletti, M., Gessaroli, E., Hithersay, R., et al. (2013). Transfer of cognitive training across magnitude dimensions achieved with concurrent brain stimulation of the parietal lobe. *Journal of Neuroscience*, **33**, 14899–14907.

Carp, J. (2012). On the plurality of (methodological) worlds: estimating the analytic flexibility of FMRI experiments. *Frontiers in Neuroscience*, **6**, 149.

Carskadon, M. A. & Dement, W. C. (2011). Monitoring and staging human sleep. In M. H. Kryger, T. Roth & W. C. Dement (Eds.), *Principles and practice of sleep medicine*, 5th edn. (pp 16–26). St. Louis: Elsevier Saunders.

Catania, K. C. (2016). Leaping eels electrify threats, supporting Humboldt's account of a battle with horses. *Proceedings of the National Academy of Sciences of the United States of America*, **113**, 6979–6984.

Caton, R. (1875). Electrical currents of the brain. *The Journal of Nervous and Mental Disease*, **2**, 610.

Chalmers, D. J. (1996). *The Conscious Mind: In Search of a Fundamental Theory*. Oxford: Oxford University Press.

Champollion, J. F. (2009). *The Code-Breaker's Secret Diaries: Rediscovering Ancient Egypt*, London: Gibson Square Books. The original French manuscript was written around 1828. The translation to English was done by M. Rynja in 2009.

Churchland, P. (2007). *Neurophilosophy at Work*. Cambridge: Cambridge University Press.

Churchland, P. S. & Sejnowski, T. J. (1988). Perspectives on cognitive neuroscience. *Science*, **242**, 741–745.

Cichy, R. M., Pantazis, D. & Oliva, A. (2014). Resolving human object recognition in space and time. *Nature Neuroscience*, **17**, 455–462.

Clark, V. P. & Hillyard, S. A. (1996). Spatial selective attention affects early extrastriate but not striate components of the visual evoked potential. *Journal of Cognitive Neuroscience*, **8**, 387–402.

Cohen, D. (1968). Magnetoencephalography: evidence of magnetic fields produced by alpha rhythm currents. *Science*, **161**, 784–786.

(2004). Boston and the history of biomagnetism. *Neurology and Clinical Neurophysiology*, **114**, 1933–1266.

Cohen Kadosh, R., Soskic, S., Iuculano, T., Kanai, R. & Walsh, V. (2010). Modulating neuronal activity produces specific and long-lasting changes in numerical competence. *Current Biology*, **20**, 2016–2020.

Conway, B., Halliday, D., Farmer, S., et al. (1995). Synchronization between motor cortex and spinal motoneuronal pool during the performance of a maintained motor task in man. *The Journal of Physiology*, **489**, 917–924.

Cooley, J. W. & Tukey, J. W. (1965). An algorithm for the machine calculation of complex Fourier series. *Mathematics of Computation*, **19**, 297–301.

Cordes, D., Haughton, V. M., Arfanakis, K., et al. (2001). Frequencies contributing to functional connectivity in the cerebral cortex in "resting-state" data. *American Journal of Neuroradiology*, **22**, 1326–1333.

Corkin, S. (2002). What's new with the amnesic patient H.M.? *Nature Reviews Neuroscience*, **3**, 153–160.

Coutanche, M. N., Solomon, S. H. & Thompson-Schill, S. L. (2016). A meta-analysis of fMRI decoding: quantifying influences on human visual population codes. *Neuropsychologia*, **82**, 134–141.

Cox, D. D. & Savoy, R. L. (2003). Functional magnetic resonance imaging (fMRI) "brain reading": detecting and classifying distributed patterns of fMRI activity in human visual cortex. *Neuroimage*, **19**, 261–270.

Cox, R. W., Chen, G., Glen, D. R., Reynolds, R. C. & Taylor, P. A. (2017). fMRI clustering in AFNI: false-positive rates redux. *Brain Connectivity*, **7**, 152–171.

Craver, C. F. (2007). *Explaining the Brain: Mechanisms and the Mosaic Unity of Neuroscience*. New York: Oxford University Press.

Dale, A. M. & Buckner, R. L. (1997). Selective averaging of rapidly presented individual trials using fMRI. *Human Brain Mapping*, **5**, 329–340.

Damoiseaux, J. S. & Greicius, M. D. (2009). Greater than the sum of its parts: a review of studies combining structural connectivity and resting-state functional connectivity. *Brain Structure and Function*, **213**, 525–533.

de-Wit, L., Alexander, D., Ekroll, V. & Wagemans, J. (2016). Is neuroimaging measuring information in the brain? *Psychonomic Bulletin & Review*, **23**, 1415–1428.

Deuschl, G., Schade-Brittinger, C., Krack, P., et al. & German Parkinson Study Group, Neurostimulation Section. (2006). A randomized trial of deep-brain stimulation for Parkinson's disease. *New England Journal of Medicine*, **355**, 896–908.

Deyoung, C. G., Hirsh, J. B., Shane, M. S., Papademetris, X., Rajeevan, N. & Gray, J. R. (2010). Testing predictions from personality neuroscience. Brain structure and the big five. *Psychological Science*, **21**, 820–828.

Di Martino, A., Yan, C. G., Li, Q., et al. (2014). The autism brain imaging data exchange: towards a large-scale evaluation of the intrinsic brain architecture in autism. *Molecular Psychiatry*, **19**, 659–667.

Diener, E. (2010). Neuroimaging: voodoo, new phrenology, or scientific breakthrough? Introduction to special section on fMRI. *Perspectives on Psychological Science*, **5**, 714–715.

Dobbs, D. (2005). Fact or phrenology? *Scientific American Mind*, **16**, 24–31.

Donders, F. C. (1969). On speed of mental processes. *Acta Psychologica*, **30**, 412–431.

Dössel, O., David, B., Fuchs, M., Krüger, J., Kullmann, W. & Ludeke, K. (1991). A modular approach to multichannel magnetometry. *Clinical Physics and Physiological Measurement*, **12**, 75.

Dubois, J., De Berker, A. O. & Tsao, D. Y. (2015). Single-unit recordings in the macaque face patch system reveal limitations of fMRI MVPA. *Journal of Neuroscience*, **35**, 2791–2802.

Dumoulin, S. O. & Wandell, B. A. (2008). Population receptive field estimates in human visual cortex. *Neuroimage*, **39**, 647–660.

Eklund, A., Nichols, T. E. & Knutsson, H. (2016). Cluster failure: why fMRI inferences for spatial extent have inflated false-positive rates. *Proceedings of the National Academy of Sciences of the United States of America*, **113**, 7900–7905.

Ellison-Wright, I. & Bullmore, E. (2009). Meta-analysis of diffusion tensor imaging studies in schizophrenia. *Schizophrenia Research*, **108**, 3–10.

Farah, M. J. (2014). Brain images, babies, and bathwater: critiquing critiques of functional neuroimaging. *Hastings Center Report,* Spec No, S19–S30.

Formisano, E., De Martino, F., Bonte, M. & Goebel, R. (2008). "Who" is saying "what"? Brain-based decoding of human voice and speech. *Science*, **322**, 970–973.

Fornito, A., Zalesky, A. & Bullmore, E. T. (2016). *Fundamentals of Brain Network Analysis*. Amsterdam: Elsevier/Academic Press.

Fotopoulou, A. (2012). Towards psychodynamic neuroscience. In A. Fotopoulou, D. Pfaff & M. A. Conway (Eds.), *From the Couch to the Lab: Trends in Psychodynamic Neuroscience*. Oxford: Oxford University Press.

Fox, M. D., Snyder, A. Z., Vincent, J. L., Corbetta, M., Van Essen, D. C. & Raichle, M. E. (2005). The human brain is intrinsically organized into dynamic, anticorrelated functional networks. *Proceedings of the National Academy of Sciences of the United States of America*, **102**, 9673–9678.

Fox, P. T., Miezin, F. M., Allman, J. M., Van Essen, D. C. & Raichle, M. E. (1987). Retinotopic organization of human visual cortex mapped with positron-emission tomography. *Journal of Neuroscience*, **7**, 913–922.

Fraga González, G., Van der Molen, M. J. W., Žarić, G., et al. (2016). Graph analysis of EEG resting state functional networks in dyslexic readers. *Clinical Neurophysiology*, **127**, 3165–3175.

Frangou, S., Chitins, X. & Williams, S. C. (2004). Mapping IQ and gray matter density in healthy young people. *Neuroimage*, **23**, 800–805.

Freeman, J., Brouwer, G. J., Heeger, D. J. & Merriam, E. P. (2011). Orientation decoding depends on maps, not columns. *Journal of Neuroscience*, **31**, 4792–4804.

Fries, P. (2009). Neuronal gamma-band synchronization as a fundamental process in cortical computation. *Annual Review of Neuroscience*, **32**, 209–224.

Fries, P., Reynolds, J. H., Rorie, A. E. & Desimone, R. (2001). Modulation of oscillatory neuronal synchronization by selective visual attention. *Science*, **291**, 1560–1563.

Friston, K., Stephan, K. M., Heather, J., et al. (1996). A multivariate analysis of evoked responses in EEG and MEG data. *Neuroimage*, **3**, 167–174.

Friston, K. J., Buechel, C., Fink, G. R., Morris, J., Rolls, E. & Dolan, R. J. (1997). Psychophysiological and modulatory interactions in neuroimaging. *Neuroimage*, **6**, 218–229.

Friston, K. J., Holmes, A. P., Poline, J. B., et al. (1995). Analysis of fMRI time-series revisited. *Neuroimage*, **2**, 45–53.

Friston, K. J., Holmes, A., Worsley, K. J., Poline, J. P., Frith, C. D. & Frackowiak, R. S. (1994). Statistical parametric maps in functional imaging: a general linear approach. *Human Brain Mapping*, **2**, 189–210.

Friston, K. J., Price, C. J., Fletcher, P., Moore, C., Frackowiak, R. S. J. & Dolan, R. J. (1996). The trouble with cognitive subtraction. *Neuroimage*, **4**, 97–104.

Friston, K. J., Rotshtein, P., Geng, J. J., Sterzer, P. & Henson, R. N. (2006). A critique of functional localisers. *Neuroimage*, **30**, 1077–1087.

Gabor, D. (1946). Theory of communication. Part 1: the analysis of information. *Journal of the Institution of Electrical Engineers – Part III: Radio and Communication Engineering*, **93**, 429–441.

Gandiga, P. C., Hummel, F. C. & Cohen, L. G. (2006). Transcranial DC stimulation (tDCS): A tool for double-blind sham-controlled clinical studies in brain stimulation. *Clinical Neurophysiology*, **117**, 845–850.

Gao, R. X. & Yan, R. (2010). *Wavelets: Theory and Applications for Manufacturing.* Berlin: Springer Science & Business Media.

Garrity, A. G., Pearlson, G. D., McKiernan, K., Lloyd, D., Kiehl, K. A. & Calhoun, V. D. (2007). Aberrant "default mode" functional connectivity in schizophrenia. *The American Journal of Psychiatry*, **164**, 450–457.

Gazzaniga, M. S. (1995). *The Cognitive Neurosciences.* Cambridge, MA: MIT Press.

Genovese, C. R., Lazar, N. A. & Nichols, T. (2002). Thresholding of statistical maps in functional neuroimaging using the false discovery rate. *Neuroimage*, **15**, 870–878.

Gervain, J., Mehler, J., Werker, J. F., et al. (2011). Near-infrared spectroscopy: a report from the McDonnell infant methodology consortium. *Developmental Cognitive Neuroscience* **1**, 22–46.

Gillebert, C. R. & Mantini, D. (2013). Functional connectivity in the normal and injured brain. *Neuroscientist*, **19**, 509–522.

Gitelman, D. R., Penny, W. D., Ashburner, J. & Friston, K. J. (2003). Modeling regional and psychophysiologic interactions in fMRI: the importance of hemodynamic deconvolution. *Neuroimage*, **19**, 200–207.

Glasser, M. F., Coalson, T. S., Robinson, E. C., et al. (2016). A multi-modal parcellation of human cerebral cortex. *Nature*, **536**, 171–178.

Gloor, P. (1969). Hans Berger on electroencephalography. *American Journal of EEG Technology*, **9**, 1–8.

Goesaert, E. & Op de Beeck, H. P. (2010). Continuous mapping of the cortical object vision pathway using traveling waves in object space. *Neuroimage*, **49**, 3248–3256.

Govindaraju, V., Young, K. & Maudsley, A. A. (2000). Proton NMR chemical shifts and coupling constants for brain metabolites. *NMR in Biomedicine*, **13**, 129–153.

Granger, C. W. (1969). Investigating causal relations by econometric models and cross-spectral methods. *Econometrica: Journal of the Econometric Society*, **37**, 424–438.

Greenberg, B. D., Malone, D. A., Friehs, G. M., et al. (2006). Three-year outcomes in deep brain stimulation for highly resistant obsessive-compulsive disorder. *Neuropsychopharmacology*, **31**, 2384–2393.

Greicius, M. D., Flores, B. H., Menon, V., ET AL. (2007). Resting-state functional connectivity in major depression: abnormally increased contributions from subgenual cingulate cortex and thalamus. *Biological Psychiatry*, **62**, 429–437.

Greve, D. N. (2011). An absolute beginner's guide to surface- and voxel-based morphometric analysis. *Proceedings of the International Society of Magnetic Resonance in Medicine*, **19**.

Grill-Spector, K. & Malach, R. (2001). fMR-adaptation: a tool for studying the functional properties of human cortical neurons. *Acta Psychologica*, **107**, 293–321.

Grinvald, A. & Hildesheim, R. (2004). VSDI: a new era in functional imaging of cortical dynamics. *Nature Reviews Neuroscience*, **5**, 874–885.

Groppa, S., Oliviero, A., Eisen, A., et al. (2012). A practical guide to diagnostic transcranial magnetic stimulation: report of an IFCN committee. *Clinical Neurophysiology*, **123**, 858–882.

Gross, J., Baillet, S., Barnes, G. R., et al. (2013). Good practice for conducting and reporting MEG research. *Neuroimage*, **65**, 349–363.

Grützner, C., Wibral, M., Sun, L., et al. (2013). Deficits in high- (>60 Hz) gamma-band oscillations during visual processing in schizophrenia. *Frontiers in Human Neuroscience*, **7**.

Hamalainen, M. S. & Ilmoniemi, R. J. (1994). Interpreting magnetic-fields of the brain – Minimum norm estimates. *Medical & Biological Engineering & Computing*, **32**, 35–42.

Hampson, M., Driesen, N., Roth, J. K., Gore, J. C. & Constable, R. T. (2010). Functional connectivity between task-positive and task-negative brain areas and its relation to working memory performance. *Magnetic Resonance Imaging*, **28**, 1051–1057.

Hansen, P. C., Kringelbach, M. L. & Salmelin, R. (2010). *MEG: An Introduction to Methods*. New York: Oxford University Press.

Haxby, J. V., Ishai, I. I., Chao, L. L., Ungerleider, L. G. & Martin, I. I. (2000). Object-form topology in the ventral temporal lobe. Response to I. Gauthier (2000). *Trends in Cognitive Sciences*, **4**, 3–4.

Haynes, J. D. & Rees, G. (2005). Predicting the orientation of invisible stimuli from activity in human primary visual cortex. *Nature Neuroscience*, **8**, 686–691.
  (2006). Decoding mental states from brain activity in humans. *Nature Reviews Neuroscience*, **7**, 523–534.

Herwig, U., Satrapi, P. & Schönfeldt-Lecuona, C. (2003). Using the international 10–20 EEG system for positioning of transcranial magnetic stimulation. *Brain Topography*, **16**, 95–99.

Hillebrand, A. & Barnes, G. (2002). A quantitative assessment of the sensitivity of whole-head MEG to activity in the adult human cortex. *Neuroimage*, **16**, 638–650.

Hillyard, S. A. & Anllo-Vento, L. (1998). Event-related brain potentials in the study of visual selective attention. *Proceedings of the National Academy of Sciences*, **95**, 781–787.

Hillyard, S. A., Hink, R. F., Schwent, V. L. & Picton, T. W. (1973). Electrical signs of selective attention in the human brain. *Science*, **182**, 177–180.

Hinojosa-Rodriguez, M., Harmony, T., Carrillo-Prado, C., et al. (2017). Clinical neuroimaging in the preterm infant: diagnosis and prognosis. *Neuroimage Clinical*, **16**, 355–368.

Hubbard, B. B. (1996). *The World According to Wavelets: The Story of a Mathematical Technique in the Making*. Natick, MA: A. K. Peters, Ltd.

Huettel, S. A., Song, A. W. & McCarthy, G. (Eds.). (2004). *Functional Magnetic Resonance Imaging*. Sunderland, MA: Sinauer Associates.

Humboldt, A. V. (2007). *Jaguars and Electric Eels*, trans. J. Wilson. London: Penguin.

Hyvarinen, A. (1999). Fast ICA for noisy data using Gaussian moments. *Proceedings of the 1999 IEEE International Symposium on IEEE*, 57–61.

ICNIRP. (2010). Guidelines for limiting exposure to time-varying electric and magnetic fields (1 Hz to 100 kHz). *Health Physics*, **99**, 818–836.

(2004). ICNIRP statement on medical magnetic resonance (MR) procedures: protection of patients. *Health Physics*, **87**, 197–216.

Inanaga, K. (1998). Frontal midline theta rhythm and mental activity. *Psychiatry and Clinical Neurosciences*, **52**, 555–566.

Issa, E. B., Papanastassiou, A. M. & Dicarlo, J. J. (2013). Large-scale, high-resolution neurophysiological maps underlying FMRI of macaque temporal lobe. *The Journal of Neuroscience*, **33**, 15207–15219.

Jasper, H. H. (1958). Report of the Committee on Methods of Clinical Examination in Electroencephalography. *Electroencephalography and Clinical Neurophysiology*, **10**, 370–371.

Jensen, A. R. (2006). *Clocking the Mind: Mental Chronometry and Individual Differences*. Amsterdam: Elsevier.

Joel, D., Berman, Z., Tavor, I., et al. (2015). Sex beyond the genitalia: the human brain mosaic. *Proceedings of the National Academy of Sciences of the United States of America*, **112**, 15468–15473.

Johnson, K. A., Minoshima, S., Bohnen, N. I., et al. (2013). Appropriate use criteria for amyloid PET: a report of the Amyloid Imaging Task Force, the Society of Nuclear Medicine and Molecular Imaging, and the Alzheimer's Association. *Journal of Nuclear Medicine*, **54**, 476–490.

Jung, T.-P., Makeig, S., Humphries, C., et al. (2000). Removing electroencephalographic artifacts by blind source separation. *Psychophysiology*, **37**, 163–178.

Jutten, C. & Herault, J. (1991). Blind separation of sources, part I: an adaptive algorithm based on neuromimetic architecture. *Signal Processing*, **24**, 1–10.

Kajikawa, Y. & Schroeder, C. E. (2011). How local is the local field potential? *Neuron*, **72**, 847–858.

Kamitani, Y. & Tong, F. (2005). Decoding the visual and subjective contents of the human brain. *Nature Neuroscience*, **8**, 679–685.

Kanai, R., Bahrami, B., Roylance, R. & Rees, G. (2012). Online social network size is reflected in human brain structure. *Proceedings of the Royal Society B-Biological Sciences*, **279**, 1327–1334.

Kanai, R. & Rees, G. (2011). The structural basis of inter-individual differences in human behaviour and cognition. *Nature Reviews Neuroscience*, **12**, 231–242.

Kanal, E., Barkovich, A. J., Bell, C., et al. & ACR Blue Ribbon Panel on MR Safety. (2007). ACR guidance document for safe MR practices: 2007. *American Journal of Roentgenology*, **188**, 1447–1474.

Kanwisher, N., McDermott, J. & Chun, M. M. (1997). The fusiform face area: a module in human extrastriate cortex specialized for face perception. *Journal of Neuroscience*, **17**, 4302–4311.

Kanwisher, N., Woods, R. P., Iacoboni, M. & Mazziotta, J. C. (1997). A locus in human extrastriate cortex for visual shape analysis. *Journal of Cognitive Neuroscience*, **9**, 133–142.

Kappenman, E. S. & Luck, S. J. (2010). The effects of electrode impedance on data quality and statistical significance in ERP recordings. *Psychophysiology*, **47**, 888–904.

Kassraian-Fard, P., Matthis, C., Balsters, J. H., Maathuis, M. H. & Wenderoth, N. (2016). Promises, pitfalls, and basic guidelines for applying machine learning classifiers to psychiatric imaging data, with autism as an example. *Frontiers in Psychiatry*, **7**, 177.

Kay, K. N., Naselaris, T., Prenger, R. J. & Gallant, J. L. (2008). Identifying natural images from human brain activity. *Nature*, **452**, 352–355.

Kellaway, P. & Crawley, J. (1964). A primer of electroencephalography of infants. Sections I and II. In P. Kellaway (Ed.), *Methodology and Criteria of Normality*, 3rd edn. Houston, TX: Baylor University College of Medicine.

Kessler, K. & Muckli, L. (2011). Reading others' minds by measuring their brains: fascinating and challenging for science, but ready for use in court? *Cortex*, **47**, 1240–1242.

Khaligh-Razavi, S. M. & Kriegeskorte, N. (2014). Deep supervised, but not unsupervised, models may explain IT cortical representation. *PLOS Computational Biology*, **10**, e1003915.

Kidwell, C. S., Chalela, J. A., Saver, J. L., et al. (2004). Comparison of MRI and CT for detection of acute intracerebral hemorrhage. *JAMA*, **292**, 1823–1830.

Kim, D.-H., Lu, N., Ma, R., et al. (2011). Epidermal electronics. *Science*, **333**, 838–843.

Kolossa, A. & Kopp, B. (2018). Data quality over data quantity in computational cognitive neuroscience. *Neuroimage*, **172**, 775–785.

Kolster, H., Peeters, R. & Orban, G. A. (2010). The Retinotopic Organization of the Human Middle Temporal Area MT/V5 and Its Cortical Neighbors. *Journal of Neuroscience*, **30**, 9801–9820.

Korhonen, O., Palva, S. & Palva, J. M. (2014). Sparse weightings for collapsing inverse solutions to cortical parcellations optimize M/EEG source reconstruction accuracy. *Journal of Neuroscience Methods*, **226**, 147–160.

Kosslyn, S. M. (1999). If neuroimaging is the answer, what is the question? *Philosophical Transactions of the Royal Society of London. Series BBiological Sciences*, **354**, 1283–1294.

Kotchoubey, B., Lang, S., Bostanov, V. & Birbaumer, N. (2002). Is there a mind? Electrophysiology of unconscious patients. *Physiology*, **17**, 38–42.

Krekelberg, B., Boynton, G. M. & Van Wezel, R. J. (2006). Adaptation: from single cells to BOLD signals. *Trends in Neurosciences*, **29**, 250–256.

Kriegeskorte, N., Goebel, R. & Bandettini, P. (2006). Information-based functional brain mapping. *Proceedings of the National Academy of Sciences of the United States of America*, **103**, 3863–3868.

Kriegeskorte, N., Mur, M. & Bandettini, P. (2008). Representational similarity analysis – Connecting the branches of systems neuroscience. *Frontiers in Systems Neuroscience*, **2**, 4.

Kriegeskorte, N., Mur, M., Ruff, D. A., et al. (2008). Matching categorical object representations in inferior temporal cortex of man and monkey. *Neuron*, **60**, 1126–1141.

Kriegeskorte, N., Simmons, W. K., Bellgowan, P. S. & Baker, C. I. (2009). Circular analysis in systems neuroscience: the dangers of double dipping. *Nature Neuroscience*, **12**, 535–540.

Krizhevsky, A., Sutskever, L. & Hinton, G. (2012). ImageNet classification with deep convolutional neural networks. *Advances in Neural Information Processing Systems*, **25**, 1090–1098.

Kubilius, J., Bracci, S. & Op de Beeck, H. P. (2016). Deep neural networks as a computational model for human shape sensitivity. *PLOS Computational Biology*, **12**, e1004896.

Kubilius, J., Wagemans, J. & Op de Beeck, H. P. (2011). Emergence of perceptual gestalts in the human visual cortex: the case of the configural-superiority effect. *Psychological Science*, **22**, 1296–1303.

Lachaux, J.-P., Rodriguez, E., Martinerie, J. & Varela, F. J. (1999). Measuring phase synchrony in brain signals. *Human Brain Mapping*, **8**, 194–208.

Le Van Quyen, M., Foucher, J., Lachaux, J.-P., et al. (2001). Comparison of Hilbert transform and wavelet methods for the analysis of neuronal synchrony. *Journal of Neuroscience Methods*, **111**, 83–98.

Lebby, P. C. (2013). *Brain Imaging: A Guide for Clinicians*. Oxford: Oxford University Press.

Lecun, Y., Bengio, Y. & Hinton, G. (2015). Deep learning. *Nature*, **521**, 436–444.

Lee, J. E., Bigler, E. D., Alexander, A. L., et al. (2007). Diffusion tensor imaging of white matter in the superior temporal gyrus and temporal stem in autism. *Neuroscience Letters*, **424**, 127–132.

Lee, J. H., Durand, R., Gradinaru, V., et al. (2010). Global and local fMRI signals driven by neurons defined optogenetically by type and wiring. *Nature*, **465**, 788–792.

Lee, W., Kim, H. C., Jung, Y., et al. (2016). Transcranial focused ultrasound stimulation of human primary visual cortex. *Scientific Reports*, **6**, Article ID 34026.

Legon, W., Sato, T. F., Opitz, A., et al. (2014). Transcranial focused ultrasound modulates the activity of primary somatosensory cortex in humans. *Nature Neuroscience*, **17**, 322–329.

Liao, Y., Huang, X., Wu, Q., et al. (2013). Is depression a disconnection syndrome? Meta-analysis of diffusion tensor imaging studies in patients with MDD. *Journal of Psychiatry & Neuroscience*, **38**, 49–56.

Lieberman, M. D. & Cunningham, W. A. (2009). Type I and Type II error concerns in fMRI research: re-balancing the scale. *Social Cognitive and Affective Neuroscience*, **4**, 423–428.

Lipton, R. B., Dodick, D. W., Silberstein, S. D., et al. (2010). Single-pulse transcranial magnetic stimulation for acute treatment of migraine with aura: a randomised, double-blind, parallel-group, sham-controlled trial. *Lancet Neurology*, **9**, 373–380.

Liu, S., Cai, W., Liu, S., et al. (2015). Multimodal neuroimaging computing: a review of the applications in neuropsychiatric disorders. *Brain Informatics*, **2**, 167–180.

Liu, S., Liu, S., Cai, W., et al. & ADNI. (2015). Multimodal neuroimaging feature learning for multiclass diagnosis of Alzheimer's disease. *IEEE Transactions on Biomedical Engineering*, **62**, 1132–1140.

Logothetis, N. K., Pauls, J., Augath, M., Trinath, T. & Oeltermann, A. (2001). Neurophysiological investigation of the basis of the fMRI signal. *Nature*, **412**, 150–157.

Lopes Da Silva, F. & Storm Van Leeuwen, W. (1977). The cortical source of the alpha rhythm. *Neuroscience Letters*, **6**, 237–241.

Makeig, S., Bell, A. J., Jung, T.-P. & Sejnowski, T. J. (1996). Independent component analysis of electroencephalographic data. *Advances in Neural Information Processing Systems*, 145–151.

Makeig, S., Debener, S., Onton, J. & Delorme, A. (2004). Mining event-related brain dynamics. *Trends in Cognitive Sciences*, **8**, 204–210.

Makeig, S. & Inlow, M. (1993). Lapse in alertness: coherence of fluctuations in performance and EEG spectrum. *Electroencephalography and Clinical Neurophysiology*, **86**, 23–35.

Makeig, S., Westerfield, M., Jung, T.-P., et al. (2002). Dynamic brain sources of visual evoked responses. *Science*, **295**, 690–694.

Malach, R., Reppas, J. B., Benson, R. R., et al. (1995). Object-related activity revealed by functional magnetic resonance imaging in human occipital cortex. *Proceedings of the National Academy of Sciences of the United States of America*, **92**, 8135–8139.

Malmivuo, J. (2012). Comparison of the properties of EEG and MEG in detecting the electric activity of the brain. *Brain Topography*, **25**, 1–19.

Mayberg, H. S., Lozano, A. M., Voon, V., et al. (2005). Deep brain stimulation for treatment-resistant depression. *Neuron*, **45**, 651–660.

Meeren, H. K., Hadjikhani, N., Ahlfors, S. P., Hämäläinen, M. S. & De Gelder, B. (2008). Early category-specific cortical activation revealed by visual stimulus inversion. *PLoS One*, **3**, e3503.

Meindl, T., Teipel, S., Elmouden, R., et al. (2010). Test-retest reproducibility of the default-mode network in healthy individuals. *Human Brain Mapping*, **31**, 237–246.

Meyer, B. U., Kloten, H., Britton, T. C. & Benecke, R. (1990). Technical approaches to hemisphere-selective transcranial magnetic brain stimulation. *Electromyography and Clinical Neurophysiology*, **30**, 311–318.

Mikl, M., Marecek, R., Hlustik, P., et al. (2008). Effects of spatial smoothing on fMRI group inferences. *Magnetic Resonance Imaging*, **26**, 490–503.

Millett, D. (2001). Hans Berger: from psychic energy to the EEG. *Perspectives in Biology and Medicine*, **44**, 522–542.

Miyapuram, K. (2008). Introduction to fMRI: experimental design and data analysis. Chapter from an unpublished Ph.D. thesis, University of Cambridge.

Monti, M. M. (2011). Statistical analysis of fMRI time-series: a critical review of the GLM approach. *Frontiers in Human Neuroscience*, **5**, 28.

Morgan, S., Hansen, J. & Hillyard, S. (1996). Selective attention to stimulus location modulates the steady-state visual evoked potential. *Proceedings of the National Academy of Sciences*, **93**, 4770–4774.

Mosconi, L., Tsui, W. H., Herholz, K., et al. (2008). Multicenter standardized 18F-FDG PET diagnosis of mild cognitive impairment, Alzheimer's disease, and other dementias. *The Journal of Nuclear Medicine*, **49**, 390–398.

Mountcastle, V. B. (1997). The columnar organization of the neocortex. *Brain*, **120** (Pt 4), 701–722.

Mukamel, R., Harel, M., Hendler, T. & Malach, R. (2004). Enhanced temporal non-linearities in human object-related occipito-temporal cortex. *Cerebral Cortex*, **14**, 575–585.

Mur, M., Bandettini, P. A. & Kriegeskorte, N. 2009. Revealing representational content with pattern-information fMRI – an introductory guide. *Social Cognitive and Affective Neuroscience*, **4**, 101–109.

Näätänen, R., Gaillard, A. W. & Mäntysalo, S. (1978). Early selective-attention effect on evoked potential reinterpreted. *Acta Psychologica*, **42**, 313–329.

Narasimhan, P. T. & Jacobs, R. E. (2002). Neuroanatomical micromagnetic resonance imaging. In A. W. Toga & J. C. Mazziotta (Eds.), *Brain Mapping: The Methods*. New York: Elsevier.

Naseer, N. & Hong, K. S. (2015). fNIRS-based brain-computer interfaces: a review. *Frontiers in Human Neuroscience*, **9**, 3.

Nichols, T. E. & Holmes, A. P. (2002). Nonparametric permutation tests for functional neuroimaging: a primer with examples. *Human Brain Mapping*, **15**, 1–25.

Nikouline, V. V., Linkenkaer-Hansen, K., Huttunen, J. & Ilmoniemi, R. J. (2001). Interhemispheric phase synchrony and amplitude correlation of spontaneous beta oscillations in human subjects: a magnetoencephalographic study. *Neuroreport*, **12**, 2487–2491.

Nitsche, M. A., Cohen, L. G., Wassermann, E. M., et al. (2008). Transcranial direct current stimulation: state of the art 2008. *Brain Stimulation*, **1**, 206–223.

Nunez, P. L. (1977). The dipole layer as a model for scalp potentials. *T.-I.-T. Journal of Life Sciences*, **7**, 65–72.

Ogawa, S., Lee, T. M., Kay, A. R. & Tank, D. W. (1990). Brain magnetic resonance imaging with contrast dependent on blood oxygenation. *Proceedings of the National Academy of Sciences of the United States of America*, **87**, 9868–9872.

Oosterhof, N. N., Connolly, A. C. & Haxby, J. V. (2016). CoSMoMVPA: multi-modal multivariate pattern analysis of neuroimaging data in Matlab/GNU Octave. *Frontiers in Neuroinformatics*, **10**, 27.

Op de Beeck, H. P. (2010). Against hyperacuity in brain reading: spatial smoothing does not hurt multivariate fMRI analyses? *Neuroimage*, **49**, 1943–1948.

Op de Beeck, H. P., Torfs, K. & Wagemans, J. (2008). Perceived shape similarity among unfamiliar objects and the organization of the human object vision pathway. *Journal of Neuroscience*, **28**, 10111–10123.

Op de Beeck, H. P., Vermaercke, B., Woolley, D. G. & Wenderoth, N. (2013). Combinatorial brain decoding of people's whereabouts during visuospatial navigation. *Frontiers in Neuroscience*, **7**, 78.

Osborn, A. G., Salzman, K. L. & Jhaveri, M. D. (2016). *Diagnostic Imaging: Brain, 3rd edn*. Amsterdam: Elsevier.

Owen, A. M., Coleman, M. R., Boly, M., Davis, M. H., Laureys, S. & Pickard, J. D. (2006). Detecting awareness in the vegetative state. *Science*, **313**, 1402–1403.

Parens, E. & Johnston, J. (2014). Neuroimaging: beginning to appreciate its complexities. *Hastings Center Report*, **44**, S2–S7.

Parkes, L. M., Schwarzbach, J. V., Bouts, A. A., et al. (2005). Quantifying the spatial resolution of the gradient echo and spin echo BOLD response at 3 tesla. *Magnetic Resonance in Medicine*, **54**, 1465–1472.

Parvizi, J., Jacques, C., Foster, B. L., et al. (2012). Electrical stimulation of human fusiform face-selective regions distorts face perception. *Journal of Neuroscience*, **32**, 14915–14920.

Pascual-Leone, A., Walsh, V. & Rothwell, J. (2000). Transcranial magnetic stimulation in cognitive neuroscience – virtual lesion, chronometry, and functional connectivity. *Current Opinion in Neurobiology*, **10**, 232–237.

Perera, T., George, M. S., Grammer, G., Janicak, P. G., Pascual-Leone, A. & Wirecki, T. S. (2016). The Clinical TMS Society consensus review and treatment recommendations for TMS therapy for major depressive disorder. *Brain Stimulation*, **9**, 336–346.

Perlaki, G., Orsi, G., Plozer, E., et al. (2014). Are there any gender differences in the hippocampus volume after head-size correction? A volumetric and voxel-based morphometric study. *Neuroscience Letters*, **570**, 119–123.

Pfurtscheller, G. & Da Silva, F. L. (1999). Event-related EEG/MEG synchronization and desynchronization: basic principles. *Clinical Neurophysiology*, **110**, 1842–1857.

Pfurtscheller, G., Stancak, A. & Neuper, C. (1996). Post-movement beta synchronization. A correlate of an idling motor area? *Electroencephalography and Clinical Neurophysiology*, **98**, 281–293.

Picton, T. W., Van Roon, P., Armilio, M. L., Berg, P., Ille, N. & Scherg, M. (2000). The correction of ocular artifacts: a topographic perspective. *Clinical Neurophysiology*, **111**, 53–65.

Pitcher, D., Duchaine, B., Walsh, V., Yovel, G. & Kanwisher, N. (2011). The role of lateral occipital face and object areas in the face inversion effect. *Neuropsychologia*, **49**, 3448–3458.

Pitcher, D., Garrido, L., Walsh, V. & Duchaine, B. C. (2008). Transcranial magnetic stimulation disrupts the perception and embodiment of facial expressions. *Journal of Neuroscience*, **28**, 8929–8933.

Pitcher, D., Goldhaber, T., Duchaine, B., Walsh, V. & Kanwisher, N. (2012). Two critical and functionally distinct stages of face and body perception. *Journal of Neuroscience*, **32**, 15877–15885.

Poghosyan, V. & Ioannides, A. A. (2008). Attention modulates earliest responses in the primary auditory and visual cortices. *Neuron*, **58**, 802–813.

Poldrack, R. A. (2006). Can cognitive processes be inferred from neuroimaging data? *Trends in Cognitive Sciences*, **10**, 59–63.

(2007). Region of interest analysis for fMRI. *Social Cognitive and Affective Neuroscience*, **2**, 67–70.

Poldrack, R. A., Baker, C. I., Durnez, J., et al. (2017). Scanning the horizon: towards transparent and reproducible neuroimaging research. *Nature Reviews Neuroscience*, **18**, 115–126.

Poldrack, R. A., Mumford, J. & Nichols, T. E. (2011). *Handbook of Functional MRI Data Analysis*. Cambridge: Cambridge University Press.

Posner, M. I. (2005). Timing the brain: mental chronometry as a tool in neuroscience. *Plos Biology*, **3**, 204–206.

Posner, M. I. & Raichle, M. E. (1994). *Images of Mind*. New York: Scientific American Books.

Power, J. D., Barnes, K. A., Snyder, A. Z., Schlaggar, B. L. & Petersen, S. E. (2012). Spurious but systematic correlations in functional connectivity MRI networks arise from subject motion. *Neuroimage*, **59**, 2142–2154.

Pratte, M. S., Sy, J. L., Swisher, J. D. & Tong, F. (2016). Radial bias is not necessary for orientation decoding. *Neuroimage*, **127**, 23–33.

Pravdich-Neminsky, V. V. (1913). Ein Versuch der Registrierung der Elektrischen Gehirnerscheinungen. *Zbl Physiol*, **27**, 951–960.

Purcell, E. M., Torrey, H. C. & Pound, R. V. (1946). Resonance absorption by nuclear magnetic moments in a solid. *Physical Review*, **69**, 37–38.

Puts, N. A. & Edden, R. A. (2012). In vivo magnetic resonance spectroscopy of GABA: a methodological review. *Progress in Nuclear Magnetic Resonance Spectroscopy*, **60**, 29–41.

Quiroga, R. Q., Reddy, L., Kreiman, G., Koch, C. & Fried, I. (2005). Invariant visual representation by single neurons in the human brain. *Nature*, **435**, 1102–1107.

Raghavachari, S., Kahana, M. J., Rizzuto, D. S., et al. (2001). Gating of human theta oscillations by a working memory task. *Journal of Neuroscience*, **21**, 3175–3183.

Raichle, M. E. (2000). A brief history of human functional brain mapping. In A. W. Toga & J. C. Mazziotta (Eds.), *Brain Mapping: The Systems*. New York: Academic Press.

Raichle, M. E. & Snyder, A. Z. (2007). A default mode of brain function: a brief history of an evolving idea. *Neuroimage*, **37**, 1083–1090.

Ray, S., Crone, N. E., Niebur, E., Franaszczuk, P. J. & Hsiao, S. S. (2008). Neural correlates of high-gamma oscillations (60–200 Hz) in macaque local field potentials and their potential implications in electrocorticography. *Journal of Neuroscience*, **28**, 11526–11536.

Rezayat, E. & Toostani, I. G. (2016). A review on brain stimulation using low intensity focused ultrasound. *Basic and Clinical Neuroscience*, **7**, 187–194.

Ridding, M. C. & Rothwell, J. C. (2007). Is there a future for therapeutic use of transcranial magnetic stimulation? *Nature Reviews Neuroscience*, **8**, 559–567.

Rissman, J., Gazzaley, A. & D'Esposito, M. (2004). Measuring functional connectivity during distinct stages of a cognitive task. *Neuroimage*, **23**, 752–763.

Rohde, G. K., Barnett, A. S., Basser, P. J., Marenco, S. & Pierpaoli, C. (2004). Comprehensive approach for correction of motion and distortion in diffusion-weighted MRI. *Magnetic Resonance in Medicine*, **51**, 103–114.

Rosanova, M., Gosseries, O., Casarotto, S., et al. (2012). Recovery of cortical effective connectivity and recovery of consciousness in vegetative patients. *Brain*, **135**, 1308–1320.

Rosenblatt, J. D. (2016). Multivariate revisit to "sex beyond the genitalia." *Proceedings of the National Academy of Sciences of the United States of America*, **113**, E1966–E1967.

Rossi, S., Hallett, M., Rossini, P. M., Pascual-Leone, A. & Safety of TMS Consensus Group. (2009). Safety, ethical considerations, and application guidelines for the use of transcranial magnetic stimulation in clinical practice and research. *Clinical Neurophysiology*, **120**, 2008–2039.

Roy, C. S. & Sherrington, C. S. (1890.) On the regulation of the blood-supply of the brain. *The Journal of Physiology*, **11**, 85–158.

Sadeh, B., Podlipsky, I., Zhdanov, A. & Yovel, G. (2010). Event-related potential and functional MRI measures of face-selectivity are highly correlated: a simultaneous ERP-fMRI investigation. *Human Brain Mapping*, **31**, 1490–1501.

Sadeh, B., Zhdanov, A., Podlipsky, I., Hendler, T. & Yovel, G. (2008). The validity of the face-selective ERP N170 component during simultaneous recording with functional MRI. *Neuroimage*, **42**, 778–786.

Salmelin, R. (2010). Multi-dipole modeling in MEG. In P. C. Hansen, M. L. Kringelbach & R. SALMELIN (Eds.), *MEG: An Introduction to Methods*. New York: Oxford University Press

Salvo, P., Raedt, R., Carrette, E., Schaubroeck, D., Vanfleteren, J. & Cardon, L. (2012). A 3D printed dry electrode for ECG/EEG recording. *Sensors and Actuators A: Physical*, **174**, 96–102.

Santens, S., Roggeman, C., Fias, W. & Verguts, T. (2010). Number processing pathways in human parietal cortex. *Cerebral Cortex*, **20**, 77–88.

Sawamura, H., Orban, G. A. & Vogels, R. (2006). Selectivity of neuronal adaptation does not match response selectivity: a single-cell study of the FMRI adaptation paradigm. *Neuron*, **49**, 307–318.

Saxe, R., Brett, M. & Kanwisher, N. (2006). Divide and conquer: a defense of functional localizers. *Neuroimage*, **30**, 1088–1096; discussion 1097–1099.

Schick, F. (2005). Whole-body MRI at high field: technical limits and clinical potential. *European Radiology*, **15**, 946–959.

Sengupta, B., Stemmler, M. B. & Friston, K. J. (2013). Information and efficiency in the nervous system – A synthesis. *PLOS Computational Biology*, **9**, e1003157.

Shallice, T. (1988). *From Neuropsychology to Mental Structure*. Cambridge: Cambridge University Press.

Shine, J. M., Koyejo, O. & Poldrack, R. A. (2016). Temporal metastases are associated with differential patterns of time-resolved connectivity, network topology, and attention. *Proceedings of the National Academy of Sciences of the United States of America*, **113**, 9888–9891.

Shmuel, A. & Leopold, D. A. (2008). Neuronal correlates of spontaneous fluctuations in fMRI signals in monkey visual cortex: implications for functional connectivity at rest. *Human Brain Mapping*, **29**, 751–761.

Shmuel, A., Yacoub, E., Chaimow, D., Logothetis, N. K. & Ugurbil, K. (2007). Spatio-temporal point-spread function of fMRI signal in human gray matter at 7 tesla. *Neuroimage*, **35**, 539–552.

Shmuel, A., Yacoub, E., Pfeuffer, J., et al (2002). Sustained negative BOLD, blood flow and oxygen consumption response and its coupling to the positive response in the human brain. *Neuron*, **36**, 1195–1210.

Shulman, R. G., Rothman, D. L., Behar, K. L. & Hyder, F. (2004). Energetic basis of brain activity: implications for neuroimaging. *Trends in Neurosciences*, **27**, 489–495.

Sitaram, R., Ros, T., Stoeckel, L., et al. (2017). Closed-loop brain training: the science of neurofeedback. *Nature Reviews Neuroscience*, **18**, 86–100.

Slotnick, S. D. (2017). Cluster success: fMRI inferences for spatial extent have acceptable false-positive rates. *Cognitive Neuroscience*, **8**, 150–155.

Snowball, A., Tachtsidis, I., Popescu, T., et al. (2013). Long-term enhancement of brain function and cognition using cognitive training and brain stimulation. *Current Biology*, **23**, 987–992.

Soares, J. M., Marques, P., Alves, V. & Sousa, N. (2013). A hitchhiker's guide to diffusion tensor imaging. *Frontiers in Neuroscience*, **7**, 31.

Sommer, I. E. C., Aleman, A., Bouma, A. & Kahn, R. S. (2004). Do women really have more bilateral language representation than men? A meta-analysis of functional imaging studies. *Brain*, **127**, 1845–1852.

Song, S. K., Sun, S. W., Ramsbottom, M. J., Chang, C., Russell, J. & Cross, A. H. (2002). Dysmyelination revealed through MRI as increased radial (but unchanged axial) diffusion of water. *Neuroimage*, **17**, 1429–1436.

Stagg, C. J., Bachtiar, V. & Johansen-Berg, H. (2011). What are we measuring with GABA magnetic resonance spectroscopy? *Communicative & Integrative Biology*, **4**, 573–575.

Stagg, C. J. & Rothman, D. (2014). *Magnetic Resonance Spectroscopy: Tools for Neuroscience Research and Emerging Clinical Applications*. Amsterdam: Elsevier.

Steeves, J. K., Culham, J. C., Duchaine, B. C., et al. (2006). The fusiform face area is not sufficient for face recognition: evidence from a patient with dense prosopagnosia and no occipital face area. *Neuropsychologia*, **44**, 594–609.

Steriade, M. (1997). Synchronized activities of coupled oscillators in the cerebral cortex and thalamus at different levels of vigilance. *Cerebral Cortex*, **7**, 583–604.

Stokes, P. A. & Purdon, P. L. (2017). A study of problems encountered in Granger causality analysis from a neuroscience perspective. *Proceedings of the National Academy of Sciences*, **114**, E7063–E7072.

Summerfield, C., Trittschuh, E. H., Monti, J. M., Mesulam, M. M. & Egner, T. (2008). Neural repetition suppression reflects fulfilled perceptual expectations. *Nature Neuroscience*, **11**, 1004–1006.

Sumner, P., Vivian-Griffiths, S., Boivin, J., et al. (2014). The association between exaggeration in health related science news and academic press releases: retrospective observational study. *BMJ*, **349**, 7015.

Sutton, S., Braren, M., Zubin, J. & John, E. (1965). Evoked-potential correlates of stimulus uncertainty. *Science*, **150**, 1187–1188.

Talairach, J. & Tournoux, P. (1988). *Co-planar Stereotaxic Atlas of the Human Brain: 3-Dimensional Proportional System; An Approach to Medical Cerebral Imaging*. Stuttgart: Thieme Medical Publishers.

Tallgren, P., Vanhatalo, S., Kaila, K. & Voipio, J. (2005). Evaluation of commercially available electrodes and gels for recording of slow EEG potentials. *Clinical Neurophysiology*, **116**, 799–806.

Tallon-Baudry, C. & Bertrand, O. (1999). Oscillatory gamma activity in humans and its role in object representation. *Trends in Cognitive Sciences*, **3**, 151–162.

Tallon-Baudry, C., Bertrand, O., Delpuech, C. & Pernier, J. (1996). Stimulus specificity of phase-locked and non-phase-locked 40 Hz visual responses in human. *Journal of Neuroscience*, **16**, 4240–4249.

Tanaka, K. 2003. Columns for complex visual object features in the inferotemporal cortex: clustering of cells with similar but slightly different stimulus selectivities. *Cerebral Cortex*, **13**, 90–99.

Tanner, D., Morgan-Short, K. & Luck, S. J. (2015). How inappropriate high-pass filters can produce artifactual effects and incorrect conclusions in ERP studies of language and cognition. *Psychophysiology*, **52**, 997–1009.

Tarr, M. J. & Gauthier, I. (2000). FFA: a flexible fusiform area for subordinate-level visual processing automatized by expertise. *Nature Neuroscience*, **3**, 764–769.

Terney, D., Chaieb, L., Moliadze, V., Antal, A. & Paulus, W. (2008). Increasing human brain excitability by transcranial high-frequency random noise stimulation. *Journal of Neuroscience*, **28**, 14147–14155.

Thomas, C., Humphreys, K., Jung, K. J., Minshew, N. & Behrmann, M. (2011). The anatomy of the callosal and visual-association pathways in high-functioning autism: a DTI tractography study. *Cortex*, **47**, 863–873.

Thompson, J. K., Peterson, M. R. & Freeman, R. D. (2003). Single-neuron activity and tissue oxygenation in the cerebral cortex. *Science*, **299**, 1070–1072.

Tumati, S., Martens, S. & Aleman, A. (2013). Magnetic resonance spectroscopy in mild cognitive impairment: systematic review and meta-analysis. *Neuroscience & Biobehavior Reviews*, **37**, 2571–2586.

Uttal, W. R. (2001). *The New Phrenology*. Cambridge, MA: MIT Press.

Van Den Heuvel, M. P. & Hulshoff Pol, H. E. (2010). Exploring the brain network: a review on resting-state fMRI functional connectivity. *European Neuropsychopharmacology*, **20**, 519–534.

Van Meel, C., Daniels, N., Op de Beeck, H. & Baeck, A. (2016). Effect of tDCS on task relevant and irrelevant perceptual learning of complex objects. *Journal of Vision*, **16**, 13.

Varela, F., Lachaux, J.-P., Rodriguez, E. & Martinerie, J. (2001). The brainweb: phase synchronization and large-scale integration. *Nature Reviews Neuroscience*, **2**, 229.

Vissers, M. E., Cohen, M. X. & Geurts, H. M. (2012). Brain connectivity and high functioning autism: a promising path of research that needs refined models, methodological convergence, and stronger behavioral links. *Neuroscience & Biobehavioral Reviews*, **36**, 604–625.

Volkow, N. D., Fowler, J. S., Gatley, S. J., et al. (1996). PET evaluation of the dopamine system of the human brain. *Journal of Nuclear Medicine*, **37**, 1242–1256.

Voroslakos, M., Takeuchi, Y., Brinyiczki, K., et al. (2018). Direct effects of transcranial electric stimulation on brain circuits in rats and humans. *Nature Communications*, **9**, 483.

Vul, E., Harris, C., Winkielman, P. & Pashler, H. (2009). Puzzlingly high correlations in fMRI studies of emotion, personality, and social cognition. *Perspectives in Psychological Science*, **4**, 274–290.

Weber, M. A., Zoubaa, S., Schlieter, M., et al. (2006). Diagnostic performance of spectroscopic and perfusion MRI for distinction of brain tumors. *Neurology*, **66**, 1899–1906.

Weber, M. J. & Thompson-Schill, S. L. (2010). Functional neuroimaging can support causal claims about brain function. *Journal of Cognitive Neuroscience*, **22**, 2415–2416.

Weinstein, M., Ben-Sira, L., Levy, Y., et al. (2011). Abnormal white matter integrity in young children with autism. *Human Brain Mapping*, **32**, 534–543.

Weisberg, D. S., Keil, F. C., Goodstein, J., Rawson, E. & Gray, J. R. (2008). The seductive allure of neuroscience explanations. *Journal of Cognitive Neuroscience*, **20**, 470–477.

White, B. R. & Culver, J. P. (2010). Phase-encoded retinotopy as an evaluation of diffuse optical neuroimaging. *Neuroimage*, **49**, 568–577.

Williams, M. A., Dang, S. & Kanwisher, N. G. (2007). Only some spatial patterns of fMRI response are read out in task performance. *Nature Neuroscience*, **10**, 685–686.

Woolrich, M. W., Jbabdi, S., Patenaude, B., et al. (2009). Bayesian analysis of neuroimaging data in FSL. *Neuroimage*, **45**, S173–S186.

Worsley, K. J., Marrett, S., Neelin, P., Vandal, A. C., Friston, K. J. & Evans, A. C. (1996). A unified statistical approach for determining significant signals in images of cerebral activation. *Human Brain Mapping*, **4**, 58–73.

Yamamoto, Y. (2003). *Jiryoku to Juryoku no hakken [Discovery of magnetic power and gravity]*. Tokyo, Japan: Misuzu shobo.

Yarkoni, T., Poldrack, R. A., Nichols, T. E., Van Essen, D. C. & Wager, T. D. (2011). Large-scale automated synthesis of human functional neuroimaging data. *Nature Methods*, **8**, 665–670.

Yoon, J. H., Maddock, R. J., Rokem, A.,et al. (2010). GABA concentration is reduced in visual cortex in schizophrenia and correlates with orientation-specific surround suppression. *Journal of Neuroscience*, **30**, 3777–3781.

Yordanova, J., Kolev, V., Wagner, U., Born, J. & Verleger, R. (2012). Increased alpha (8–12 Hz) activity during slow wave sleep as a marker for the transition from implicit knowledge to explicit insight. *Journal of Cognitive Neuroscience*, **24**, 119–132.

Yovel, G. & Kanwisher, N. (2005). The neural basis of the behavioral face-inversion effect. *Current Biology*, **15**, 2256–2262.

Zangen, A., Roth, Y., Voller, B. & Hallett, M. (2005). Transcranial magnetic stimulation of deep brain regions: evidence for efficacy of the H-coil. *Clinical Neurophysiology*, **116**, 775–779.

Zevin, J. D., Datta, H., Maurer, U., Rosania, K. A. & McCandliss, B. D. (2010). Native language experience influences the topography of the mismatch negativity to speech. *Frontiers in Human Neuroscience*, **4**.

Zhao, F., Jin, T., Wang, P. & Kim, S. G. (2007). Improved spatial localization of post-stimulus BOLD undershoot relative to positive BOLD. *Neuroimage*, **34**, 1084–1092.

Index